Mandibular Suction Effective Denture Fabrication Technique

Mandibular Suction-effective Denture

"The Professional"

-Clinical and Laboratory Technique for Class I/ II/ III with Aesthetics-

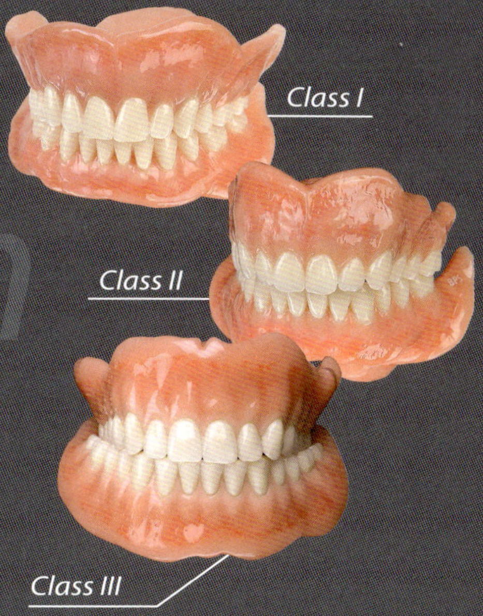

Jiro Abe, D.D.S.
Kenji Iwaki, R.D.T.
Tetsuya Sudo, R.D.T.
Kyoko Kokubo, R.D.T.

The Professional

QUINTESSENCE PUBLISHING

Berlin, Barcelona, Chicago, Istanbul, London, Milan, Moscow, New Delhi, Paris, Prague, São Paulo, Seoul, Singapore, Tokyo, Warsaw

Preface

4 Step from start to finish "Mandibular Suction-Effective Denture and BPS" : A Complete Guide (Quintessence Publishing) was published right after the Great East Japan earthquake on March 11, 2011 with the purpose to encourage the dental professionals who were affected by the disaster. This publication has been quite memorable to me since I put a strong emphasis to raise positive awareness for emotional recovery for those who have been affected by the disaster even though there was an atmosphere that it is quite inappropriate to publish the book then to respect the feeling of those who have been affected by the disastrous environment.

This book has been translated in English, Korean and Chinese and has been widely acclaimed by the dentists and denturists all over the world.

The reason for the high acclamations came from the dentists who couldn't believe that they can actually fabricate the Mandibular denture with this technique that actually stays in with the strong suction. This book was revolutionary to the dentists and their patients. Mandibular Suction-Effective Denture and BPS technique has been attributed to the great influences in the dental school faculty members' teaching motivation, skill level of the general dentists and high patients' treatment satisfaction. Patient's satisfaction leads to more new patients' referral to the dental professional ; therefore, there is quite positive economically effect to the dentists. In the aging society, aging population have a lot of fear for acquiring heart disease, blood disease, pulmonary disease, Alzheimer disease and so on. The dentists should be able to provide the non-surgical treatment by avoiding implant treatment for those elderly patients who request non-surgical approach. Thus, Mandibular Suction-Effective Denture has been on demand in this aging society.

After publication of 4 Step from start to finish "Mandibular Suction-Effective Denture and BPS" : A Complete Guide, so many followers are claiming that this book is the denture revolution. Also a lot of dental professionals start to attending the author's lectures and hands on courses to improve their clinical skills. The author started to have more opportunities to give lectures all over the world. Also the author's trained protege begin to give lectures and courses all over the world. This gives me a great satisfaction to prove that Japanese technique has been accepted and spread to all over the world. However, this is just the beginning and surely not the end. I strongly wish that my protege and students in the world will improve and enhance this technique to spread all over the world.

Next step to those who mastered the basic Mandibular Suction-Effective Denture technique is to acquire the higher successful technique to apply to more advanced and complicated cases. Nowadays I get a lot of questions about the treatment concept for the diagnosis and technique such as tooth set up and anatomical surface texture for ClassII,III cases. Since each patient has unique anatomical feature and difference case acceptance, so it is very difficult to achieve 100% patient's satisfaction every time but it may be possible to achieve 80% patient's satisfaction. There is a huge demand from the dental professional to acquire the basic laboratory technique to achieve this constant 80% patient's satisfaction.

3 renowned dental technicians ; Mr. Kenji Iwaki, Mr. Tetsuya Sudo and Ms. Kyoko Kokubo, who are all

BPS Technical Instructors, agreed to participate to share their expertise. They have their own opinions for the denture fabrication technique, but all of them posses high knowledge of overall denture fabrication technique. It is a great pleasure to show their knowledge and techniques in this book. Also it is a big responsibility for me to convey their detail techniques in this book. It is a mutual technical and mental improvement for dentists to collaborate with high skilled dental technicians. I would sincerely hope that those dental technicians will keep collaborating with the respected dentists and improve their techniques and skills in order to contribute on the development of complete denturs.

The technique described in this book has been following with BPS (Biofunctional Prosthetic System) created by Ivoclar Vivadent. This technique is believed to be the most accurate system in regards to creating the most accurate and comfortable interocclusal relationship with dentures. Needless to say, the international company support will prevail this technique all over the world. I would like to express my sincere appreciation for the support to Mr. Cristoph Linder/ Senior Asia Sales Manager Japan/Korea and Dr. Frank Zimmerling and Mr. Matteus Boxhoorn / Top instructors in the main office at Liechtenstein.

Also, I would like to extend my appreciation to Dr. Yukio kameda, Dr. Katsushi Sato, Dr.Yoshihiro Saito and Dr. Fumiaki Yamazaki who have been helping to prosper Mandibular Suction-Effective Denture technique and JPDA(Japan Plate Denture Association), denturists; Mr.Stephen McGlynn, Mr. Arnold Jabour, Mr. Carl Fenwick, Mr.John Wibberley, Mr.Paul McNally, Mr.Markus Fischer, Ms.Esther Slovak-Schwenning, Ms. Erika Colebank and dentists; Dr. Noh Kwantae, Dr.Andrew Zhao Long, Dr. Kelvin Khng, Dr. Jonathan Shen.

This is the last but not the least, I would extend my sincere appreciation to Mr. Shigeki Wakabayashi / QDT Editorial Chief at Quintessence Publishing Japan for the detail advice for this publication. His strong will to publish the book that will inspire dental professionals of all over the world and consequently help edentulous patients, motivated me to put this book together.

Autumn, 2017, Jiro Abe

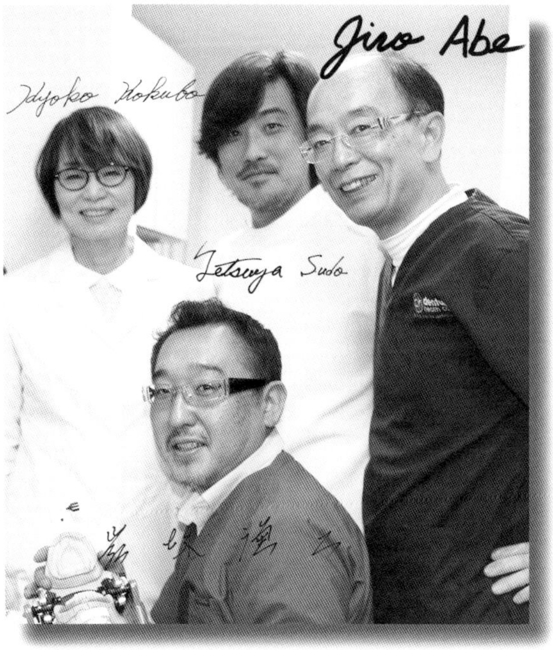

Profiles

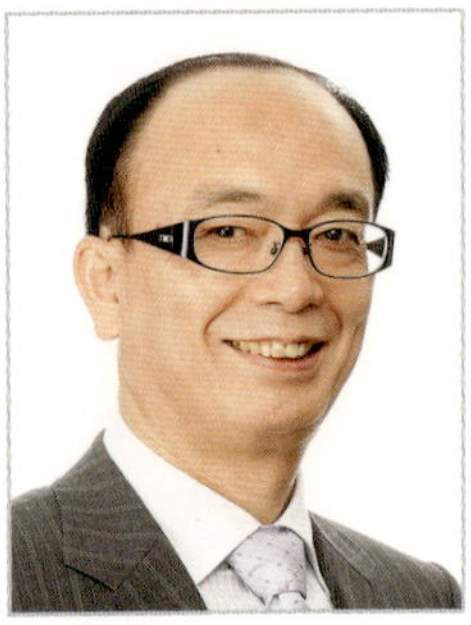

Jiro Abe D.D.S.,Ph. D.

1955	Born at Sendai city, Miyagi prefecture, Japan
1981	Graduated from Tokyo Dental College
2001~present	Lecturer of GC's complete denture seminar
2006~2015	President of Japan Denture Association
2008~present	Ivoclar Vivadent BPS International Instructor
2010~present	Lecturer of Morita's complete denture seminar
2012~present	Clinical professor at the Tohoku university graduate school of dentistry
	Visiting professor at the Kanagawa Dental College
2015~present	International comitee member of the American Prosthodontic Society

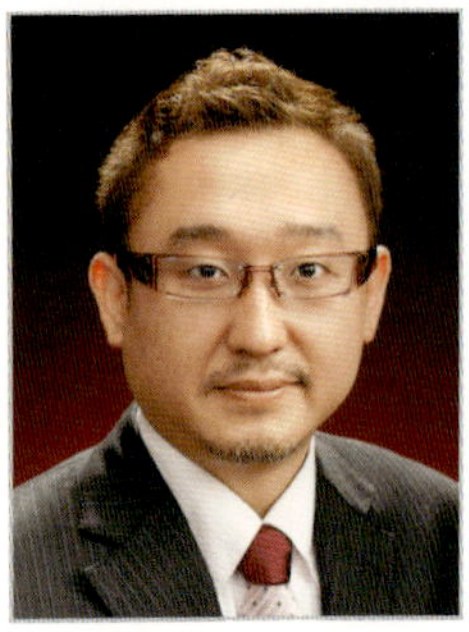

Kenji Iwaki R.D.T.

1994	Graduated from Department of Dental Technology, Nippon Dental University College at Tokyo
2000	Established I.D.T Dental Labortatory
2010~Present	Board member of Gotanda Denture Association
2014~Present	Ivoclar Vivadent BPS International Technical Instructor
2016	Reorganization I.D.T Dental Labortatory to Dental Labor IDT
2016~Present	Board member of Japan Plate Denture Association

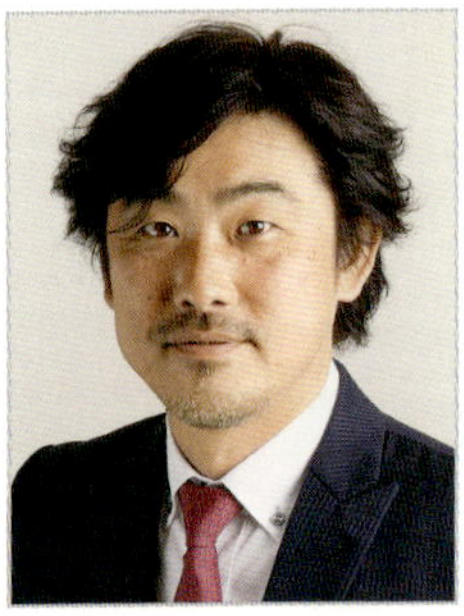

Tetsuya Sudo R.D.T.

1993	Graduated from Aishi College of Dental Technology
1993~2011	Managed marketing division of Kyowa Dental Laboratory
2005	Technical Instructor of Morita's Mandibular suction effective denture seminar
2011	Established Defy (Dental laboratory)
2014~Present	Ivoclar Vivadent BPS International Technical Instructor
2016~Present	Board member of Japan Plate Denture Association

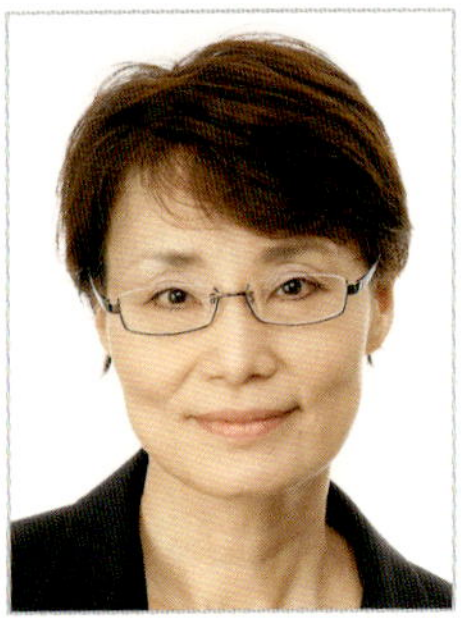

Kyoko Kokubo R.D.T.

1976	Graduated from Department of Dental Technology, Toho Dental College
1982	Chief of Ace Dental(Dental laboratory) plate denture division
2010~Present	Ivoclar Vivadent BPS International Technical Instructor
2012~2015	Lecturer of the Kanagawa Dental College
2015~Present	Certified teaching dental technician of the Japan Academy of Clinical Dentistry
2016~Present	Auditor of Japan Plate Denture Association
2017~Present	Regular member Teaching technician Japan Plate Denture Association

Part 1

Introduction

1 Suction Magic

After publishing 4 Step from start to finish "Mandibular Suction-Effective Denture and BPS" : A Complete Guide in 2011, a lot of people have attended lectures and seminars to learn suction denture technique[1]. I received a lot of positive review comments such as " I couldn't believe that the mandibular denture can actually have a great suction to the ridge." " I sincerely appreciate that a lot of my patients can be treated without implant treatments." " I get a lot of patients referral with the reputation of Suction Denture." Even on the Facebook, a lot of dentists and denturists all over the world are posting treatment videos and pictures and course informations. The author is proud of the publication of 4 Step from start to finish "Mandibular Suction-Effective Denture and BPS" : A Complete Guide. Moreover, in Japan the suction denture has not only improved success rate of home dental care treatment in edentulous patients[2,3] but also extended to the treatment application for the edentulous sleep apnea patients[4-6].

At the same time, I received other comments such as " I would like to improve my suction denture technique to be able to treat more complicated cases." " I would like to learn the laboratory technique to improve suction strength." In order to fulfill those requests, the clinical and laboratory techniques for basic to complicated denture cases following BPS(Biofunctional Prosthetic System) will be described in this book.[7-10]

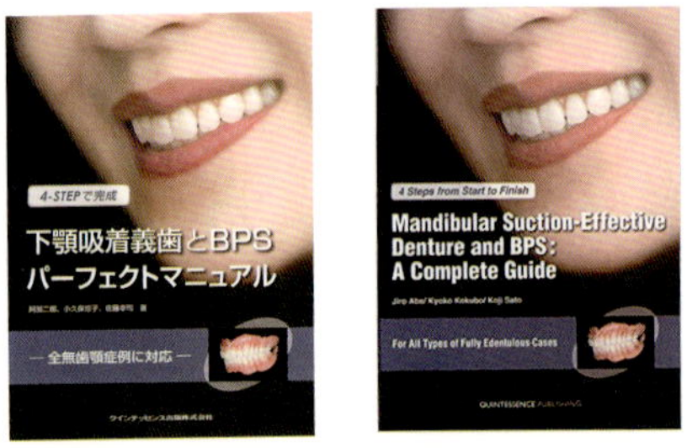

Fig 1a,b Japanese version and English version of Mandibular Suction-Effective Denture and BPS : A Complete Guide.

2 Difference between the conventional denture treatment and the Mandibular Suction-Effective Denture treatment combined with BPS

First of all, I would like to express the importance to learn the conventional denture treatment method in order to establish the fundamental concept of the denture treatment. It is important for the readers to understand that I have no intention to dismiss the conventional denture treatment method just because I advocate Mandibular suction effective denture technique. By stating this, I would like to describe the differences as follows.

(1)General concept of denture fabrication (Table1)

Conventional denture fabrication technique with stick compound advocated by Dr. Boucher CO in the 1960's is far different from Mandibular Suction-Effective Denture technique advocated by the author. This conventional treatment theory is that denture flange should extend to the muscle attachment to cover the maximum ridge surfaces in order to get a denture stabilization. This is a

Table 1 Difference between Conventional denture fabrication technique and Suction effective denture technique

	Conventional technique	Suction effective denture technique
Mandibular denture fabrication concept	Maximize denture surface stress-bearing area	Tightly sealed denture base entire border
Treatment target	muscle	oral mucosa
Treatment goal	Mandibular denture stability and retention	Mandibular denture suction with strong retention

Table 2 Preliminary impression technique difference

	Conventional technique	Suction effective denture technique
Preliminary impression technique	**Purpose : Clear identification of muscle attachment** By applying stress, mucosa is extended. Therefore, anatomical features of muscle attachment become clear Pressure loaded impression Opened mouth impression	**Purpose : Impression should reproduce the intra oral anatomical features of the closed mouth rest position with minimum distortion** Least pressure loading impression Closed mouth impression

correct theory. However, lately there are not many dentists who can teach accurate compound technique; therefore, this compound technique became less popular. The detailed compound technique is not well described even in the popular denture book " Prosthodontic Treatment for Edentulous Patients".[12-13]

On the other hand, no matter it is maxillary or mandibular denture fabrication, the suction effective denture treatment emphasis should be paid attention to the oral mucosa. The maximum suction will be acquired by having tight contact between denture base and oral mucosa and creating negative pressure between mucosa and the denture base during swallowing. Once main focus for the treatment has changed, obviously the focus for the preliminary impression, custom tray fabrication method and shape of custom tray and method of final impression will be changed accordingly. The clinical success will be achieved without mixing up those two different concepts together.

(2) Preliminary impression dissimilarity (Table 2)

For the conventional denture treatment, the preliminary impression should be performed to capture muscle attachments clearly by applying positive pressure on the mucosa. The custom tray is fabricated by having landmark of muscle attachments through preliminary impression process. On the other hand, the preliminary impression for the suction effective denture fabrication technique is performed by using a frame cut back tray (YDM, Morita) that will prevent deformation around the retro-molar pad area. This tray allows to capture not only the natural retro-molar pad anatomy but also entire edentulous ridge with low pressure on the mucosa at the resting position of the mandible. Then the custom tray for final closed-mouth functional impression to be able to achieve mandibular denture suction can be fabricated.[14]

Table 3 Final impression technique difference between conventional denture fabrication technique and suction effective denture fabrication technique

	Conventional technique	Suction effective denture technique
Final impression	Dentist oriented method	Patient oriented method
	Mostly opened mouth impression	Mostly closed mouth impression
	Functional impression controlled by the dentist	Dynamic functional impression
	Repeat impression partially until completion	One time total impression
	Impression outcome changes depending on the dentist, even though the same custom tray is used	Impression outcome is consistent with the same custom tray no matter who the dentist is

(3) The elements of custom tray fabrication influenced by 2 different denture fabricating concepts

Let's evaluate Fig 2,3 by considering the matter that has been explained so far. Fig 2 shows the denture surrounding muscles but no tongue and mucosal tissue. Fig 3 shows usual intra-oral view with the denture in.

Suction effective denture custom tray becomes smaller than the custom tray made with the conventional method preliminary impression that emphasize muscle attachment than mucosal landmark.

(4) Final impression technique

The conventional final impression method is opened-mouth technique. The dentist softens the stick compound and takes impression. If the dentist changes, there is a chance that same impression cannot be reproduced due to the change of the applied pressure on the lips or cheek or different softening point of the compound. Therefore, the conventional final impression method outcome may vary depending on the dentist's clinical experience or technical skill levels. (Table 3).
On the other hand, the suction effective denture impression technique is closed mouth technique that is mainly performed by using patient's functional movements. The outcome of the final impression depends on how correctly the preliminary impression and custom tray fabrication procedures have been carried out.

(5) Custom tray positioning

For the simple denture treatment, either methods would produce the successful denture with high patient's satisfaction. However, the difficult case involving severe ridge resorption would create a difficulty for the dentist to even place the custom tray in the correct position. During the conventional final impression taking with compound, most of the dentists would have experienced to lose the correct custom tray positioning by repeating border moulding with compound multiple times.

On the other hand, suction effective denture BPS impression technique requires to insert maxillary tray connected with mandibular tray and take closed-mouth functional final impression; therefore,

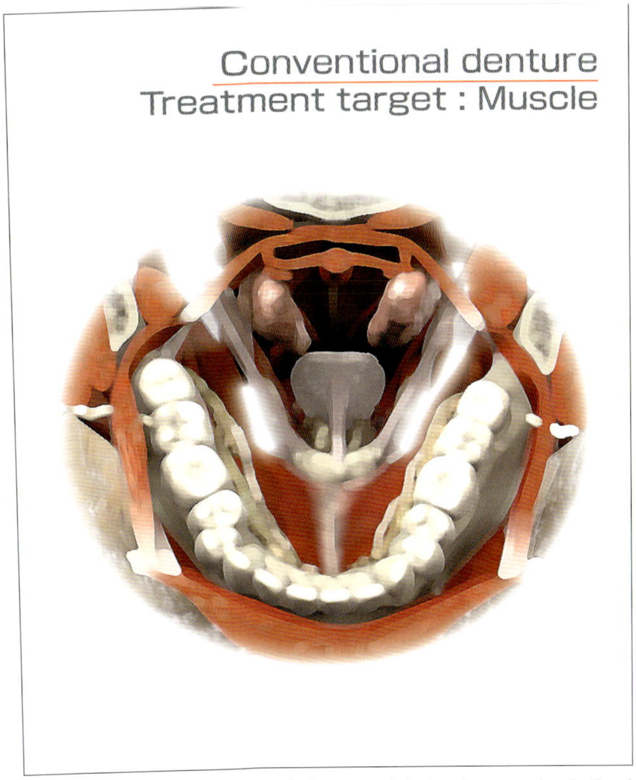

Fig 2 In the conventional denture fabrication method, final impression for the retention and support is done by targeting muscle features.

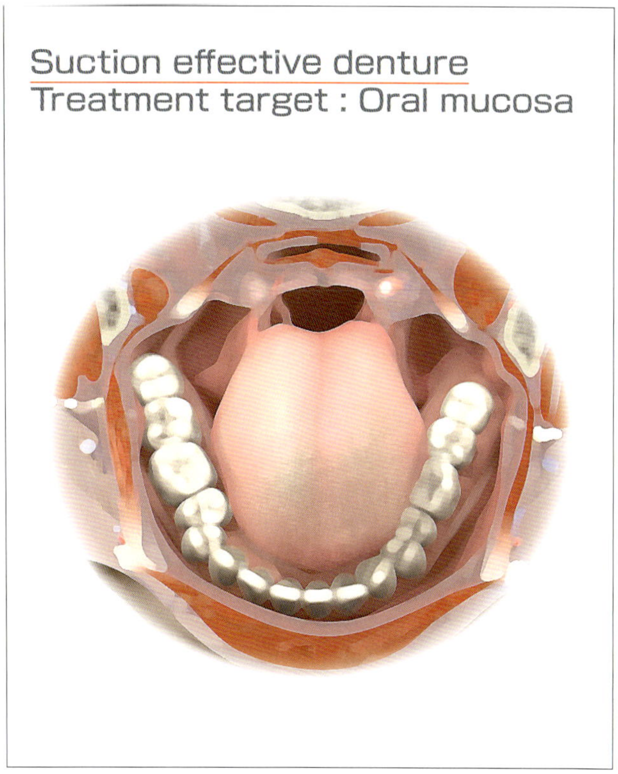

Fig 3 In the suction effective denture fabrication method, suction effective final impression for maximum total denture base border closure is done by targeting oral mucosa's features.

possibility of tray displacement is very low and the accurate functional final impression can be acquired.

3 Summary

The Mandibular suction effective denture is "the denture that the patient will feel resistance due to negative pressure when removing the denture." And this type denture should be fabricated by the dentist who fully understand the fabrication mechanism (Fig 4). Mr. Sato quoted in his book "What is Suction Denture?" (2014, Dental Diamond) that the suction denture is the denture never comes out[1]. My initial advise to the reader is to start with trying to take an accurate final impression that all the impression border should be well surrounded by the oral mucosa without having any air leak from the border.

I would like for the readers to understand that suction effective denture fabrication process is completely different from the conventional denture fabrication method, such as method of taking preliminary impression, custom tray designing line and fabrication mechanism, the final impression should be taken with closed-mouth technique and tooth set up and final polish should be designed for the denture to be wrapped around by the oral mucosa.

Suction mechanism of mandibular complete dentures

It is very important to fully understand the mechanism of total denture border seal in order to fabricate suction effective denture.

①Complete and total seal of the interior denture base surface and oral mucosa in the retromolar pad region (Primary seal)

The retromolar pad must be totally covered by the denture base. Initial process should start with preliminary impression with the frame cut back tray

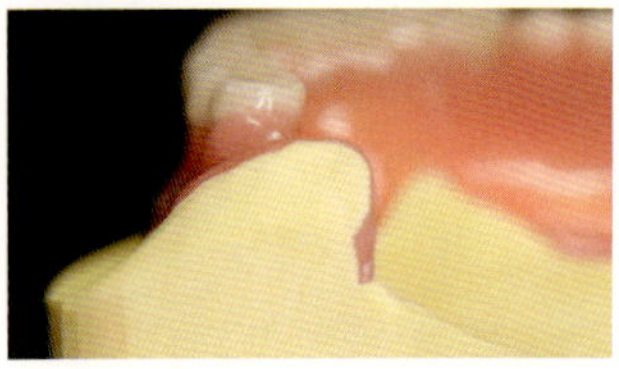

②Seal above the retromolar pad (Secondary closure)

The posterior border seal can be achieved by having contact between the buccal mucosa and the side of the tongue above the denture base where covers retromolar pad. This contact point is called BTC point

※BTC point : Buccal mucosa, Tongue side wall, Contact point

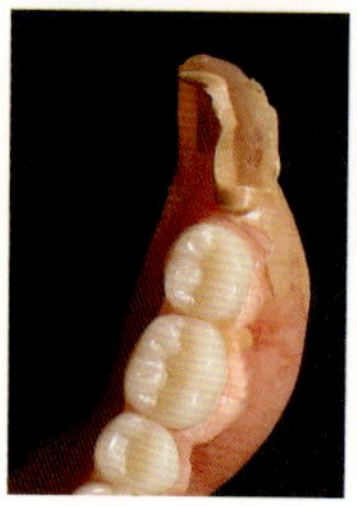

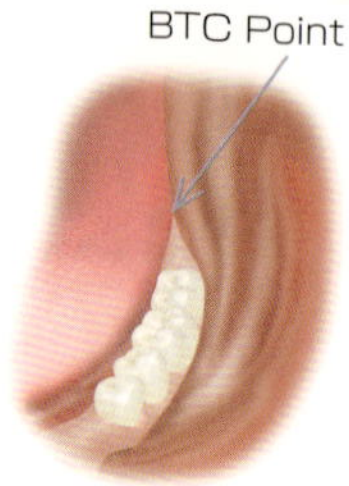

③Compensatory closure in the retromylohyoid muscle fossa region

A wall must be created to resist tongue pressure applied when tongue root presses against the lingual policed surface. This wall can be created by extending the denture border by 2-3mm beyond the mylohyoid ridge

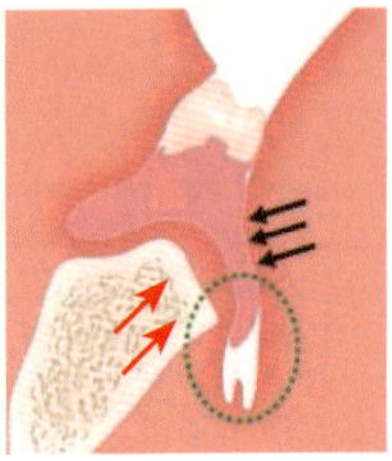

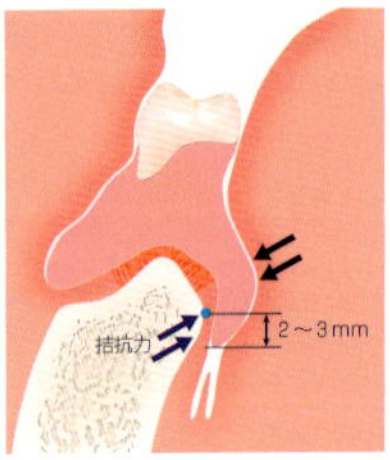

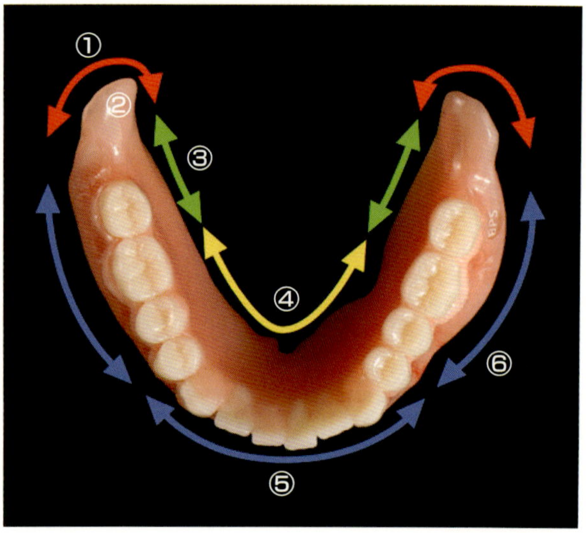

④Interior/exterior double closure in the sublingual fold region

With an abundance of spongy tissue, the contact between the denture border and mucosa in the sublingual fold region is maintained to provide a stable and strong seal

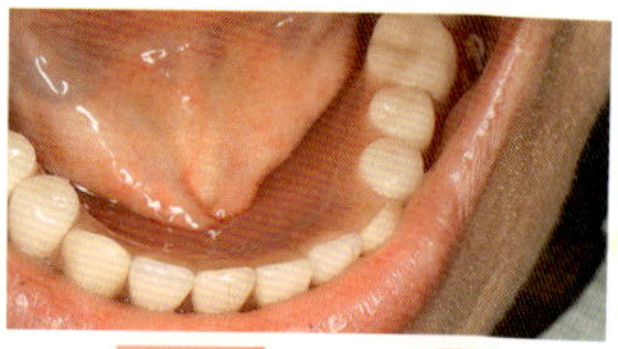

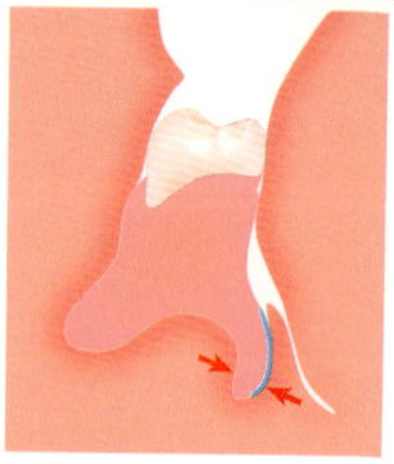

⑤Interior/exterior double closure in the labial area

A labial seal is created with the lower lip in contact with the exterior denture base surface and alveolar mucosa in contact with the interior denture base surface

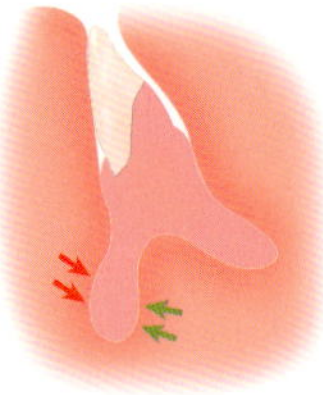

⑥Interior/exterior double closure in the buccal area

A buccal seal is created with the buccal mucosa in contact with the exterior denture base surface and alveolar mucosa in contact with the interior denture base surface

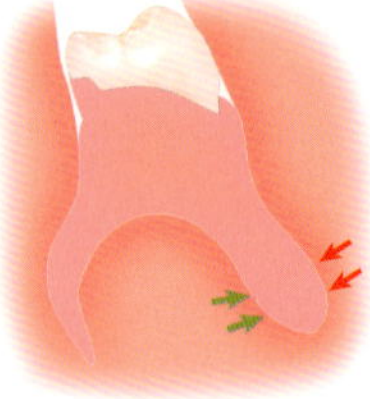

Fig 4 Suction mechanism of mandibular complete dentures[16-17].

Part 2

Everything starts from the simple intra-oral examination

Intra-Oral Examination

1 Sharing the examination of mandibular suction potential among the clinical and lab side

This oral examination sheet (Fig 1)[18-19] is developed for suction-effective denture with minimum check items stressing on clinical practice. It allows the practitioner to evaluate the patient if suction-effective denture could be fabricated or not in 10 minutes at the first visit. Successful suction-effective impression will be achieved by utilizing the appropriate impression technique according to the result of this examination (refer to Part 5 P74).

Success rate of achieving satisfactory suction-effective denture is considered to be about 87% by the well trained dentist[20-21]. Successfully screening the rest of 13%, which is considered as difficult case, utilizing this examination sheet allows the initial consultation to be more effective and specific (Fig 2).

This examination result is shared with the technician allowing him/her to consider about fabrication of the custom tray or denture teeth setting, thus being able to work with the dentist collaboratively sharing the same treatment goal from the start (refer to Part 5 P75).

2 Suction inhibiting factor

Utilization of this examination sheet is as follows. At first, check (✔) where it applies (Fig 3).

Suction inhibiting factor is categorized into two groups, anatomical factor and mandibular jaw position factor. They are all measured by Qualitative Analysis, which does not require measuring equipment.

Anatomical factor is divided to 5 items and it is considered as difficult case if there are more than two ✔ are marked as poor. Mandibular jaw position factor is divided to 3 items and it is considered as difficult case if ✔ is marked in any of the right most column (Class 3, unstable, severe).

It is retromolar pad area where accurate diagnosis is most difficult to make. There are four specific examination items, which is shown in the middle portion of the sheet. Expression of the evaluation result is different from other factors, but they all mean good, fair, poor in order from the left. It is marked as fair in [4. Pear shaped retromolar pad], if only one item is marked as poor and it is marked as poor, if more than two items are marked as poor in this section.

Following suction inhibiting factors, considered to be mandibular position factors, tend to be more significant to make suction of the mandibular denture difficult than anatomical factors, because occlusal interference due to unstable occlusion causes movement of the denture on the ridge breaking border seal.

Examination items for mandibular complete denture

Suction inhibiting factor	Right			Left		
	Good	Fair	Poor	Good	Fair	Poor
1. Ridge form						
2. Spongy tissue in sublingual fold region						
3. Space for denture extension in retromylohyoid fossa region						
4. Pear-like shaped retromolar pad						

Retromolar pad (one risk is ☑ as Fair, ☑ as Poor, if more than two risks are marked)

	Right	Left
1. The presence of firm fibrous tissue in anterior half	(Yes slightly No)	(Yes slightly No)
2. Size	(Large Moderate Small)	(Large Moderate Small)
3. Tilt angle	(Shallow Moderate Steep)	(Shallow Moderate Steep)
4. Change during open and close movement	(Small Moderate Large)	(Small Moderate Large)

5. Tongue retraction upon opening mouth	☐ Normal (less than 2cm)	☐ Further retraction (2〜4cm)	☐ Even further retraction (more than 4cm)
6. Jaw relationship	☐ Class I	☐ Class II	☐ Class III
7. Mandibular jaw position	☐ Guided position and habitual occlusal position coincide or within 2mm of discrepancy	☐ More than 2mm of discrepancy	☐ More than mm of discrepancy and unstable tapping point
8. Temporomandibular joint function	☐ Normal	☐ Disfunction	☐ Severe disfunction with pain

Special Note :
Wearing time of the denture, (Maxillary) Flabby tissue, Tori (Mandibular) Flabby tissue, Genial tubercle shallow labial vestibule in mandibular anterior region, etc →

Fig 1 Examination sheet for suction-effect of the mandibular complete denture.

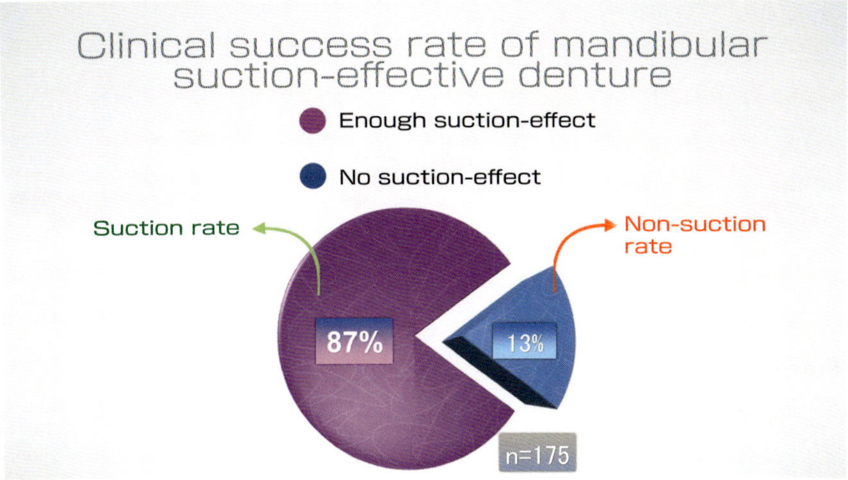

Fig 2 Clinical success rate of mandibular suction-effective denture (this figure is based on the reference 20).

[Anatomical suction inhibiting factor]

① Extensive ridge resorption

If the ridge is resorbed extensively, border seal tends to break due to air invasion by movement of the denture on the ridge during occlusion. It is considered Good if the amount of the bone above mental foramen is equal or more than that below. It is considered Fair if it is less and Poor if the bone loss is right above the mental foramen.

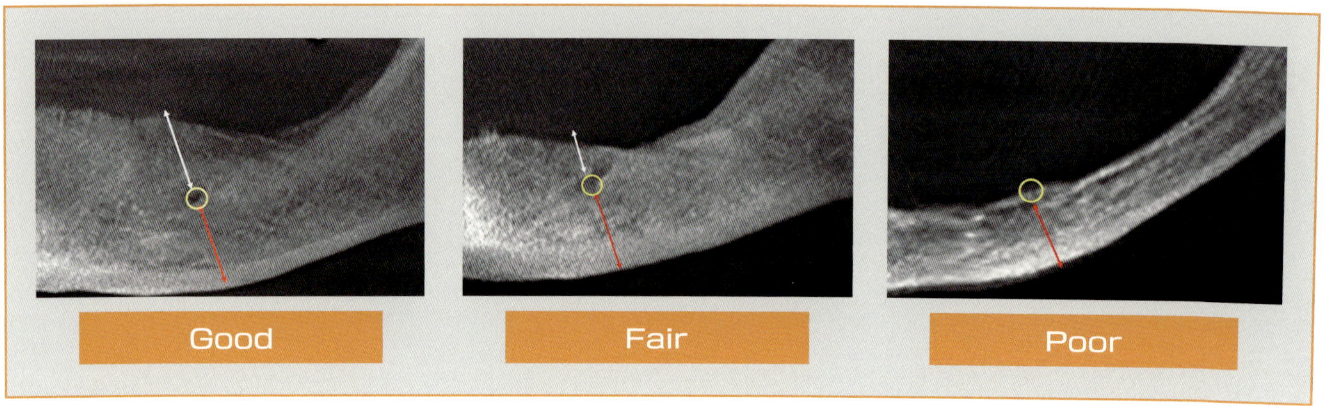

If the condition is poor: Accuracy of every step of preliminary impression, fabrication of custom tray and final impression is critical.

② Lack of spongy tissue of sublingual fold area

Strong border seal is generated by lingual flange being engaged in spongy tissue[22]. It is considered as Good if bulging spongy tissue is appreciated when the patient is asked to close the mouth slowly from the open position. It is considered as Fair if the bulge is minimum and as Poor if it is firm in tent-like shape.

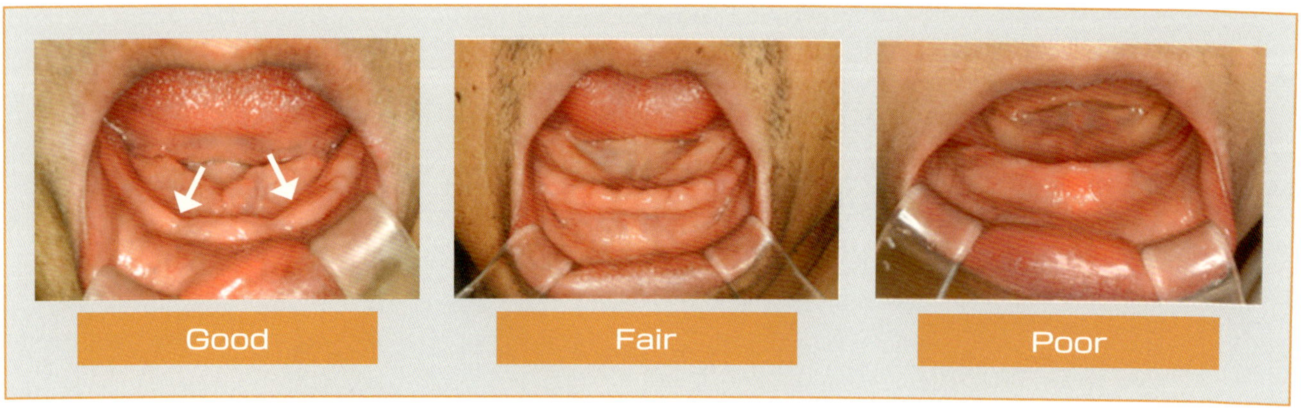

If the condition is poor: Optional impression technique to acquire lingual border seal utilizing silicone putty is required. ➩Refer to Fig 40, 41 in Part 5

③ Shallow retromylohyoid space

Complete seal is not accomplished unless the denture border is extended at least 2mm below this area of sublingual aspect of the retromolar pad. It is considered as Good if the retromylohyoid space, which allows extension of the denture border at least 2mm below the mylohyoid ridge, is confirmed by using the dental mirror. If it is shallow, it is considered as Fair and Poor if there is no space for extension.

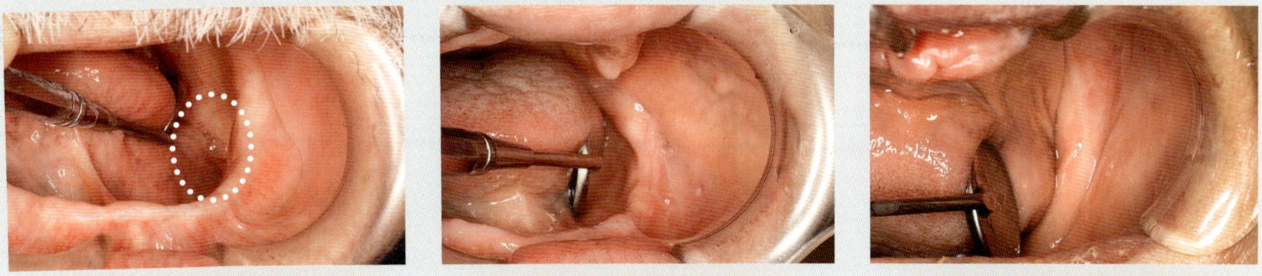

Enough space | Shallow space | No space

If the condition is poor: The custom tray is fabricated after modifying the study model by preparing the retromylohyoid space so that the denture border is extended below the mylohyoid ridge at least 2mm even only in the undercut area of the lingual posterior portion of the retromolar pad.

④ Strong retraction of the tongue upon opening the mouth

If the patient retracts the tongue strongly and unconsciously when opening the mouth, air gets in from the lingual flange edge of the denture and breaks border seal[23-26]. The position of the tip of the tongue in relation to anterior area of the ridge is checked at the rest position of the mandible or at the position with the mouth slightly open. If retraction of the tongue is less than 2cm, it is considered as Normal, 2~4cm as Further retraction and more than 4cm as even further retraction.

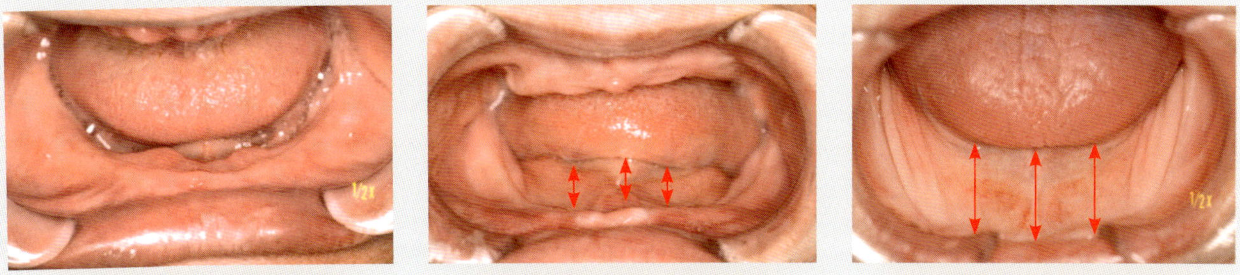

Retraction less than 2cm | Retraction between 2~4cm | Retraction more than 4cm

If the condition is poor: Lingual sealing technique using silicone putty is required. ➩Refer to Fig 40, 41 in Part 5.

⑤ Unfavorable shape of the retromolar pad

Retromolar pad is considered to be the most difficult part to establish good border seal, due to change of the shape of it during open and close motion of the mouth. There are four examination items and each side is examined. ① Is there any firm fibrous tissue in anterior region? ② Size (large or small). ③ Tilt angle of the retromolar pad (shallow or steep). ④ Change of the the shape during open and close motion of the mouth (large or small). If there is no check in Poor, it is considered overall as Good. It is considered as Fair, if there is one check in Poor and as Poor, if there are more than two checks in Poor. It is recorded in [4. Pear-like shaped retromolar pad].

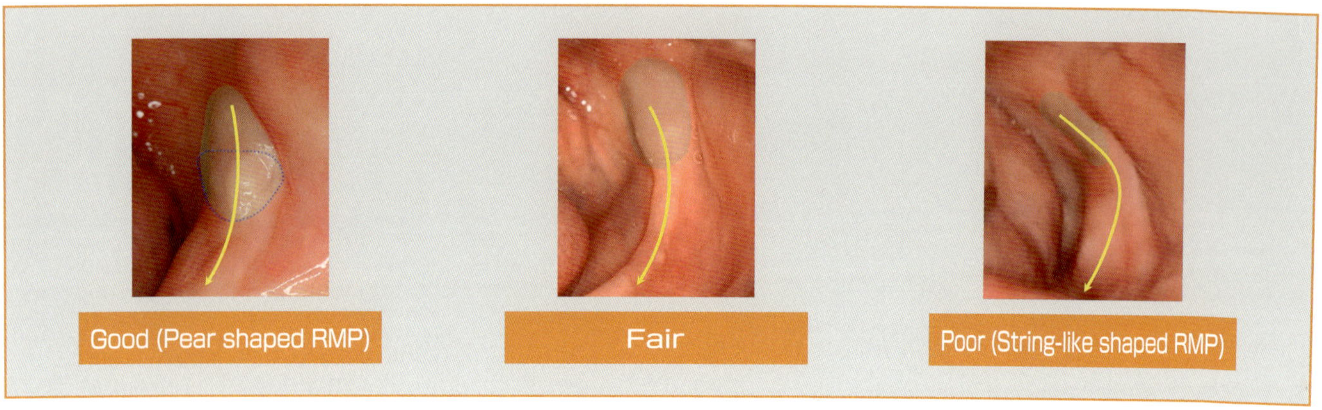

If the condition is poor: Fit of the custom tray is required to be improved before the final impression using self-cure acrylic resin.⇨Refer to Fig 33 in Part 5.

[Suction inhibiting factor due to mandibular position]

① Problematic jaw relationship of Class II or Class III

Large overjet tends to be provided in Class II case resulting in allowing large play in forward-backward direction. As a result, border seal breaks by air invasion due to sliding movement of the denture on the ridge. Low tongue posture is often found in Clas III jaw relationship, which makes lingual border seal difficult. Strong Opening Reaction by lower lip during opening the mouth contributes to dislodgment of the denture in Class III as well.

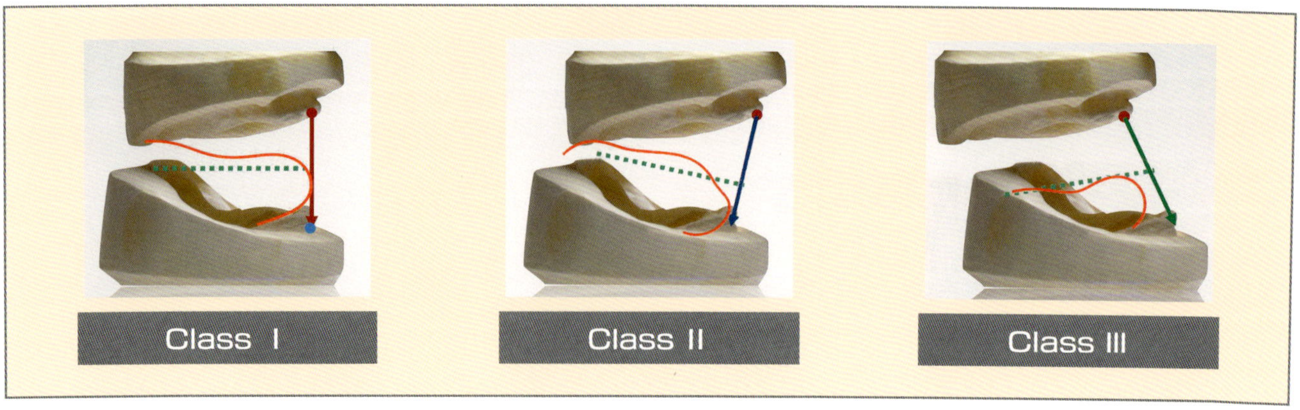

Class II Division 1 (Refer to Part 6) and Class III (Refer to Part 7) require special attention.

② Unstable mandibular position

If mandibular position is unstable, the border seal breaks as air invades from the border due to the movement of the denture on the ridge caused by occlusal interference. In this case, discrepancy between the guided position and patient's habitual occlusal position is checked by guiding the mandible backward with the existing denture in the mouth. Another guiding method is first to have the patient open his/her mouth touching the posterior region of the palate with tip of the tongue. The dentist stands in front of the patient and hold lateral side of mandibular denture teeth and then ask the patient to close the mouth keeping tip of the tongue touching the palate. The mandible is guided backward and the discrepancy can be observed.

If the discrepancy is more than 2mm, it is considered that discrepancy exists between the guided position and habitual occlusal position. If tapping point is unstable at guided position, it is considered that mandibular position is unstable.

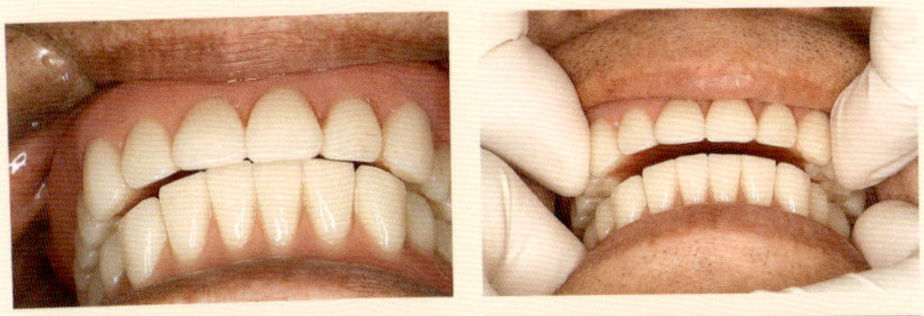

Patient' s habitual occlusal position

Guided mandibular position by the dentist

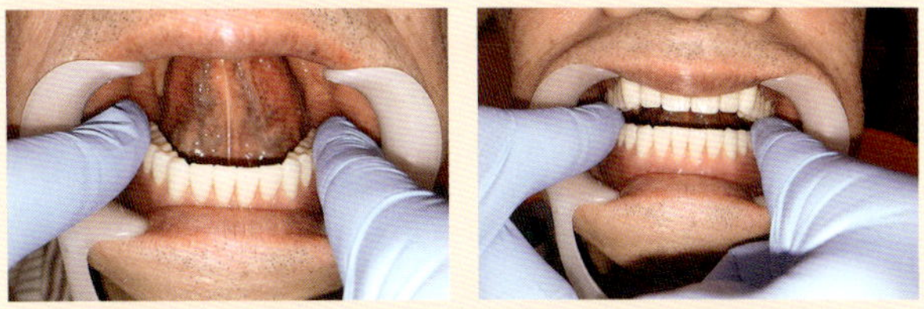

Mandibular denture teeth are held and the patient is asked to close the mouth with tip of the tongue touching the palate

③ Extensive temporomandibular functional disorder

Drastic displacement of mandibular jaw position, which induce click sound, could generate occlusal interference breaking the seal between mucosa and the denture.

Palpate about 13mm in front of the ear hole asking the patient open and close the mouth. It is considered as Good, if both condyles move simultaneously and smoothly. It is considered as Functional Problem, if one condyle precedes the other or one of the condyle deviates belatedly when it moves. It is considered Sever Functional Problem, if click sound caused by abnormal movement of condylar disc or pain accompanies the symptoms above.

The treatment denture to correct mandibular position is indicated if strong suction inhibiting factors due to mandibular jaw position are observed[31, 32]. Implant supported oeverdenture sometimes would be indicated if strong functional disorder such as click sound of temporomandibular joint is observed.

If the condition is poor: The treatment denture is indicated to stabilize the mandibular position.

Soft liner is recommended for the sensitive mucosa. Cream type denture adhesive is recommended for the patient with dementia or dry mouth.

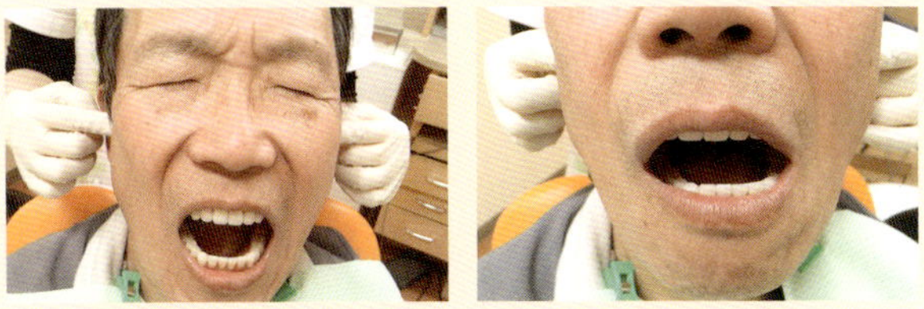

Strong temporomandibular functional disorder

3 Summary

Pretreatment intra-oral examination is not only for evaluation of potential for suction-effective denture, but also provides valuable information for the dentist about appropriate impression technique and for the dental technician about necessary contrivance at each fabrication step for achieving successful suction-effect. The treatment plan is made according to the findings of the intra-oral examination, which should be accessible anytime. Specific procedure is discussed in Part 5.

Part 3

Inviolable rules for success in complete denture treatment

1 Inviolable rules for success in complete denture treatment

Success in complete denture treatment is defined as follows,

[Maxillary complete denture never dislodges]

[To achieve suction-effect for mandibular complete denture]

Top priority is prevention of dislodgment of maxillary complete denture. It is required to "find optimum vertical dimension of occlusion and take maxillary and mandibular suction-effective impression under stable occlusion" in order to achieve above two objectives. Patient's satisfaction is obtained as a result[33-37].

Even if great suction-effective impression is taken, patient would have hard time to chew if the denture moves on the ridge due to poor intermaxillary record. On the other hand, the denture would function well enough even without suction-effect as long as occlusal position is stable at one point (Fig1). Intermaxillary record is the most important step and BPS system offers predictable result[38].

2 The reason to recommend impression procedure at closed position

It is important for mandibular suction-effective impression to take both preliminary and final impression at closed position. The condition that negative pressure inside the denture base generates is at the moment the patient bites in from mandibular rest position.

Saliva under the denture base is discharged at that biting moment generating negative pressure by sealing the denture border all around[39].

Fit of the denture around the retromolar pads and retruction of the tongue while opening the mouth are the anatomical suction inhibiting factors of mandibular complete denture, which are difficult to manage. The space created at the lingual denture border due to retruction of the tongue is often manageable to be sealed by utilizing optional seal-effective impression technique using silicone putty, which is described in Fig 41, 42 in Part 5. Border seal at the retromolar pad area, which changes its form easily during open and close motion, can be achieved only during preliminary and final impression procedure (Refer to Fig 33 in Part 5).

Fig 2 Upper illustrates relationship of the retromolar pad and the denture border when the denture is fabricated at closed mouth condition. The retromolar pad is stretched posteriorly changing the shape thinner when the mouth is opened and it contracts and gets shortend and rounded when the mouth is closed.

Impression is taken at closed position covering the retromolar pad with the denture base completely. Deformation of the retromolar pad upon opening the mouth is controlled by the denture base, since posterior part of the retromolar pad consists of soft glandular tissue. Lack of direct muscle attachment to the area

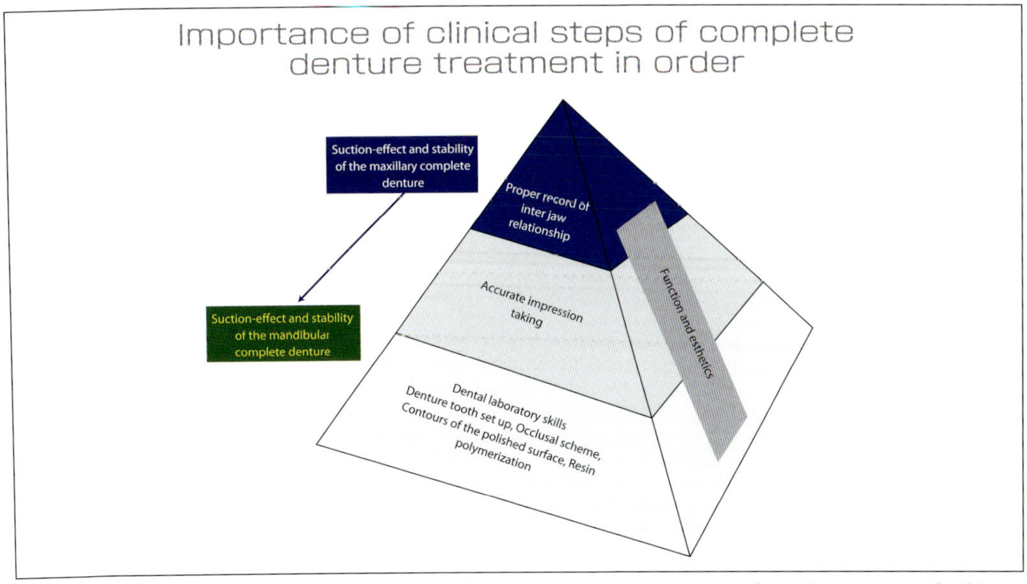

Fig 1 Importance of clinical steps of complete denture treatment in order. Proper record of inter jaw relationship is considered to be the most important step.

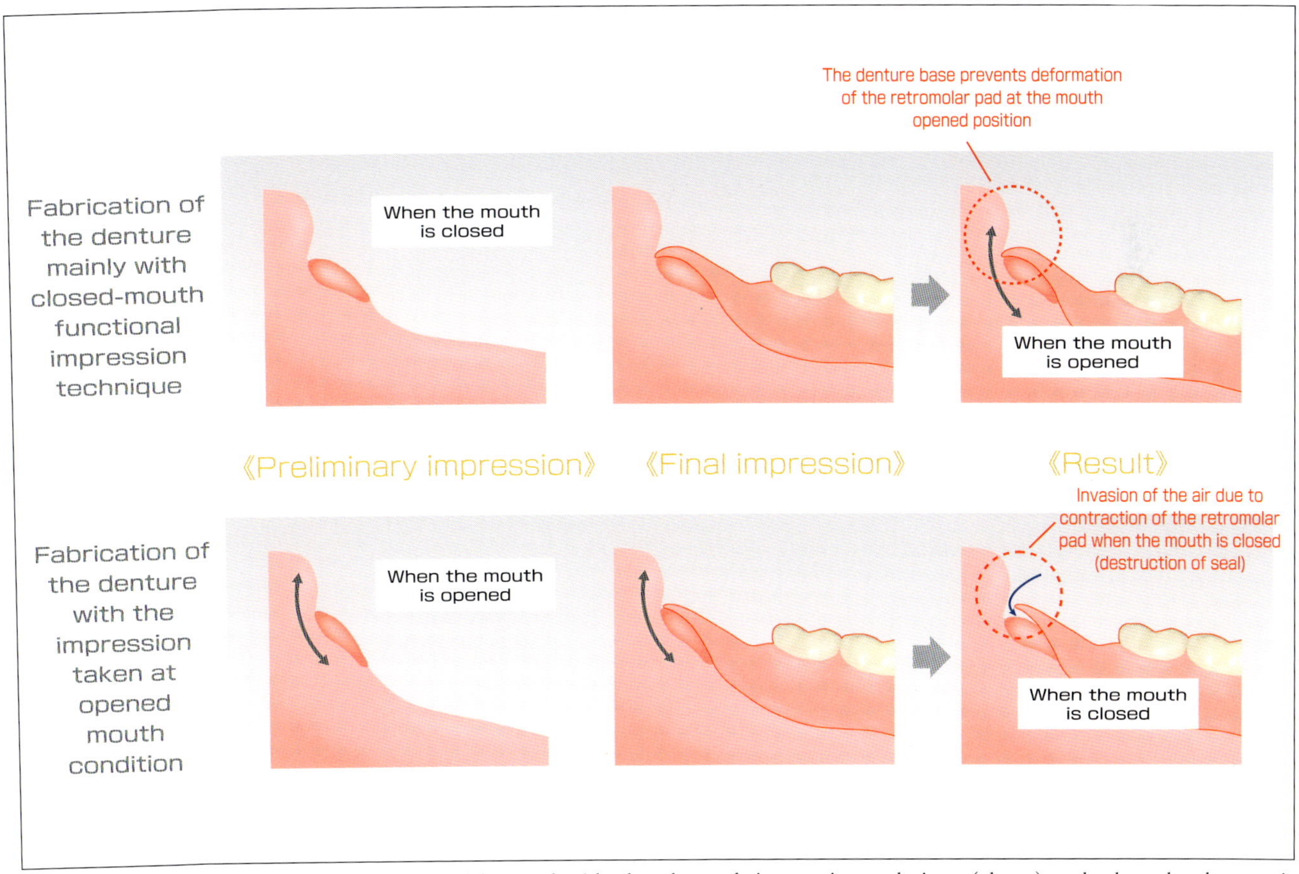

Fig 2 The illustrations when the denture is fabricated with closed-mouth impression technique (above) and when the denture is fabricated with opened-mouth impression technique (below).

is another reason that the denture base covering retromolar pad completely could prevent deformation of the retromolar pad.

Fig 2 Lower illustrates fabrication of the denture at opened mouth condition. If the impression is taken at opened mouth condition with the retromolar pad stretched and thinned, it creates space underneath the denture base once the retromolar pad contracts when the mouth is closed breaking the border seal.

The principle for suction-effect of maxillary and mandibular denture is complete border seal of the entire denture borders. The maxillary denture would fall down and the mandibular denture would lift up if there is even one spot of air leak.

Due to the reasons above, it is important to take preliminary and final impression mainly under mouth closed condition in order to achieve mandibular suction-effective complete denture.

3 Mandibular displacement after insertion of the denture destroys suction-effect

Sustained stable occlusion is important factor for stability of maxillary and mandibular suction-effective dentures.

Change in mandibular jaw position after the denture is inserted causes deviation from occlusal position resulting in pain. Once occlusal balance is lost, border seal breaks and the mandibular denture starts to lift up.

(1)The anterior space, which is lost in short period of time

Sustained stable occlusion of the dentures contributes to comfortable suction-effective denture. It is the theory for complete denture to provide 1.5 ~ 2.0mm of anterior clearance to avoid anterior occlusal interference (Fig 3). It is believed to prevent falling of the maxillary denture by eliminating anterior sole contact during excursive movement.

Clinically speaking however, provided anterior clearance often diminishes in short period of time resulting in maxillary and mandibular anterior teeth contact (Fig 4). Patients suffer from pain or instability of dentures due to this occlusal discrepancy.

(2) The cause of loss of the space

Denture teeth on the market nowadays would not wear down in such a short period to time. Hence, it is conceivable that this space loss is due to shift of the mandible (Fig 5). Why would this phenomena happen?

Anterior space is about 0 ~ 0.2mm, which is considered to be almost contacting, in most of healthy dentate people (Fig 6). This condition is created by the body to determine the Anterior Stop of the mandible by the contact against maxillary anterior teeth. Rather straight mandibular closing movement, which is

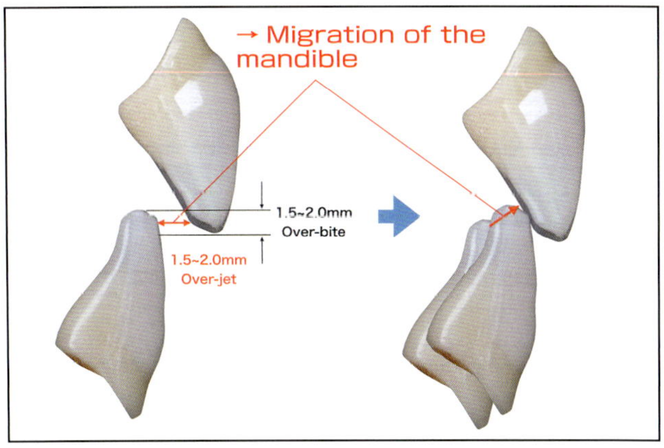

Fig 3 It is the general theory in complete denture prosthetics to provide 1.5～2.0mm of anterior clearance (horizontal overlap) in order to avoid anterior occlusal interference. Maxillary and mandibular anterior teeth end up with contacting in many cases once the anterior space is lost just in several months after delivery of dentures.

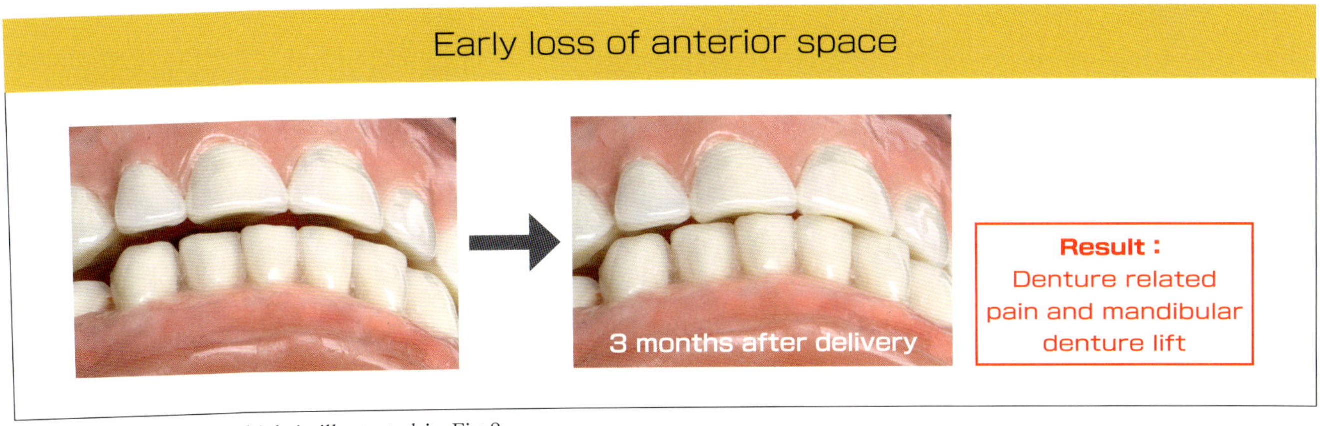

Fig 4 Clinical case, which is illustrated in Fig 3.

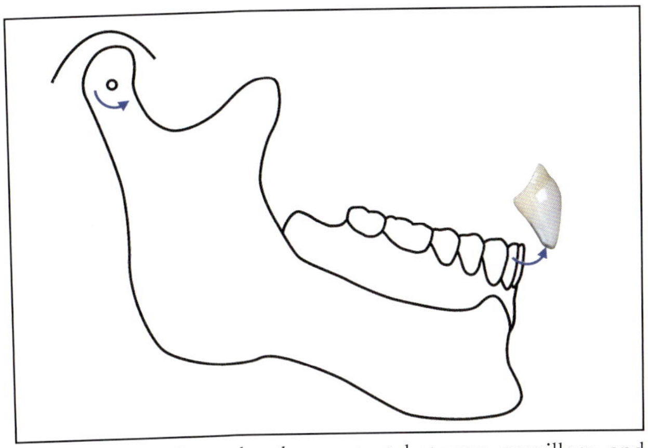

Fig 5 Our body seeks the contact between maxillary and mandibular anterior teeth regardless of the condition if it is dentate or edentulous. The edentulous mandible especially tends to rotate by the joint in counter-clockwise rotation until anterior teeth come into contact if large anterior clearance is provided to the complete dentures.

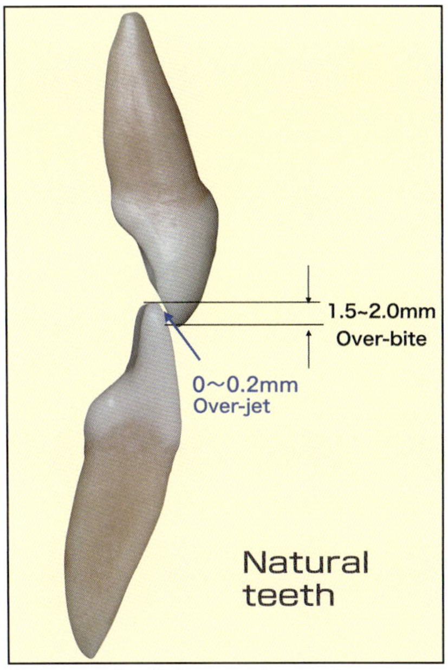

Fig 6 As little as 0～0.2mm of anterior space, which is considered as almost contacting, is observed in most of healthy dentate people.

Anterior clearance in Class I

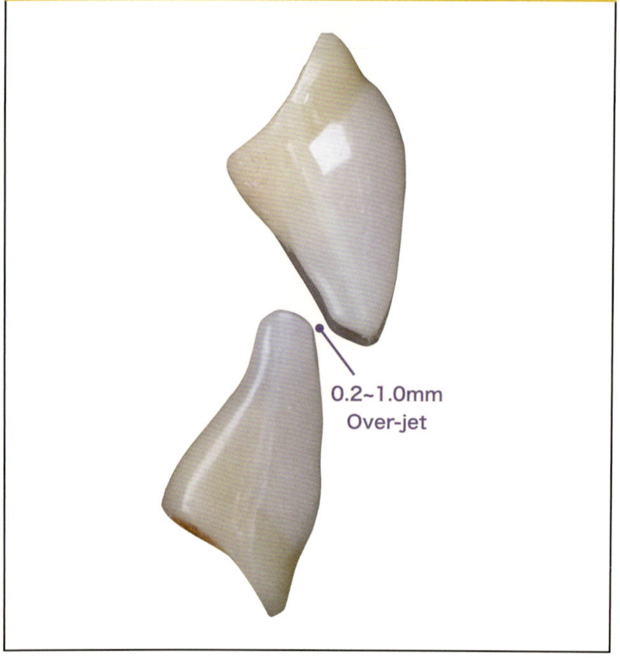

Fig 7 Anterior tooth relationship of Class I. 0.2mm of space is not large enough to eliminate the anterior interference by adjustment on the articulator. Realistically, an effort should be made to keep anterior clearance within 1.0mm.

Anterior clearance in Class II - 2 with maxillary flabby ridge

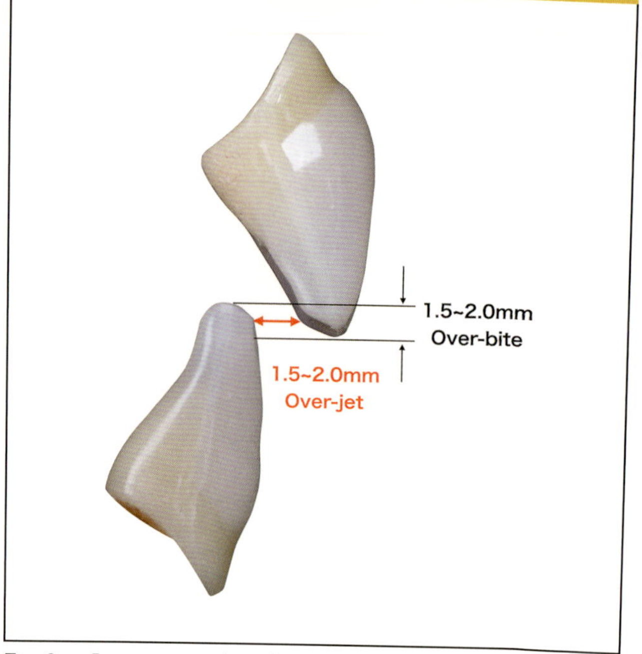

Fig 8 Larger anterior clearance is provided intentionally to prevent maxillary denture fall in the case with maxillary flabby ridge.

determined by mandibular anterior terminal position, allows reasonable function. Excessive contact between maxillary and mandibular teeth is prevented by providing slight space inbetween[40].

Similarly, many edentulous patients tend to move their jaw forward to close the space between maxillary and mandibular teeth to create anterior stop. In other words, it is quite natural for our body to seek for anterior stop regardless it is dentate or edentulous[41].

Early loss of the anterior clearance due to anterior migration of the mandible failing to sustain the mandibular jaw position, which was registered as "right position" is not desirable for the clinician. Providing right amount of anterior clearance for each Class of Occlusion (Class I, II, III) is important to stabilize the mandibular position for the sake of "prevention of the maxillary denture from falling".

(3) Optimum anterior space for each Class of Occlusion

Cases of Class I, Class II Division 2 with maxillary flabby ridge, Class II Division 1, which has tendency of developing large anterior space, are presented in this section. Please note that anterior clearance, created by denture tooth set up, is provided in specific way for each case.

Anterior clearance in Class II - 1

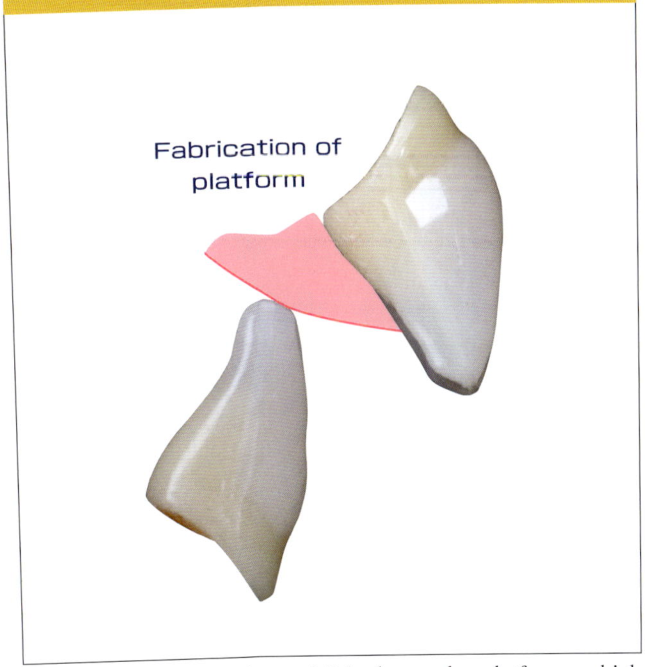

Fig 9 Anterior stop is established on the platform, which is created to fill large anterior space generated by maxillary protrusion in Class II - 1 case (refer to Fig 11 in p.157 Part 6).

Anterior clearance in Class III

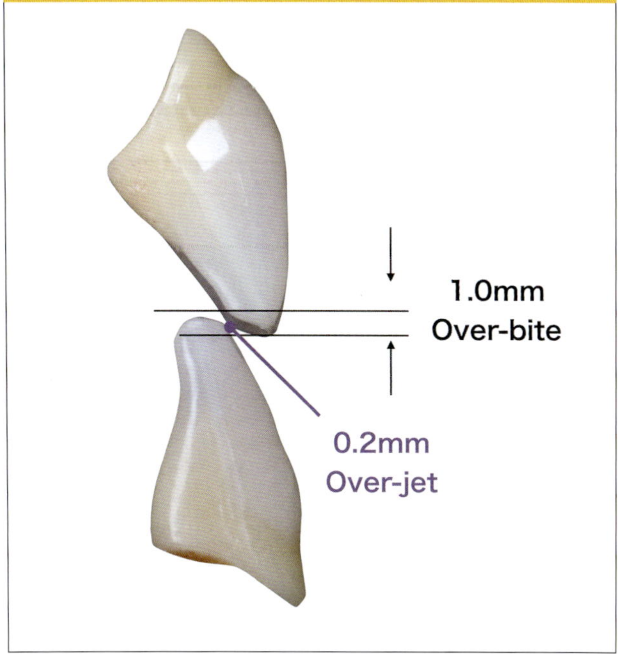

Fig 10 Anterior teeth relationship of Class III. Slight anterior space or slight contact of maxillary and mandibular anterior teeth is provided as well as shallow 0.5mm of Over-bite.

1) CLASS I (Fig 7, refer to Part 4)

Occlusal relationship is maintained by providing minimum amount of anterior clearance and preventing migration of the mandibular jaw position. It is important to keep the space within 1mm on the articulator.

2) Class II -2 (Maxillary flabby ridge, Fig 8, refer to Part 5)

Anterior clearance of less than 1mm, same as Class I, is provided for usual Class II- 2 case. However, tendency of the body to seek the contact against maxillary anterior teeth should be ignored in the case of maxillary anterior flabby ridge in order to prevent maxillary denture fall, which is patient's biggest complaint. Larger anterior space is provided to avoid anterior interference for the sake of controlling inflammation of flabby ridge as well as preventing maxillary denture fall. Occlusion is adjusted periodically to maintain the mandibular position preventing the maxillary denture from falling.

3) Class II - 1 (Fig 9, refer to Part 6)

Anterior stop is established on the platform, which is created to fill large anterior space generated by maxillary protrusion.

4) Class III (Fig 10, refer to Part 7)

Most of the class III patients want to have a facial appearance of class I individual. Slight anterior contact or slight anterior clearance with shallow over-bite of 0.5mm is provided, which prevents anterior interference during functional movement and tendency of mandibular protrusive migration.

4 Summary

Key elements for success of complete denture treatment are to establish stable occlusion, to put first priority on stability of maxillary denture and to establish suction-effect of the mandibular denture to the ridge to improve patient's satisfaction. Closed mouth impression technique must be employed to achieve suction-effect of the mandibular denture.

Properly designed anterior clearance for each case is very important to facilitate maintenance of the occlusal relationship provided originally for long term patient's satisfaction.

Part 4

Clinical case 1
Easy case : The Class 1 occlusion clinical case with and ideal ridge and stable mandibular position

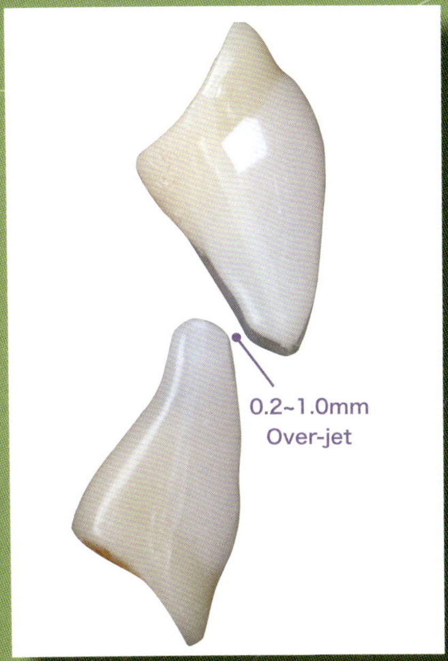

Dental Technician:
Kenji Iwaki

First of all, the basic Suction effective/ BPS denture technique that can accomplish the denture insertion with 4 clinical visits from the start to finish is introduced.

On the first visit, intra oral exam, diagnosis, Maxillary and Mandibular preliminary impressions and the preliminary interocclusal record with the centric tray are accomplished.

1 Intra oral condition diagnosis for mandibular denture suction (Intra-oral Examination)

Intra oral exam at the first visit reveals maxillary and mandibular ridge conditions are ideal and mandibular jaw position is quite stable. Except not enough spongy tissue is present in the sublingual fold region, the initial diagnosis reveals that not only the maxillary denture but also mandibular denture fabrication will be successful (Fig 1,2). For the case like this, It is very important to inform the patient the positive outcome of the successful suction effective denture fabrication.

2 Consultation : Explain the patient that maxillary and mandibular suction effective denture success rate is 90%

The patient's issues and complain with the existing denture should be well perceived and listed. Those should be reflected in the new denture fabrication process. The most important point is that the treatment process should be well explained to the patient including the possibility of the successful outcome of the suction effective denture based on the initial diagnosis.

Explanation should never be indecisive such as " I don't know that the denture fabrication can be successful unless I try." but " Your suction effective denture will be 90% successful according to my thorough diagnosis. Consequently, you will be able to eat effectively and speak clearly." This explanation will be the key for gaining the patient's confidence in you. The success rate should varies depending on the dentist's years' and numbers of suction effective denture treatment; therefore, the comment for the patient should be considered with the dentist's capability. For example, if talking about cancer treatment, the patient wouldn't decide to have a surgery by having told that it isn't sure that the surgery can cure the cancer.

The patient will decide to have a suction effective denture treatment once he/she hears the success rate of the treatment.

Also, it is important to understand that there is no treatment that possesses 100% success rate.

Class Ⅰ

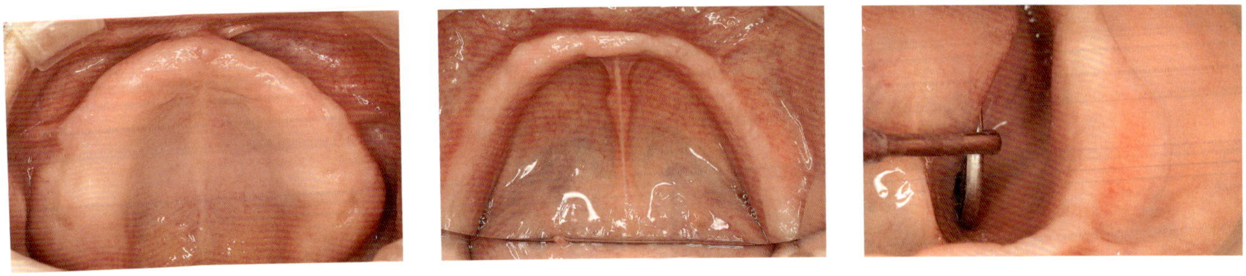

Fig 1 81yrs old male patient. Ideal alveolar ridge condition and jaw relationship. Yet, sub lingual spongy tissue has been slightly lacking.

Examination items for mandibular complete denture

Suction inhibiting factor	Right			Left		
	Good	Fair	Poor	Good	Fair	Poor
1. Ridge form	☑			☑		
2. Spongy tissue in sublingual fold region		☑			☑	
3. Space for denture extension in retromylohyoid fossa region	☑			☑		
4. Pear-like shaped retromolar pad	☑			☑		

Retromolar pad (one risk is ☑ as Fair, ☑ as Poor, if more than two risks are marked)

	Right	Left
1. The presence of firm fibrous tissue in anterior half	(✓Yes slightly No)	(✓Yes slightly No)
2. Size	(✓Large Moderate Small)	(✓Large Moderate Small)
3. Tilt angle	(✓Shallow Moderate Steep)	(✓Shallow Moderate Steep)
4. Change during open and close movement	(✓Small Moderate Large)	(✓Small Moderate Large)

5. Tongue retraction upon opening mouth	☑ Normal (less than 2cm)	☐ Further retraction (2～4cm)	☐ Even further retraction (more than 4cm)
6. Jaw relationship	☑ Class Ⅰ	☐ Class Ⅱ	☐ Class Ⅲ
7. Mandibular jaw position	☑ Guided position and habitual occlusal position coincide or within 2mm of discrepancy	☐ More than 2mm of discrepancy	☐ More than mm of discrepancy and unstable tapping point
8. Temporomandibular joint function	☑ Normal	☐ Disfunction	☐ Severe disfunction with pain

Special Note :
Wearing time of the denture, (Maxillary) Flabby tissue, Tori (Mandibular) Flabby tissue, Genial tubercle shallow labial vestibule in mandibular anterior region, etc

→ Complain of the existing denture that cannot provide the good chewing function.

Fig 2 Result of the list of the exam from the of this case.

Preliminary impression of the Maxillary ridge using the Accu-Dent XD System

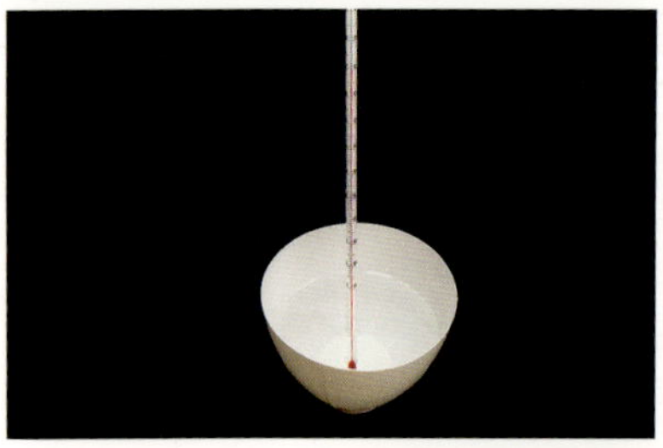
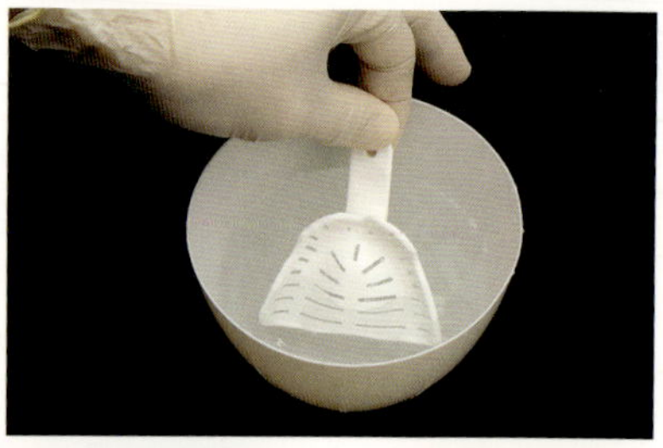
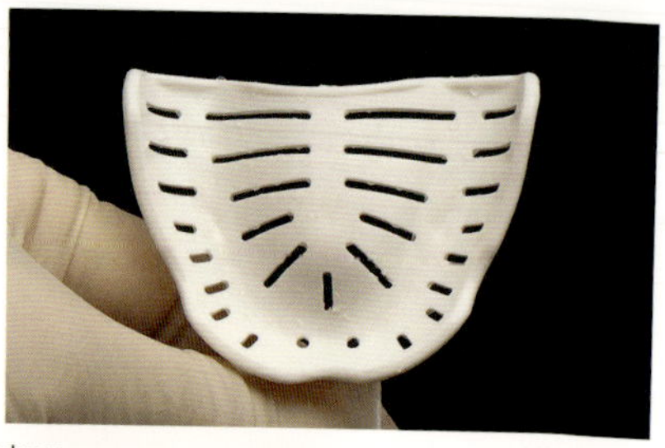

①Soak the thermoplastic tray in 70℃ warm water

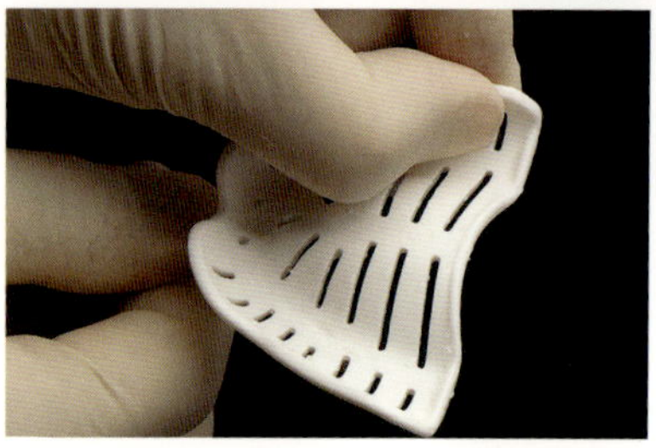

②Mold the tray according to the shape of the ridge

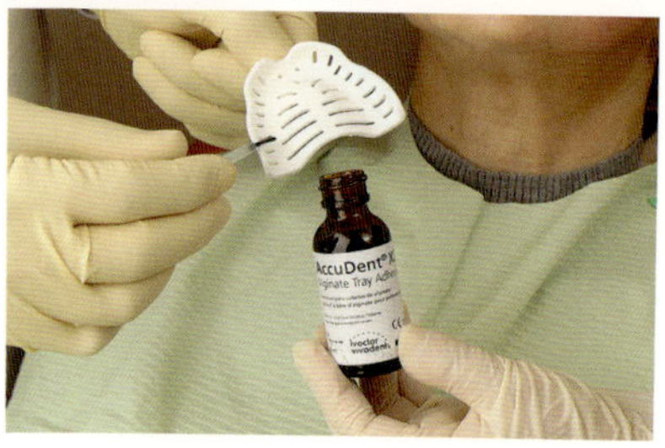

③Apply tray adhesive

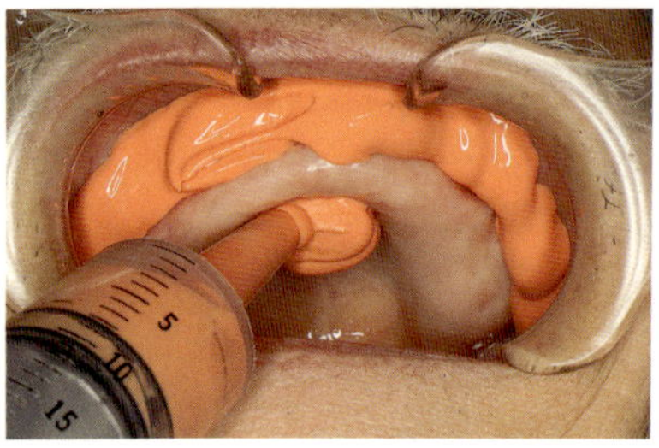

④Apply syringe Accu-Gel with the syringe tip intra-orally

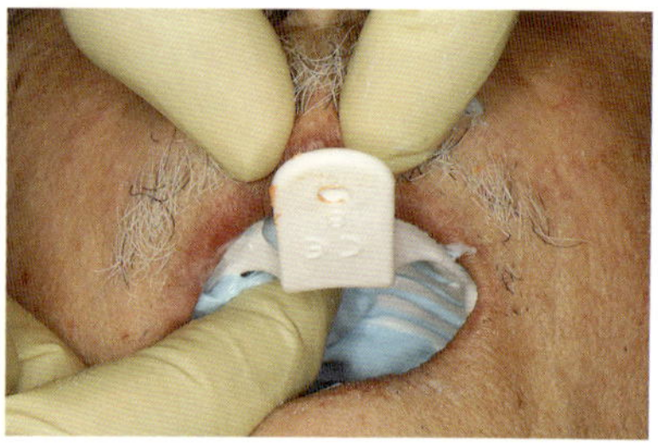

⑤Load the tray with high viscosity tray Accu-gel and insert it intra-orally

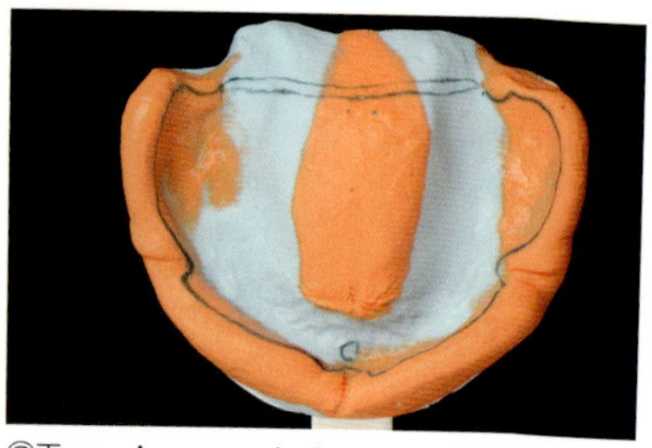

⑥Tray Accu-gel changes color from purple to blue with setting

Fig 3 Preliminary impression of the Maxillary ridge using the Accu-Dent XD System. (possible to use other company's material)

3 Maxillary preliminary impression : 2 impression materials that have different flow rate are used

First, the interview regarding gag reflex should be done with the patient. If there is no issue with the gag reflex, the preliminary impression should be performed (Fig 3).

Double impression technique by using high flow and low flow impression materials, are used to acquire maxillary and mandibular preliminary impressions. This impression should be done with non functional technique that should dictate the denture border preliminary, so it is not the functional impression that requires lip and cheek active movements.

Clean and bubbleless impression would motivate the dental technician's motivation for success. Therefore, obviously the unclear impression with a lot of bubbles would discourage the dental technician's motivation of success.

Preliminary impression of the Mandibular ridge using the Accu-Dent XD System

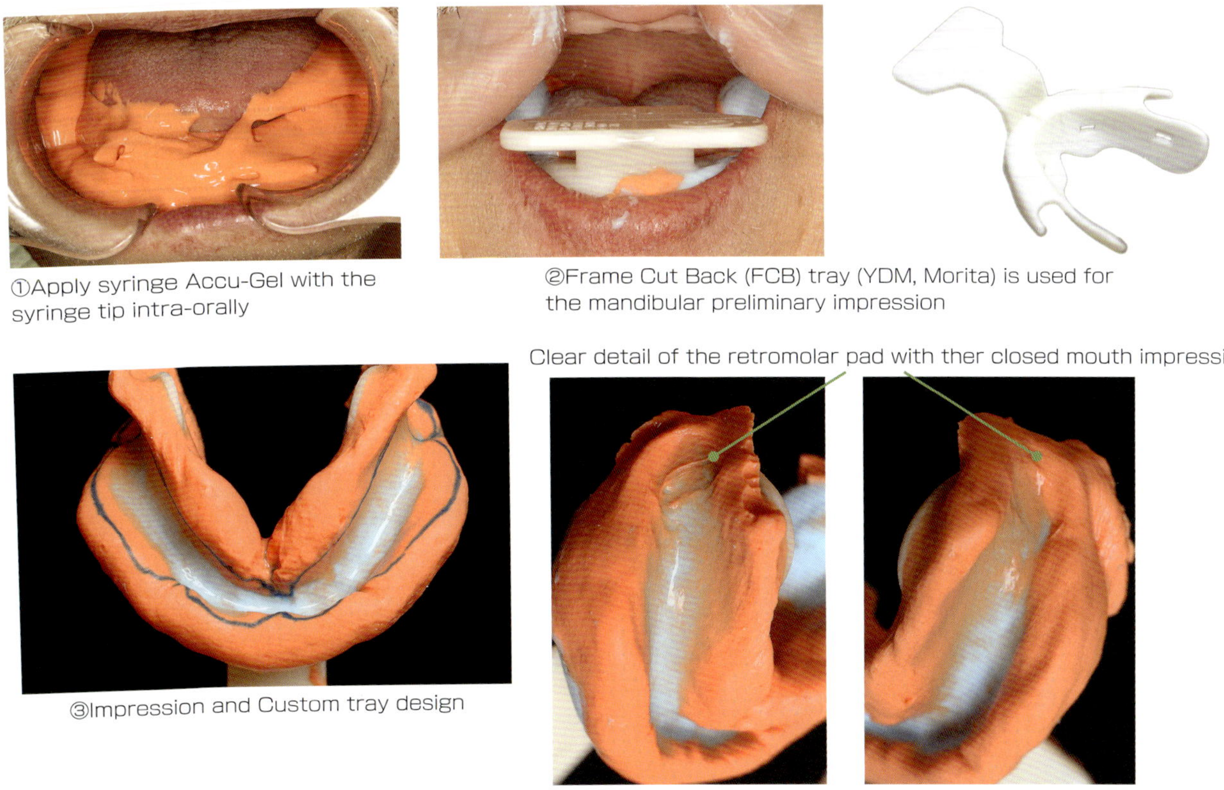

①Apply syringe Accu-Gel with the syringe tip intra-orally

②Frame Cut Back (FCB) tray (YDM, Morita) is used for the mandibular preliminary impression

Clear detail of the retromolar pad with ther closed mouth impression

③Impression and Custom tray design

Natural form of retromolar pad in rest position is reproduced

Fig 4 Mandibular preliminary impression using the Accu-Dent XD System (Ivoclar vivadent) and frame cut back tray (FCB tray). This technique allows to produce ideal border seal with the final denture by preventing to have the distortion in the impression of the retromolar pad and buccal shelf.

The several detail techniques of preliminary impression method will be discussed on Part 5 Class 2 difficult case.

4 Mandibular preliminary impression : AccuDent XD system and Frame cutback tray

Mandibular preliminary impression technique must be taken with mandibular jaw closed so that the impression will represent a natural form of the retromolar pad region and buccal shelf area in mandibular rest position (Fig 4). The most difficult area to achieve the complete denture base peripheral seal is considered to be the retromolar pad region; therefore, It is ideal to acquire the retromolar pad impression with the closed-mouth in mandibular rest position. The Frame cut back tray is that the frame of the tray is cut back in the retromolar pad and buccal shelf regions to minimize deformation of the tissue around the retromolar pads. This Frame cut back tray (YDM, Morita) should be used for the preliminary impression.[42-44]

Fundamental impression technique with the Centric tray with the silicone putty

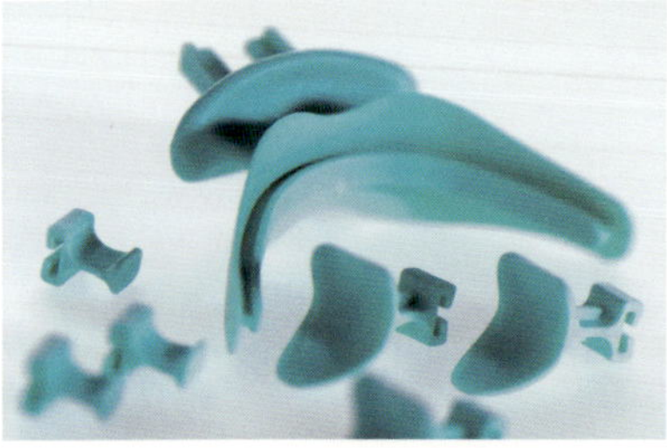

①Centric tray (Ivoclar Vivadent)

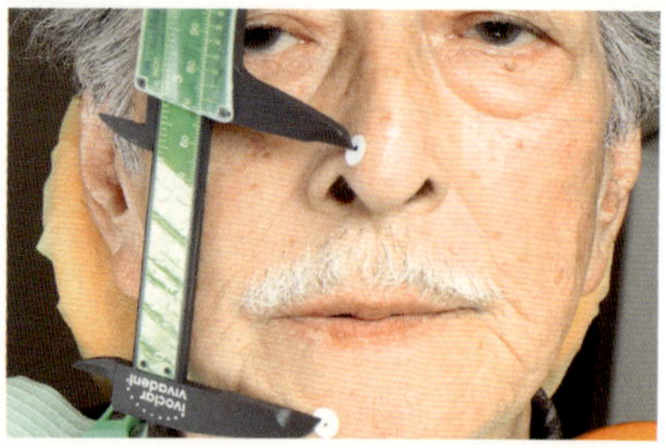

②Measuring the appropriate vertical dimension of occlusion (VDO) between the two reference points

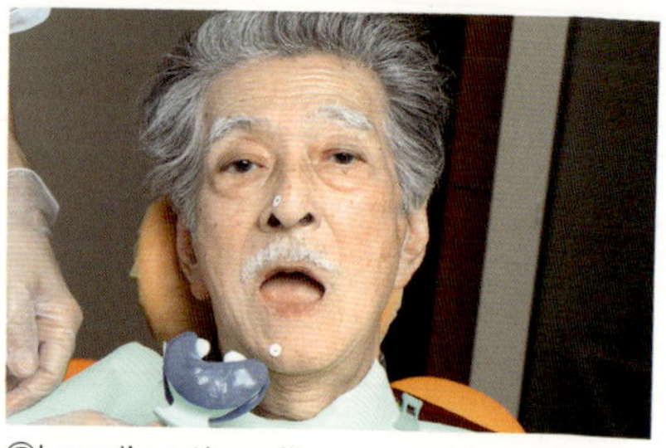

③Loading the silicone putty on the tray

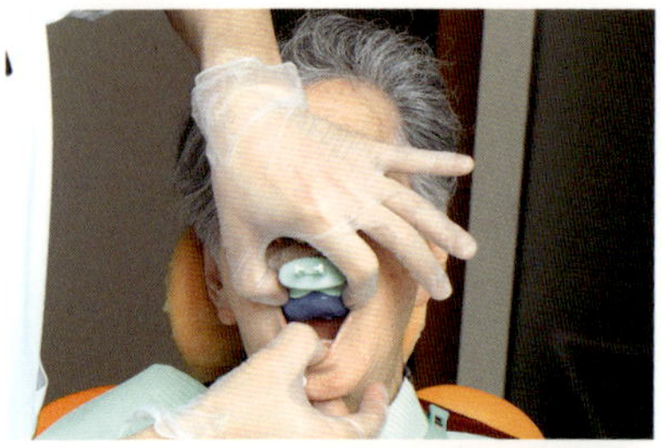

④After inserting the tray in the patient's mouth, holding the tray with the left hand and secure the tray on the maxillary arch. Then guide the mandible with right thumb to the centric position to close to the tray

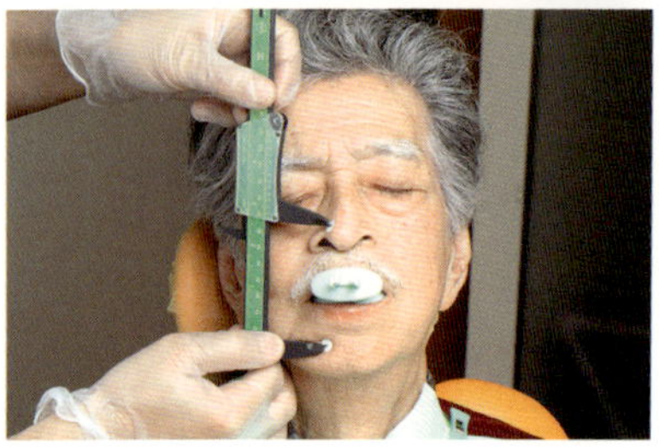

⑤Let the patient close until the VDO position that was recorded previously

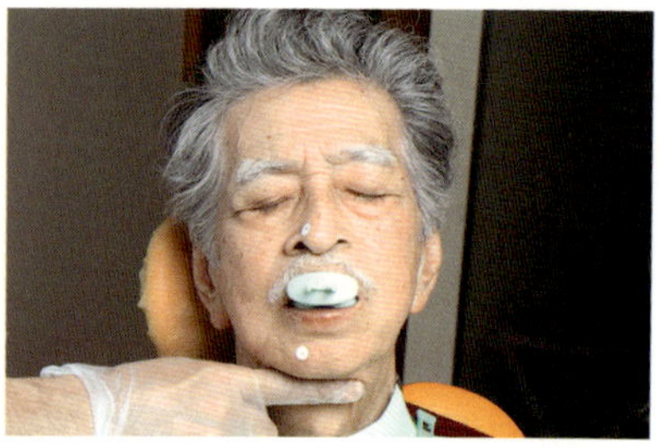

⑥Ask the patient to swallow to predetermined OVD has been reached

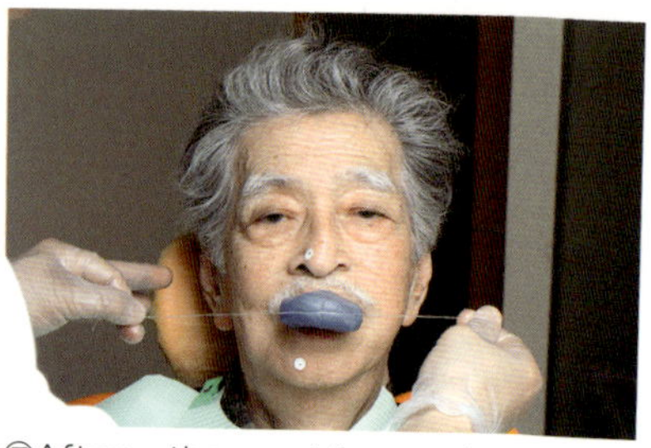

⑦After the setting, place the silicone putty on the handle in order to record the horizontal line and midline. This lines will be the reference for the mounting to the articulator

Fig 5 Fundamental impression technique with the Centric tray with the silicone putty.

5 Initial interocclusal record with the Centric tray (Basic Technique)

By using the Centric tray for the initial interocclusal record, spending time to adjust uneven wax rims during interocclusal record process can be dramatically cut short.

However this double arch impression technique to acquire impression of maxillary and mandibular arches together with silicone putty or low flow alginate impression material can be technically difficult. The dentist's hand technique is very important to acquire the accurate impression; therefore, this section will explain the basic hand technique throughly (Fig 5). Please refer Part 5 page 86-91 for the centric tray professional technique.[45]

Mounting the preliminary casts by using the Centric tray bite

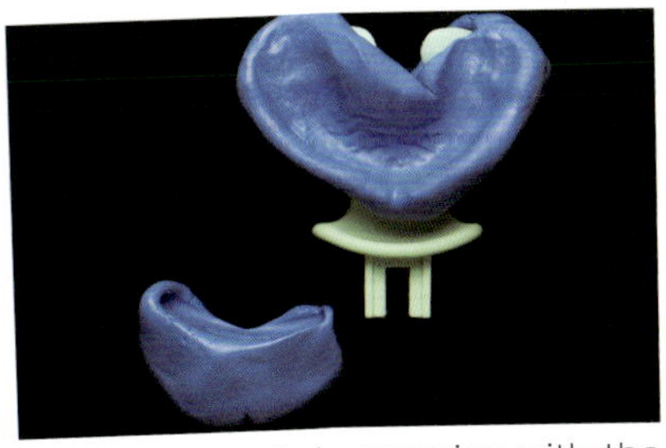

①Maxillary arch impression with the Centric tray

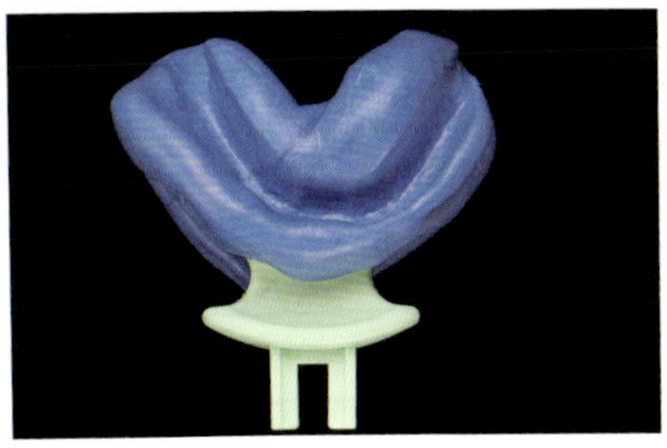

②Mandibular arch impression with the Centric tray

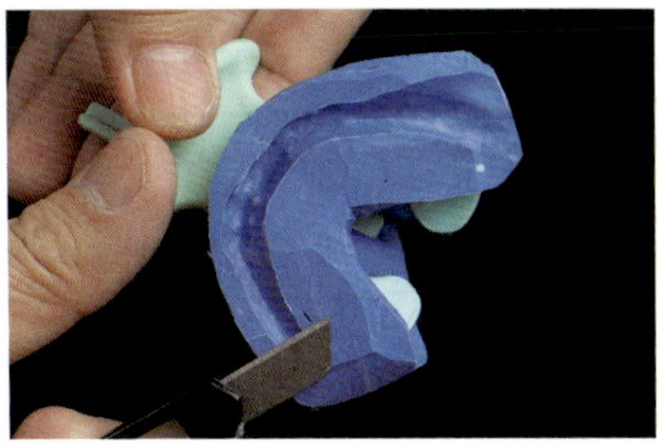

③Cut the excess material to fit the models

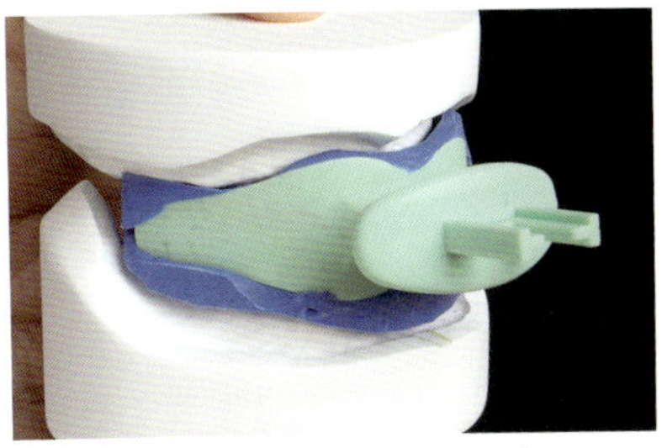

④Models are fit to the Centric tray bite

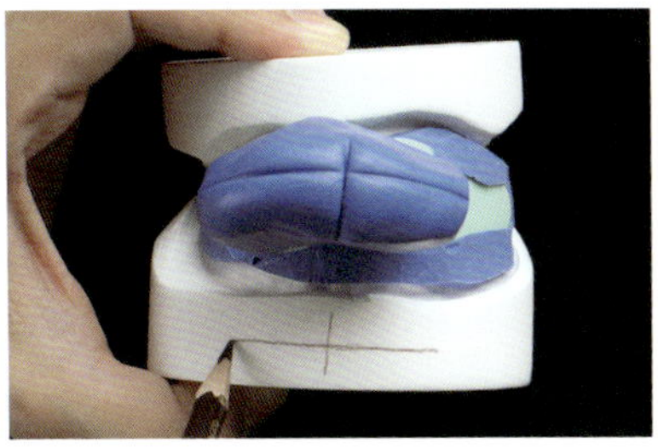

⑤Marking the horizontal line and mid line on the silicone putty to the models allows accurate model mounting

Fig 6 Mounting the preliminary casts by using the Centric tray bite.

6 Preparation for mounting with Centric tray bite

The biggest concern of the dentist is that the silicone bite can fit to the models made by the preliminary impressions. The author's experience proves that the successful Centric tray impression can fit to most of the models made by the preliminary impressions; therefore, the dentist should focus on completing the successful Centric tray impression(Fig 6, 7). Even though the slight inaccuracy with the acquired interocclusal record can be detected, the accurate final impression can be acquired if the recovery technique such as using wax during the custom tray trying in is applied. (Referred Part4, page 46, Fig 17).

The Centric tray bite is considered to be a preliminary bite registration, it is not considered to be the final accurate interocclusal record.

Mounting method using the Horizontal guide with the Centric tray bite

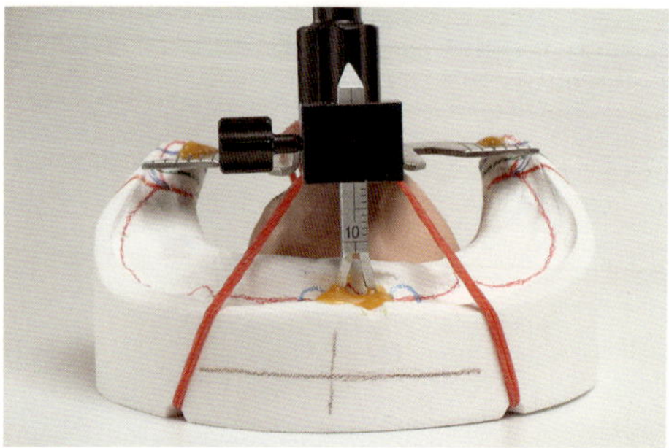

①Use a rubber band to fix the Horizontal Guide to the cast

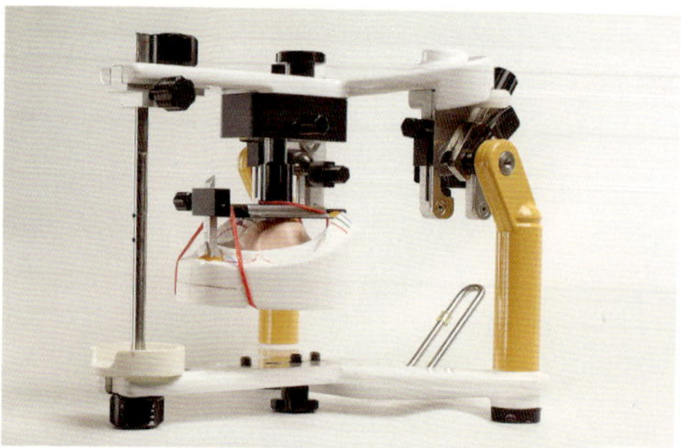

②Mount mandibular cast to Stratos articulator. The mandibular cast is mounted after the Horizontal tray's fixing pin is secured to the instrument carrier. Then mount the maxillary cast using the Centric tray bite

Fig 7 Class I case mounting method by using the Horizontal guide. Refer Part 5 page 91 Fig 15 for the class II,III case mounting method by using the Horizontal guide.

7 The custom tray design and fabrication

In this section, the fundamental maxillary custom tray design, mandibular custom tray design, method of wax block out and fabrication method of the custom trays will be explained by using the simple denture case.

It doesn't matter either it is the maxillary or mandibular denture, all the custom tray border should come in contact with the soft mucosa that is mobile. This is the most important principle to fabricate the suction effective maxillary and mandibular dentures.

(1)Maxillary custom tray design

The important concept to understand is that the maxillary mucogingival junction movement during mouth opening and closing is 1/3 of that of mandible[46-48]. Maxillary denture suction can be effective by having large contact area with the denture base and minimum displacement of mucobuccal fold.

For the case that has the ideal maxillary alveolar ridge, the buccal custom tray

Custom tray design for the Maxilla that has a good ridge condition

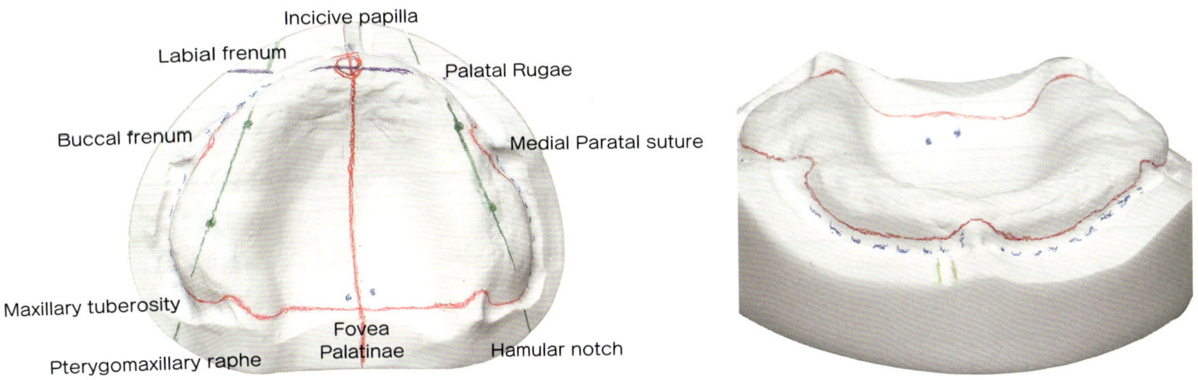

Basically, outline for the custom tray should be marked approximately 2mm above the deepest part of the mucobaccal fold.
Posterior border should be outlined with the line created by the nose blow effect and Ah-line zone.
A-Zone : When the patient is asked to say "Ah", the soft palate goes up and vibrates. This can be the determinant for posterior border
Nose blow effect method : The patient is instructed to blow air through the pinched nose, causing the soft palate to drop. The border between the soft and hard palates becomes clearer

The outline in the labial area should be drawn 3mm above the deepest part of the mucobaccal fold, because the upper lip and orbicularis oris move more than the soft tissue in the posterior area. So freedom of space should be applied

Fig 8 Custom tray design for the Maxilla that has a good ridge condition.

outline should be marked approximately 2mm above the buccal mucogingival junction and 3mm above the labial mucogingival junction. The posterior border outline should be marked 2~3mm posterior to the hard and soft palate junction that is acquired by the "Ah" line method or Nose-blowing method (Fig 8).

Also the straight line through incisive papilla and connecting line of alveolar ridge crest should be marked on the cast for mounting the Gnathometer M that is the device for BPS technique.

(2) Mandibular custom tray design for suction effective denture

Mandibular suction effective denture custom tray design should be the same no matter what kind of alveolar ridge condition the patient has[49-51]. The individual change can be applied by changing the tray thickness. This method allows for every doctor to design the appropriate custom tray.

Ideally, marking a custom tray design line directly on the impression should

Custom tray design for the mandible that has a good ridge condition

Custom tray design for the mandible is mostly uniform. The individual change can be applied by changing the tray thickness

Buccal Aspect

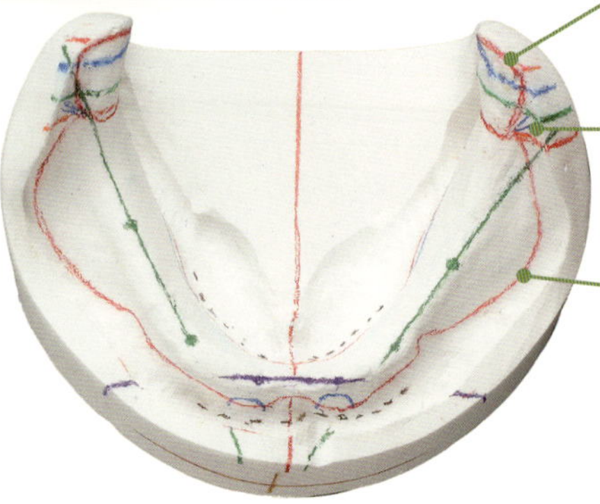

①Follow the outline of the retromolar pad

②Avoid Someya sinew string at the root of the retromolar pad

③Draw a line at the most inferior point of the mucobuccal fold

Retromylohyoid fossa region

④Enter into the retromylohyoid fossa region 2-3mm past the mylohyoid ridge

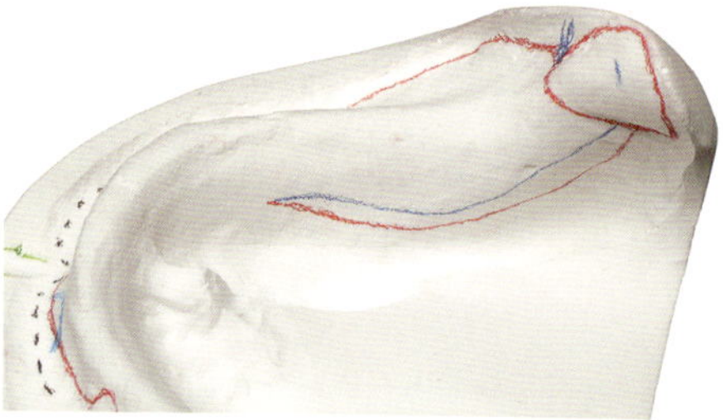

④-1 The mylohyoid ridge is headed toward the center of the lingual side of the retromolar pad

④-2 Draw a line approximately 2mm posterior to ④-1 point to enter into the retromylohyoid fossa region 2-3mm past the mylohyoid ridge

④-3 A deflection point of the S-shaped curve will be reached by going further forward

Labial aspect

⑤-1 Avoid the buccal frenum

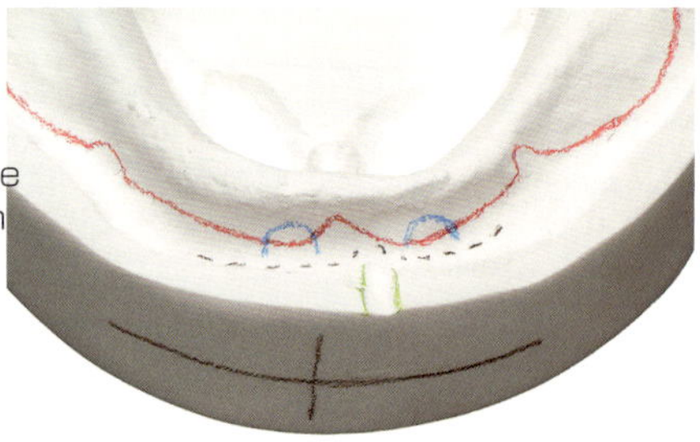

⑦Consider the movement of mucobuccal fold, draw the outline 2mm above the mucobuccal fold

⑥Mentalis muscle attachment should be blocked with wax, but mentalis muscle is not so active so it is OK to be covered by tray

⑤-2 Avoid lower labial frenum in the midline

Mandibular lingual region

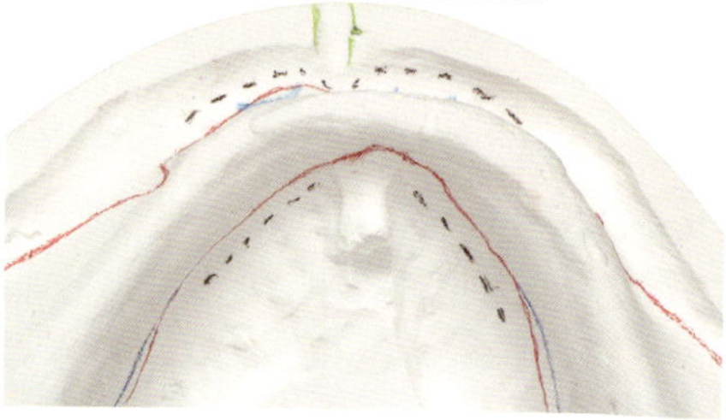

⑧Follow the most convex part of this region and completely avoid lingual frenum

Fig 9 Custom tray design for the mandible that has a good ridge condition.

Someya sinew string

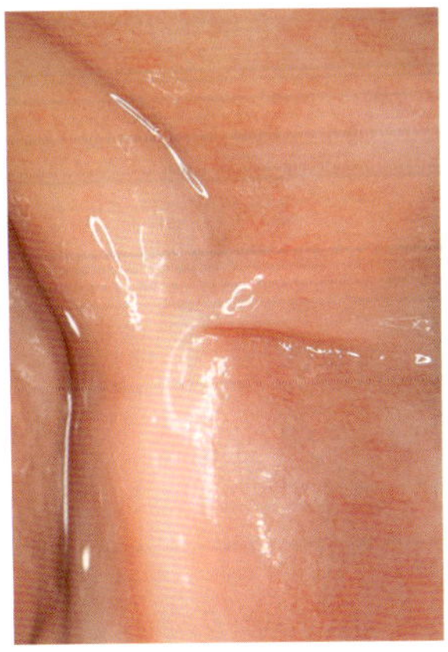

Clear Someya sinew string

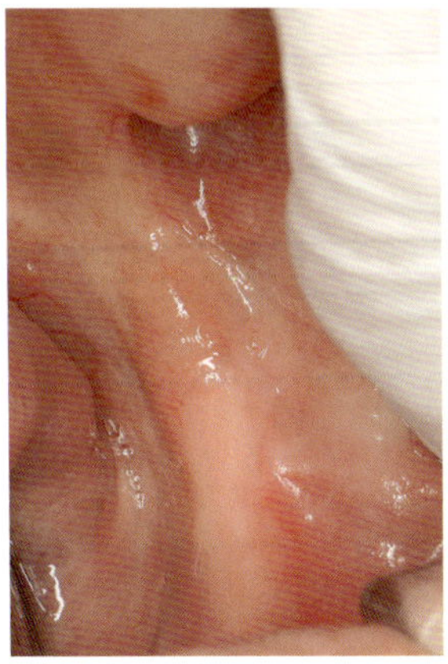

Unclear Someya sinew string

Fig 10 Someya sinew string is a mucosal sinew-like string formed under tension at the buccal root of the retromolar pad posterior to the second molar. Seiichiro Someya first discovered and reported this structure. Even though the sinew string can be visible in only 10-20% of the edentulous population, this area should be avoided at the time of custom tray fabrication. [52,53] Someya sinew string visibility improves approximately 40% by placing pressure with a dental mirror or a finger against the area buccal to the retromolar pad.

increase the accuracy; however, this line will disappear with disinfecting solution so the line needs to be marked on the model.

The mandibular custom tray design is a bit complicated compared to the maxillary custom tray design. The designing line for the mandibular custom tray should be referred to Fig 9. The model should be fabricated from the preliminary impression with a frame cut back tray in a closed mouth rest position. The satisfactory custom tray can be fabricated by following the marked designing line on the model in order to acquire the ideal suction effect, so the denture border seal theory described in Part 1 page 14 Fig 4 can be fulfilled. The custom tray design for the difficult case should be referred to Part 5 page 98~99.

(3) Wax blockout for the model

The methods of wax blockout for the model (Fig 11) are as follows,

1) Maxilla : Alveolar ridge that doesn't have compressive tissue, incisive papilla area that is the nerve opening and hard palate should be blocked out with wax.

2) Mandible : Fibrous incompressible tissue anterior to the retromolar pad, retromyohyoid fossa undercut region, alveolar ridge crest, mentalist muscle attachment area, undercut and sublingual fold area should be blocked with

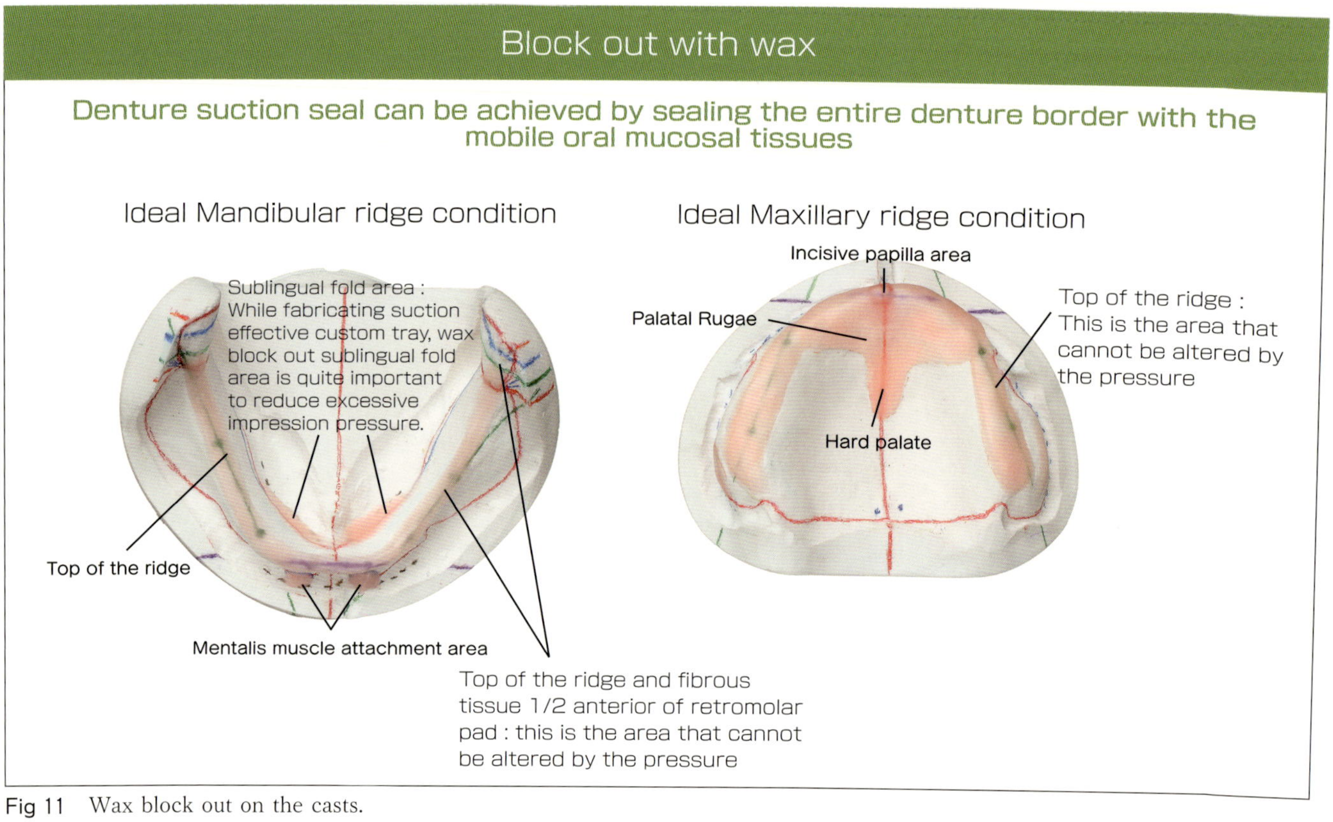

Fig 11 Wax block out on the casts.

wax. Especially, if too much pressure is applied on the sublingual fold area during the impression, this area will cause pain after the denture insertion; therefore, a sufficient block out is necessary in this region.

(4) Custom tray fabrication

Maxillary and mandibular custom tray bases should be fabricated with resin base by following the designing outline and Gnathometer M is installed (Fig 12).

Gnathometer M is a great device that allows to record Gothic arch tracing right after the final impression. Of course it is possible to fabricate the traditional waxed rim custom tray. But the big benefit for this method is that the interocclusal record can be acquired by using the final impression as the most accurate fit tray, so the error with the interocclusal record can be minimized. The installation location of Gnathometer M for Class I,II,III cases is very important at the time of final impression. There can be a anteroposterior position discrepancy compared with the maxillary and mandibular basic arch setting. Generally, for the ideal ridge relationship case, mandibular anteroposterior position should be set on the cross line of anterior alveolar ridge crest. And for the severe ridge resorption case, it should be set on the mid-cross line between anteroposterior width of the anterior alveolar ridge.

Fabrication of resin base and mounting the Gnathometer M : Class I

Gnathometer M is the device that can take final impression and gothic arch.This device allows to provide final vertical dimension of occlusion

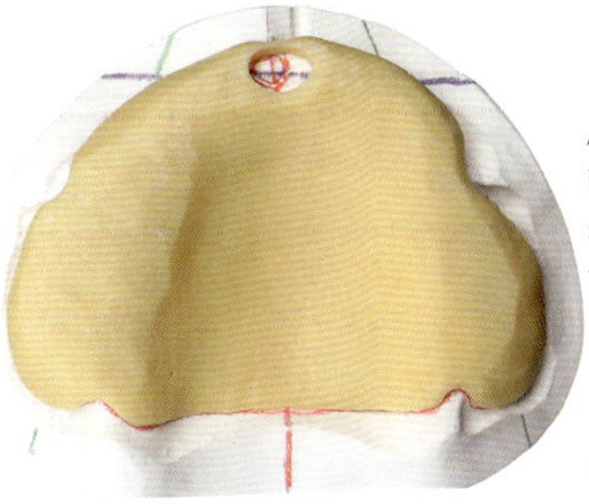

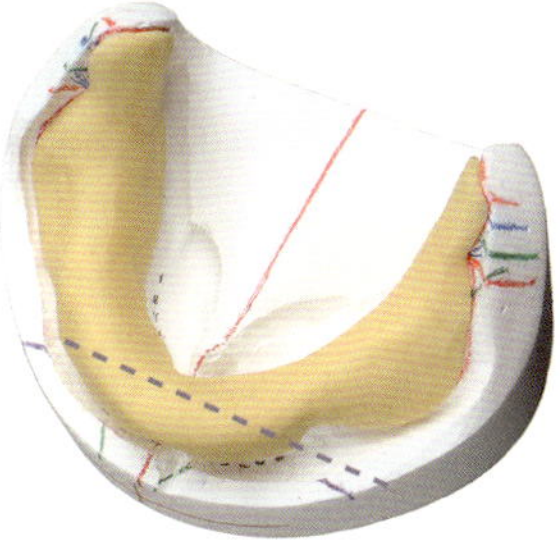

A hole around the incisive papilla area should be made on the resin base, in order to determine anteroposterior position of the Gnathometer M. Position of the basic arch 7 mm for male and 9 mm for female anterior to the incisive papilla. Mandibular basic arch position : middle line of anteroposterior width should match to the transverse line of the top of the ridge

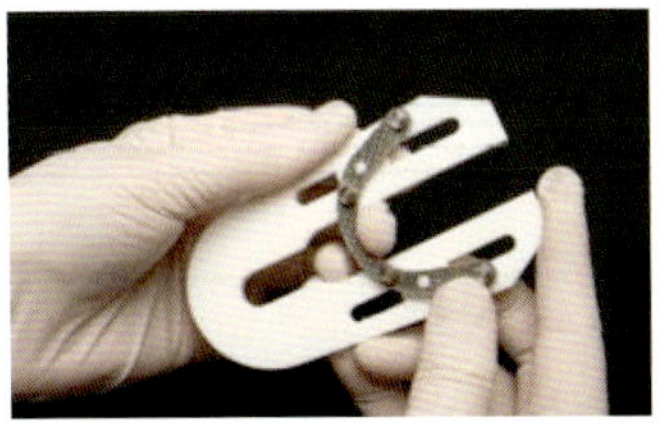

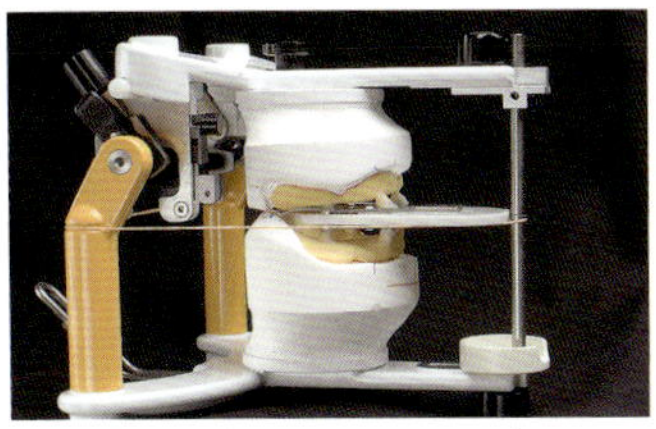

For Class I case, posterior reference point is set 1/3 superior point of the retoromolar pad. And Gnathometer M should be secured with self cure resin according to the camper's plane

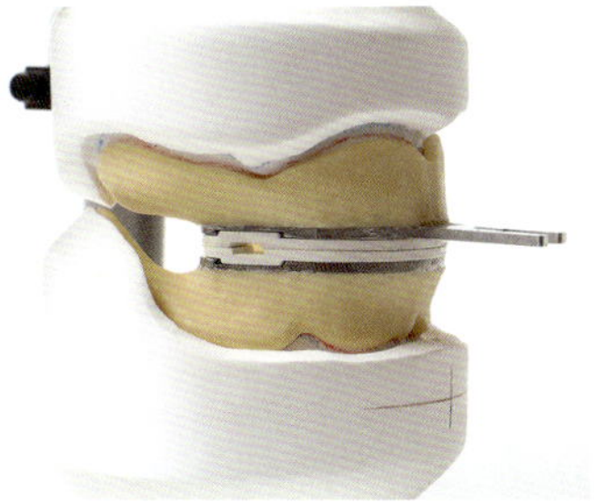

Completion of Max and Mad custom trays

Fig 12 Wax block out on the cast.

1) 7 ideas and 3 different thickness should be applied on the suction effective mandibular denture custom tray

The most important point of the mandibular custom tray fabrication is to apply 7 ideas on the occlusal surface to achieve mandibular denture suction. 6 ideas were explained in the "4 steps from start to finish. Mandibular Suction-Effective Denture and BPS: A Complete Guide" (Quintessence Pub. 2011), but one more idea that is to apply concavity on the tongue base area is added ; therefore, there are 7 ideas should be applied for custom tray fabrication. By applying those ideas on the custom tray, the border seal on the lingual fold and buccal and labial border area is enhanced. Also BTC point appears on the posterior region; therefore, the border seal becomes perfect.[54-57]

In this section, the fundamental custom tray fabrication method for the mandibular suction effective denture is explained. (Fig 13).

2) BTC point

BTC point is The Buccal Mucosa and Tongue side wall-Contact point[58] (Fig14). A posterior border seal of the mandibular complete dentures secured by the intimate contact between the buccal mucosa and tongue above the retromolar

Seven ideas for custom tray fabrication to achieve mandibular denture suction

Seven ideas need to be incorporated into the custom tray in order to achieve mandibular denture suction. This allows to provide more suction on the area of sublingual fold region and buccal mucosa. The denture suction while closing can be well achieved by facilitating BTC point with buccal mucosa and tongue

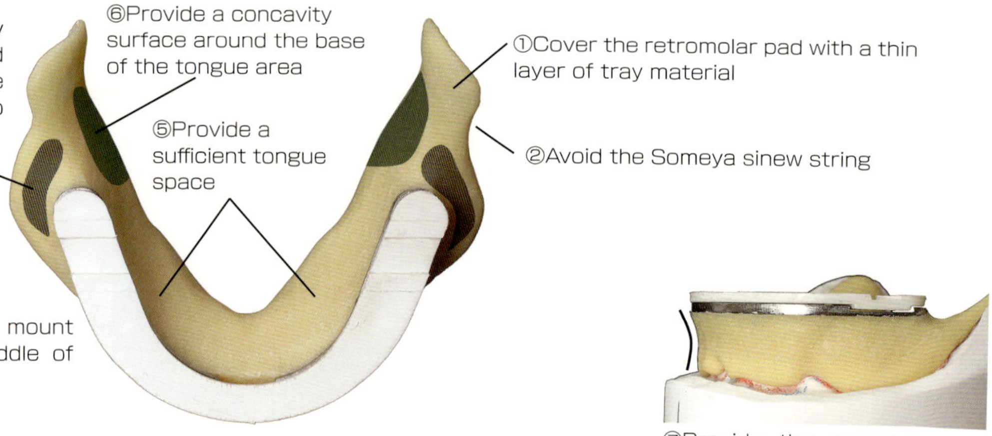

Fig 13 Seven ideas for custom tray fabrication to achieve mandibular denture suction.

pad.

If the custom tray is over extended towards to buccal shelf so the retromolar pad cannot be covered by the buccal tissue or the lingual area is overextended to the retromylohyoid fossae, BTC point cannot be formed. Also if the posterior teeth are set up too lingually or buccally, BTC point formation can be interfered. In other words, BTC point formation can be used as a check point to evaluate the appropriate denture base length or teeth set up. BTC point can be confirmed at the time of final impression or fit check during final denture insertion.

3) Variation of denture border thickness to optimize the patient's individuality

The tray design of custom tray should be uniform in any case, however, the patient's individuality can be optimized by changing the tray thickness.

In order for the mandibular suction mechanism to work efficiently, it is of particular importance to ensure adequate thickness of the tray in the sublingual fold region, for the sublingual fold region is rich in spongy tissue and can provide a strong suction(Fig 13).

It is also important to make sure that the buccal shelf area of the custom tray has a sufficient thickness, so that the final denture can be firmly supported by the buccal mucosa.

Moreover, in a case with shallow labial vestibule where the mentalis muscles are

BTC Point

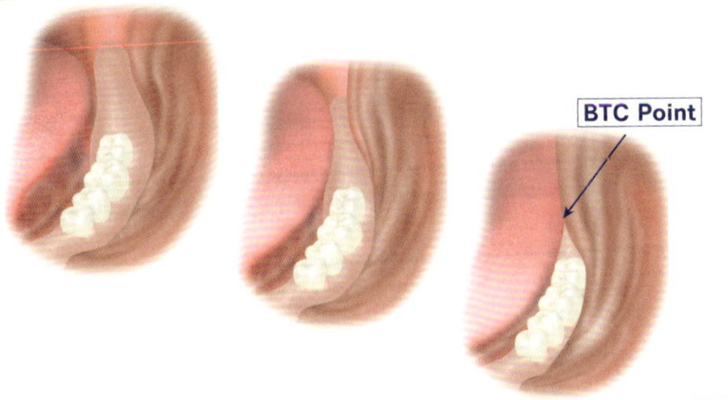

Fig 14 BTC point appears opening movement to closing movement (B: Buccal mucosa), T : (Tongue side wall) C : (Contact).

Maxillary denture custom tray thickness

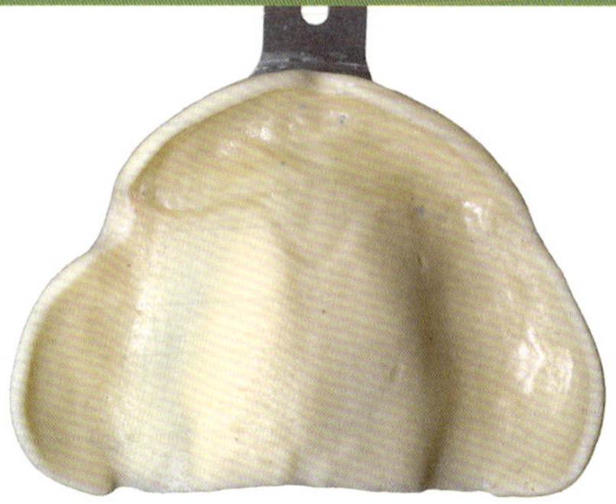

Fig 15 If the ridge condition is good, the custom tray border becomes thinner. Contrary, it the ridge resorption is severe, the custom tray border becomes thick. It is important to fabricate the custom tray with an appropriate thickness tray according to the ridge condition. This case's tray thickness is thin since the ridge condition is ideal.

Mandibular full denture custom tray thickness

The design of custom tray should be uniform in any case, however, the individuality can be optimized by changing the tray thickness. Thickness tray application can change the denture suction effect.

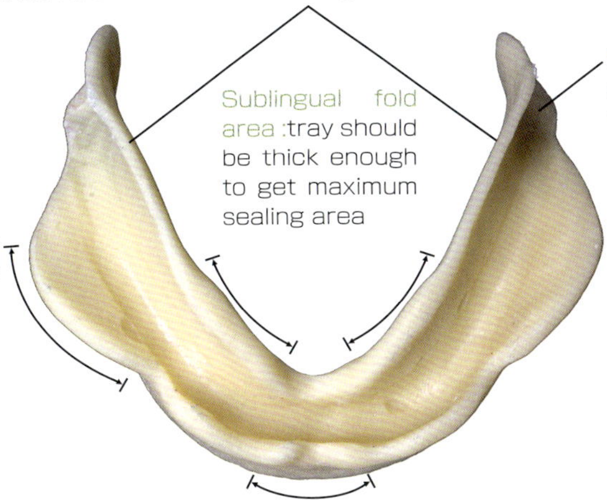

Fig 16 Mandibular full denture custom tray thickness.

attached on top of the labial ridge crest, the thickness should be provided to the labial part of the tray, so that the concavity is easily created at the labial polished surface of the mentalis part, resulting in reinforcing the lip support (Fig 15,16).

Gnathometer M' s Midline, Horizontal line, Camper line need to be checked

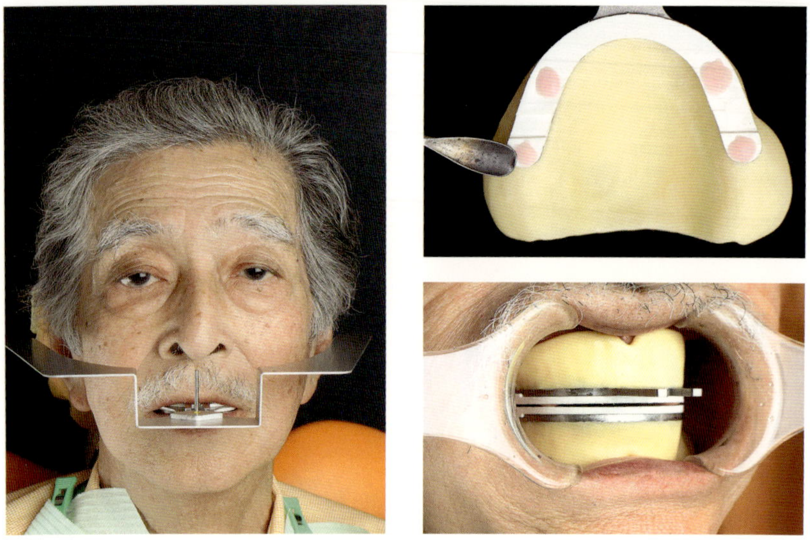

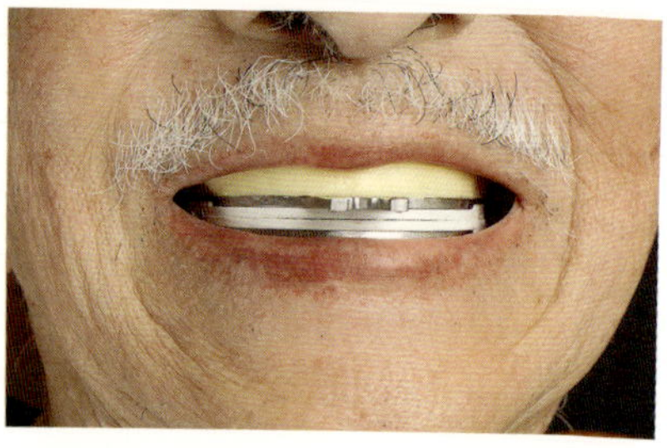

Centric tray bite is not perfect. We may not be aware that there is a large space under the tray even though the bite registration seems to be perfect. If the space between upper and lower trays seems to be small due to the error, the final impression can be proceeded with added wax in order to make even pressure toward the ridge when taking precision impressions. However the trays show large space or large discrepancy, Gnathometer M needs to be reset

Fig 17 Gnathometer M's Midline, Horizontal line, Camper line need to be checked.

Adjustment of interior surface

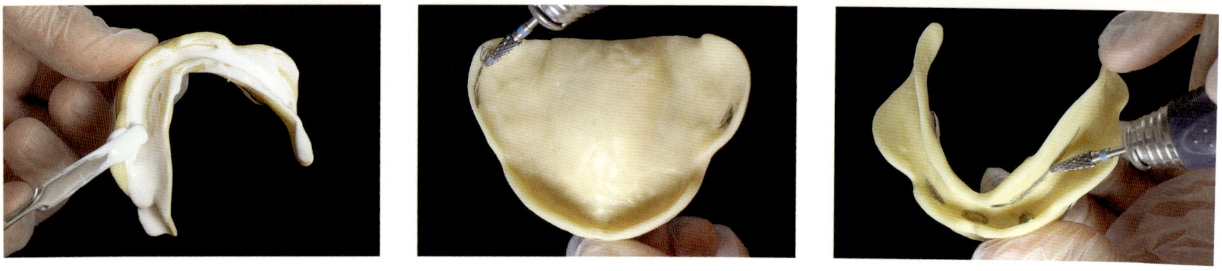

Fig 18 Adjustment of interior surface should be done by trying in the mouth using GC Fit checker by hand pressure and occlusal pressure prior to final impressions.

8 Maxillary and mandibular final impressions

Prior to the final impression, the parallelism of custom trays or side shift between maxillary and mandibular trays and pain at the time of tray insertion should be checked to make even presure toward the ridge crest when taking final impressions.

3 important check points are as follows,

1) Gnathometer M's midline and parallelism with the horizontal plane and parallelism with Camper line (Nasoauricular plane, Fig 17).

2) Bite error check with 4 point wax poles.

3) The custom tray adaptation should be checked (The dentist's finger

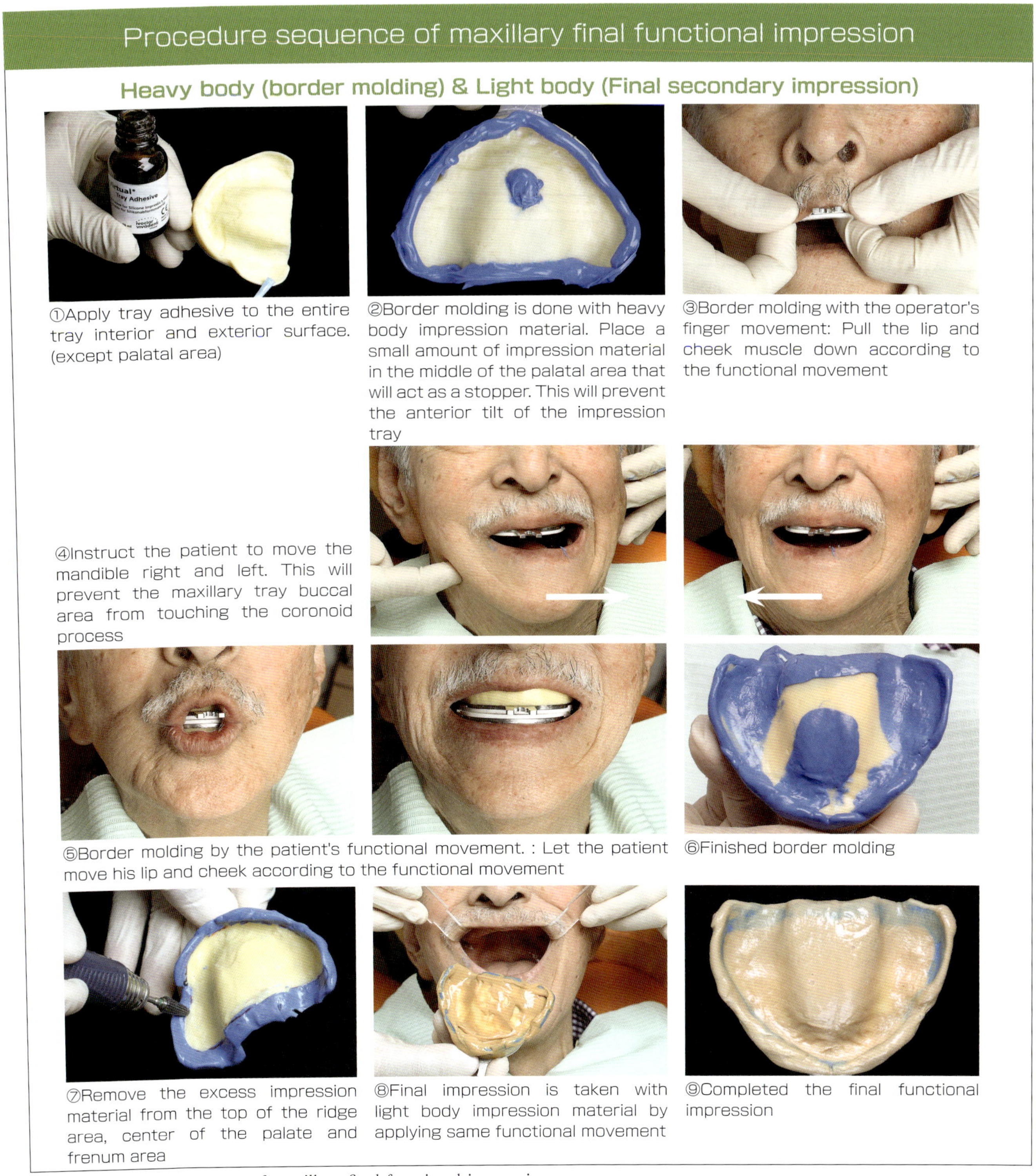

Fig 19 Procedure sequence of maxillary final functional impression.

pressure and trays in occlusion, Fig 18).

(1)The sequence of maxillary final impression technique

In this section, the fundamental maxillary impression technique will be shown (Fig 19). The detail functional impression technique will be shown in Part5 with Class

Procedure sequence of mandibular final impression

Heavy body (border molding), monophase (retromlar pad area) and light body (Final secondary impression)

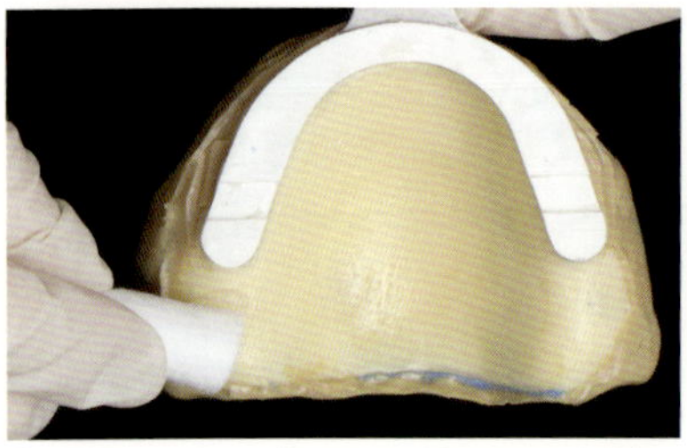

① Place vaseline on the posterior area of maxillary final impression in order for the mandibular impression not to stick together

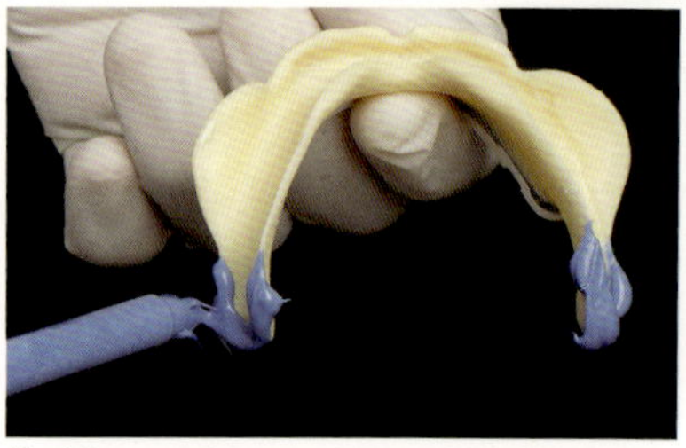

② Monophase type impression material that is more flowable than the heavy body impression material should be applied to the retromolar pad area to prevent the shape distortion

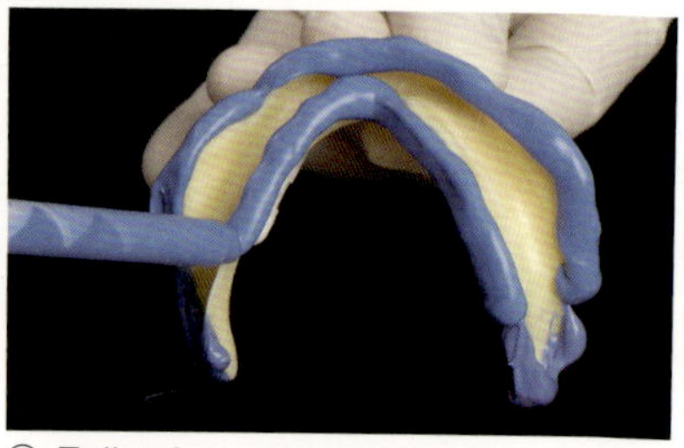

③ Following monophase impression material placement, heavy body impression material is placed on the border. After the tray is inserted, the patient is instructed to do 5 fundamental suction denture movements

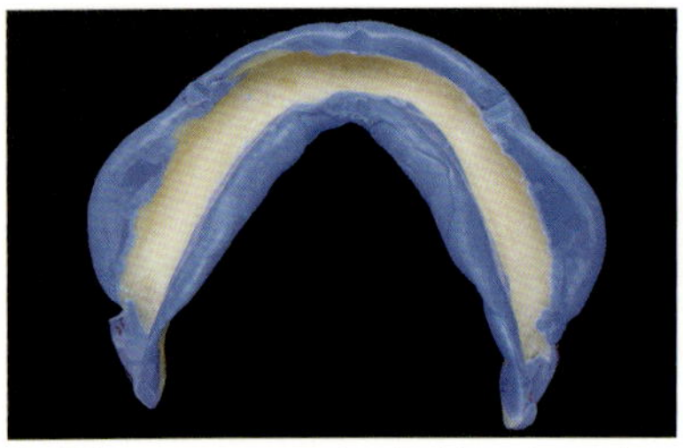

④ The removal of the border molding material from the zone of the immobile ridge mucosa will reinforce the border seal

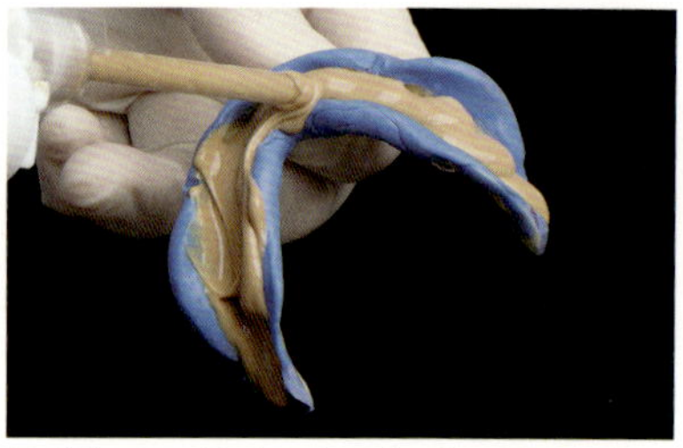

⑤ Place light body impression material to the interior surface of the tray. After the tray insertion, the patient is instructed to do 5 fundamental suction denture movements

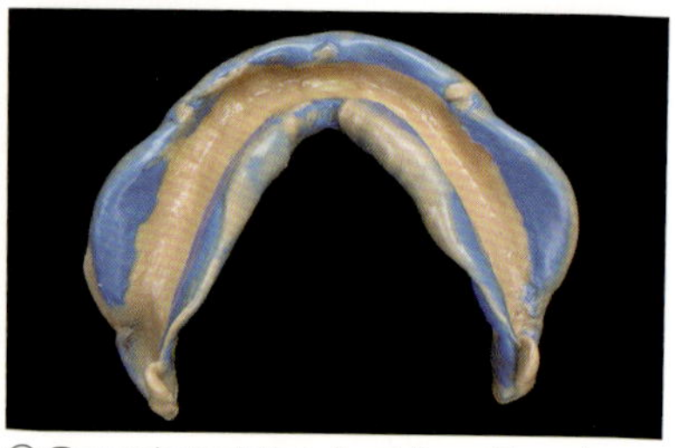

⑥ Completed the final functional impression

Fig 20 Procedure sequence of mandibular final impression.

II case and the impression technique for maxillary flabby gum will be shown with atlas.

(2)The sequence of mandibular final impression technique

1) The important points of the mandibular final impression technique

The denture sinks in slightly when the teeth come into occlusion from the mandibular rest position. Negative pressure is generated as a result. Therefore, the mandibular final impression should be taken during the patient's closed mouth functional movement. This method allows an inexperienced dentist to acquire the satisfactory final impression. Nowadays the young dentists demand the simplified and systematic method and moreover the results should be perfect. This suction effective impression technique is the predictable method that can work for everybody regardless with the experience.

Functional postdam impression

Place monophase type impression material along the posterior border of maxillary impression. After inserting this in the mouth, the patient is instructed to bite with the gentle pressure and swallow. The patient is instructed to wait by applying this gentle pressure until the impression material is completely set. This technique will allow to acquire the tight posterior seal

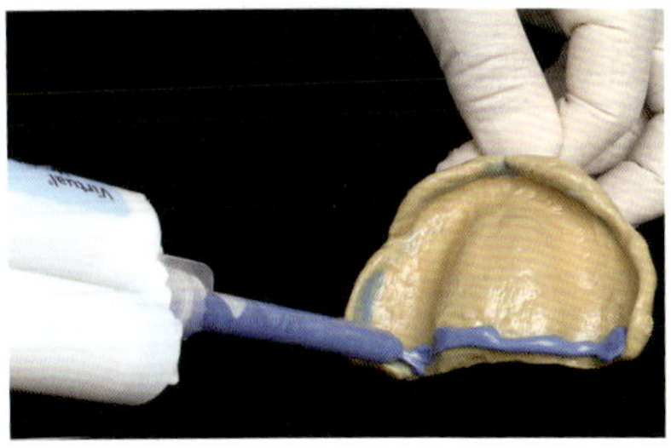

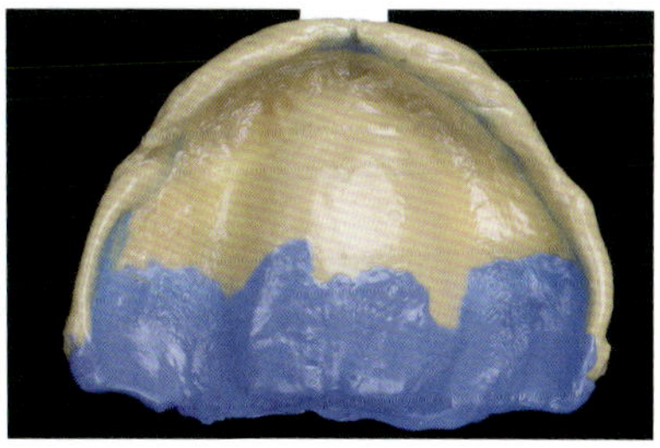

Fig 21 Functional postdam impression.

2) 5 fundamental movements

By letting the patient make those 5 fundamental movements correctly, automatically the perfect final impression can be taken (Fig 20). The suction effective final impression technique for the difficult case is referred in Part 5 page112-120.

1) Purse the lips (say"woo")
2) Retract the corners of the mouth (say "eee")
3) Move the tongue from side to side and forward with opened mouth
4) Push the back side of the tray with the tongue in closed-mouth position
5) Swallowing

The patient should repeat 2~3 times of a cycle of those 5 movements and the complete setting of impression material should be waited with the light occlusal pressure.

3) Fabrication of functional postdam

There is a tendency that maxillary impression suction becomes weaker as maxillary and mandibular impression material's setting's completed.

Asian people's maxillary arch tends to have a shorter anteroposterior length; therefore, the main stress bearing area locates more anteriorly compared to that of Caucasians'. This cause superior dislocation of the maxillary impression gradually. So the posterior border seal becomes weaker. Functional postdam impression should be taken with the monophase impression material.

Gothic arch tracing with Gnathometer M

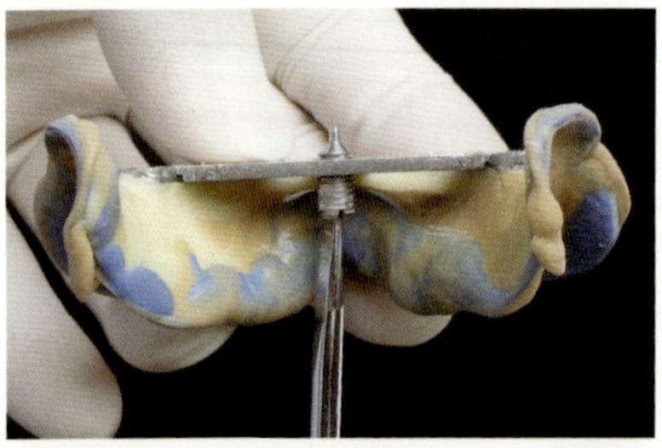

Before Gothic arch tracing with the Gnathometer M, VDO is reconfirmed by using phonation and freeway space measurement. The screw of the Gnathometer M is turned with the screw driver and the hight is secured with the sticky wax

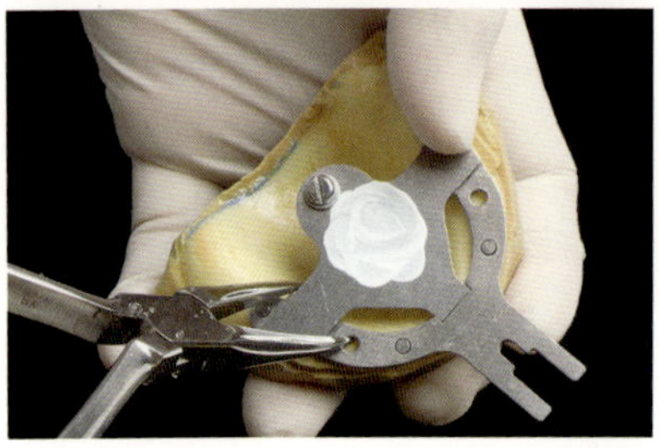

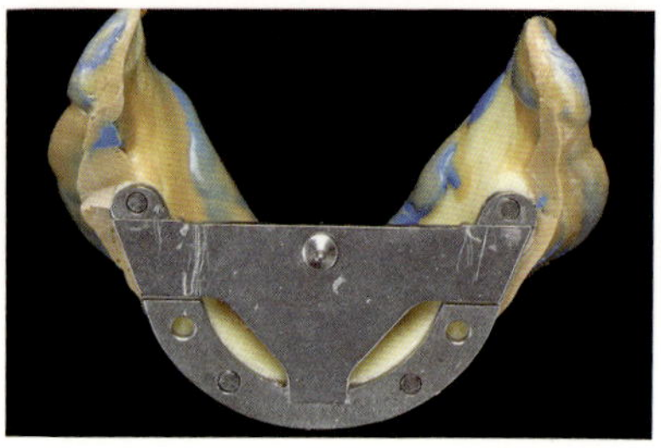

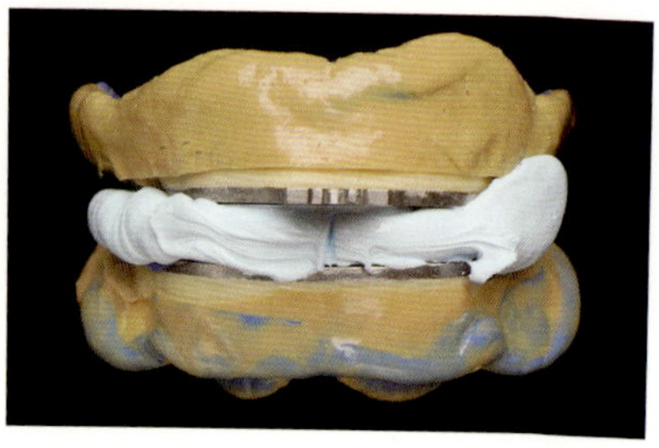

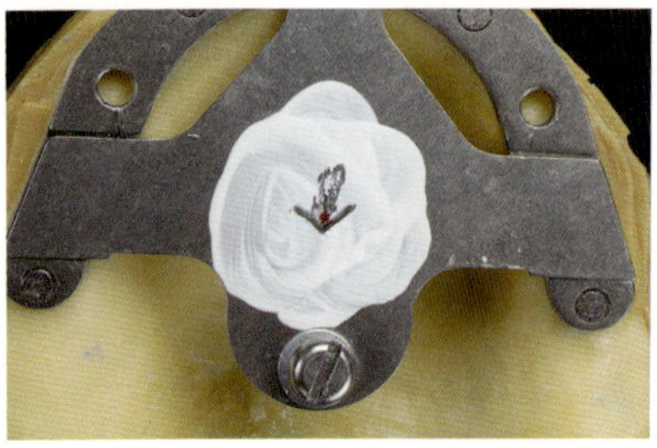

The figure shows that tapping points are observed 0.5mm anterior to the apex point. The mandibular movement disorder can be detected by relatively small gothic arch tracing figure

Fig 22 It takes one hour to acquire the final impression. During one hour, the patient's habitual mandibular position with the patient's existed dentures should be lost, the accurate mandibular position can be acquired (deprogramming). The accurate final impression would allow to register the appropriate mandibular position.

9 Gothic arch tracing with Gnathometer M coupled with deprogramming

After spending about an hour for final impression, the habitual occlusion with the patient's existing dentures has been released from the routine and the patient's authentic interocclusal record led by his/her muscle activity can be acquired easily.

First of all, the patient's OVD is checked again, the Gnathometer M's stylus is turned to adjust the hight according the patient's OVD. Then the Gothic arch is traced (Fig 22). The advantage of this method is that the patient's interocclusal relationship can be observed visually. This method determines the definitive mandibular position. If there is a case that cannot have a stable tapping point or the patient cannot figure out his/her own bite, the therapeutic dentures need to be provided.

Confirmation of maxillary ridge crest lines by the laser marker stand

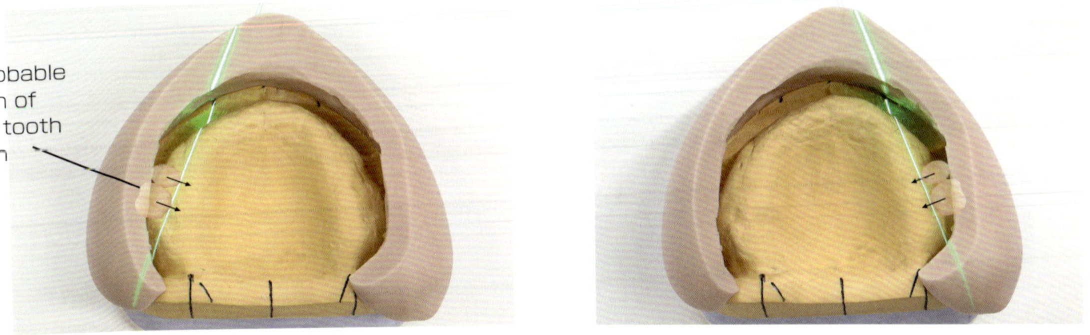

The maxillary ridge crest lines are considered to be the former location of teeth. Maxillary ridge resorption happens to inwards, therefore, if lingualized occlusion is selected as tooth set up scheme, the lingual cusp of denture teeth should be aligned to the maxillary ridge crest, if full balanced occlusion is selected as tooth set up scheme, central fossa of the denture teeth should be aligned to the maxillary ridge crest

Fig 23 Confirmation of maxillary ridge crest lines by the laser marker stand.

10 Master casts fabrication with boxing method

The master casts needs to be fabricated with the purpose to acquire the accurate resin denture border. Generally, since there is an important information around 5mm from the final impression border for the accurate denture fabrication, the model stone should be poured with the wire wax or model block boxing to preserve those information.

11 Model analysis and the landmarks for setting the denture teeth

(1)Maxillary arch landmarks

Even though mandibular alveolar ridge condition is ideal, Maxillary arch landmark for the tooth set up should be marked well so not to have an unstable maxillary denture (Fig 23,24).

Once maxilla becomes edentulous, maxillary alveolar ridge generally starts to have bone resorption buccally and the alveolar ridge becomes smaller. The trace of roots on the alveolir ridge crest is considered to be the lingual periphery of molars; therefore, this can be a landmark for denture teeth to be set up on the location where natural teeth used to exist. This set up allows not only the denture stability but also creating an appropriate space for the tongue to move freely for the speech efficiency.

The anatomical landmark in the maxillary anterior region is the Incisive papilla and the first large pair of palatene rugae (Fig 25). According the research by Watt, the

Reference lines for maxillary posterior tooth set up

Reference lines for setting posteror teeth are drawn in order to obtain final denture's retention and stability

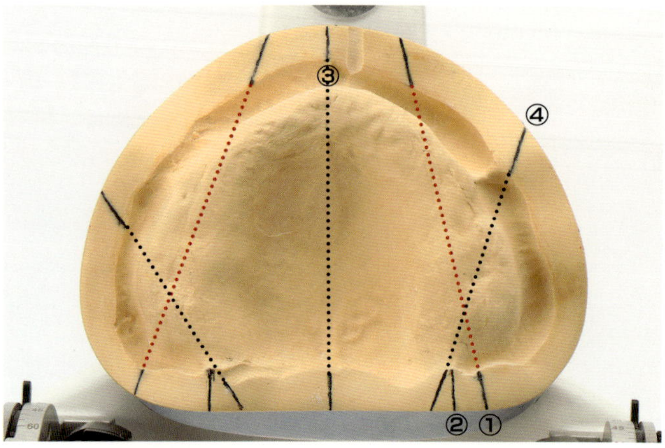

①Ridge crest line
②Hamular notches
③Median palatine raphe
④Deflection point of curve of the ridge crest line

Fig 24 Reference lines for maxillary posterior tooth set up.

Maxillary anterior area's anatomical landmarks

Draw the reference lines for Maxillary anterior teeth set up by considering esthetic and phonetics

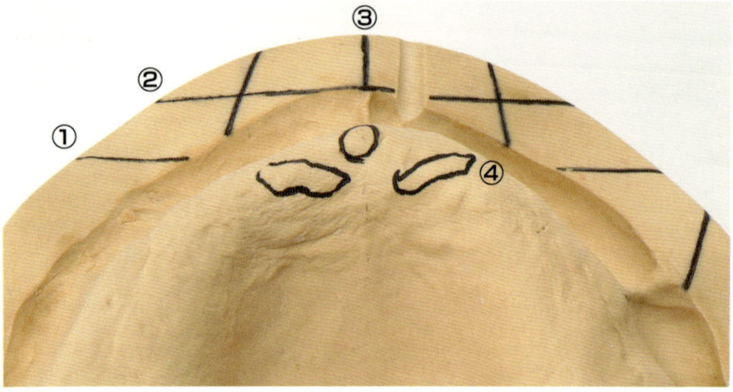

①Transverse line from the midpoint of incisive papilla
②Transverse line 7mm anterior to the midpoint of incisive papilla (Anterior tooth set up reference line), the reference line for the buccal surface of maxillary anterior teeth (male reference line is located 7mm anterior to the midpoint of incisive papilla, female reference line is located 9mm anterior)
③Midline
④The first large pair of palatine rugae

Fig 25 Maxillary anterior area's anatomical landmarks.

previous natural teeth location can be speculated by those anatomical landmarks if the patient has the ideal alveolar ridge condition[60]. However, if the patient has the sever resorbed ridge or anterior flabby gum condition, those anatomical landmarks cannot be the good reference, so the denture teeth need to be set up a few mm forward (Refer Part 5).

(2) Mandibular arch landmarks

1) Occlusal surface

Mandibular landmarks can be more complex compared with those of Maxilla,

Confirmation of mandibular ridge crest lines by the laser marker stand

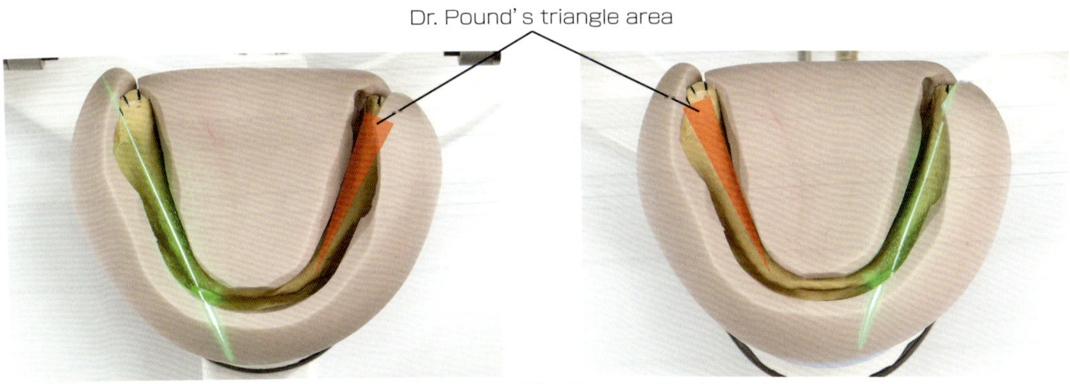

Fig 26 Confirmation of mandibular ridge crest lines by the laser marker stand.

since the surface area is limited and tongue movement needs to be taken into consideration. By marking those landmarks, the vision for teeth set up outcome becomes clear.

The mandibular posterior teeth are arranged in the bucolicgual center of the ridge where it is easier to achieve the BTC point (Fig 14, 26). Clinically, this area is considered almost as same as neutral zone or Pound Line (Pound E[61].).

After pouring stone to the impression, the silicon putty index surrounding the master cast is fabricated. This would show the neutral zone surrounded between buccal mucosa and tongue. The triangle space advocated by Dr. Pound is formed with the line between the lingual edge of the retromolar pad and canine remnant area and the line between the buccal edge of the retromolar pad and canine remnant area. This is the location for denture teeth's molar lingual cusps to be situated. This tooth set up allows the space for the tongue and also the creation of the BTC point naturally.

2) Lateral view

By using Profile compass (Candulor, Rinkai), the anatomical feature is marked on the the model's lateral surface. In order to avoid the anterior dislocation of the denture, the denture teeth should not be set up on the alveolar ridge that has steep angle more than 22.5 degree anteroposteriorly (Fig 27, Gerber A).

The area between the posterior tooth set up limit (avoiding this steep angle area) and the anterior alveolar ridge curve limit, is considered to be the stable area for the denture tooth set up, so molar denture teeth should be set up within this area.

Reference lines for mandibular posterior tooth set up

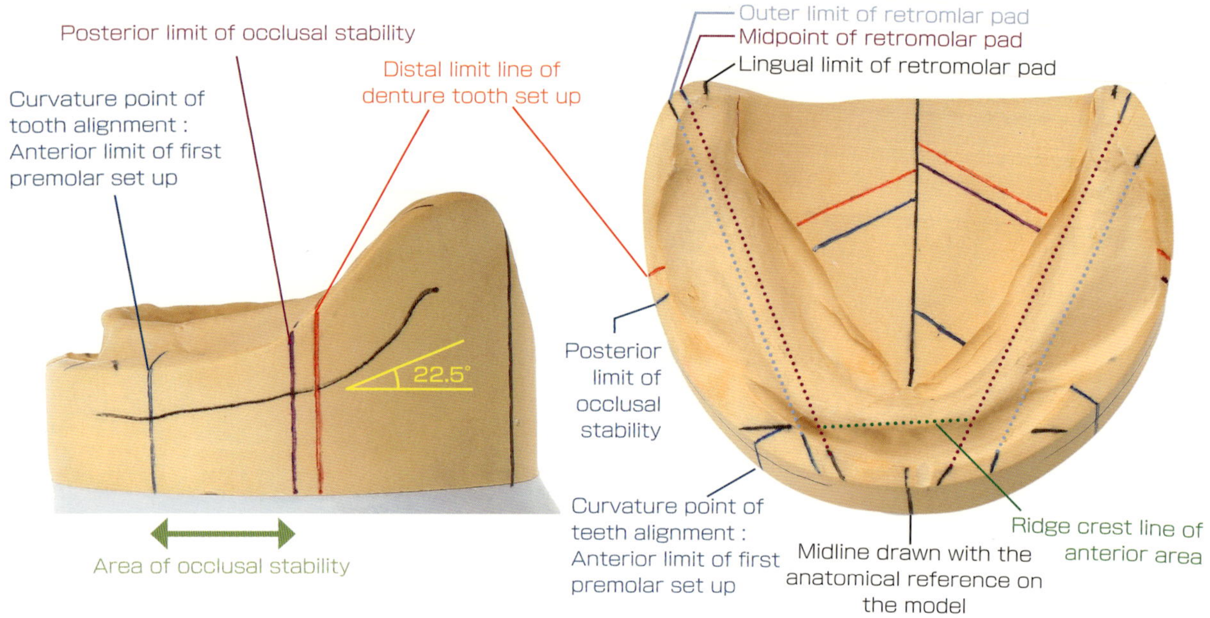

Fig 27 Posterior tooth set up reference line (midpoint of posterior ridge width). If teeth are set up too lingually, the tongue will be moved to the retruded position and cannot stay anteriorly. Therefore, the air pocket is created anterior to the tongue edge and consequently denture suction is disrupted. If teeth are set up too buccally, the denture teeth will get in the way of buccal mucosa that should cover the retromolar pad, so the denture seal of the buccal edge of the retromolar pad will be disrupted.

The reference area/ lines of Maxillary and mandibular posterior tooth setup on the master casts

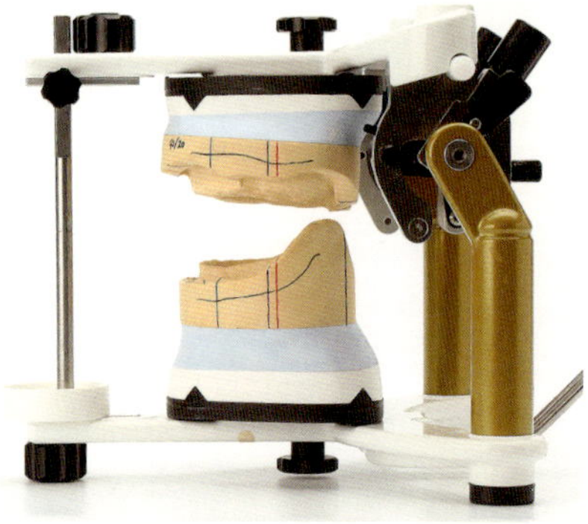

By transferring the mandibular tooth set up reference lines to the maxilla, the individual tooth set up limit can be determined

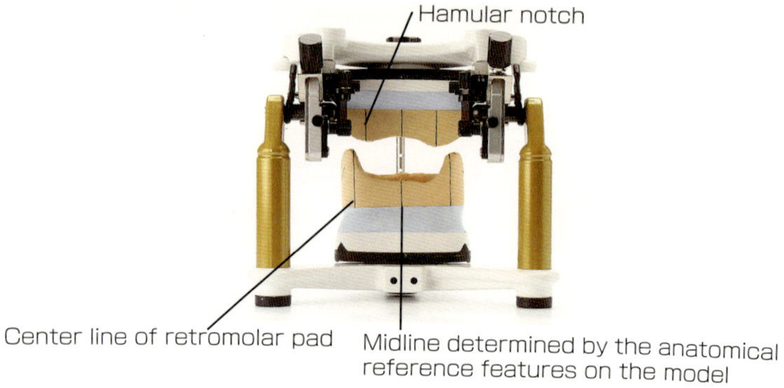

Since there is a large gap between the maxillary hamuler notch line and the center line of retromolar pad, the maxillary and mandibular jaw relationship is not ideal. In this case, it is important to set up maxillary premolars slightly palatally, so the maxillary denture dropping can be prevented

Fig 28 The reference area/ lines of Maxillary and mandibular posterior tooth setup on the master casts (Verify the jaw relationship discrepancy).

3) Posterior view

It is important to check the mounted casts posteriorly so the information of the jaw relationship can be analyzed from the different point of view (Fig 28).

Maxillary and mandibular central and canine set up

The maxillary centrals should be set up 7mm anteriorly from the center of the incisive papilla for male. Two centrals were set slightly unaligned intentionally to add individuality. When setting the maxillary canines, the buccal hight of contour should be positioned 9mm from the first large pair of palatine rugae

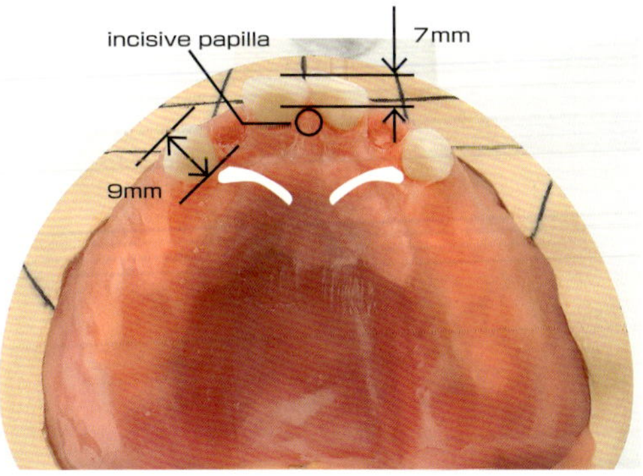

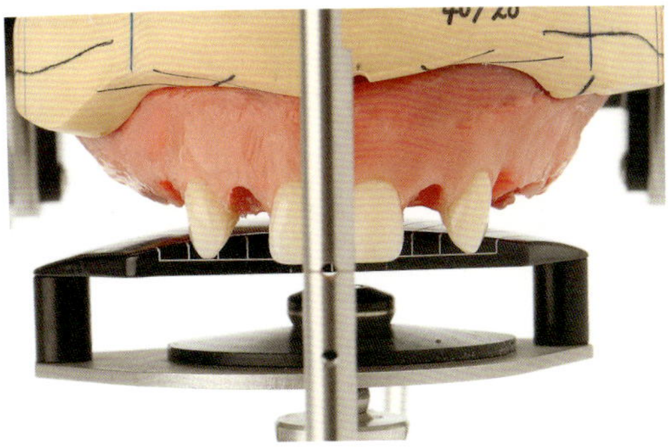

The average vertical position of centrals should be located in 1/2 of the distance between maxillary and mandibular ridge distance plus 2mm that is the vertical overlap. In this case, maxillary lip is lower, the centrals are positioned 4mm plus vertically. The canines are set as same level as the centrals

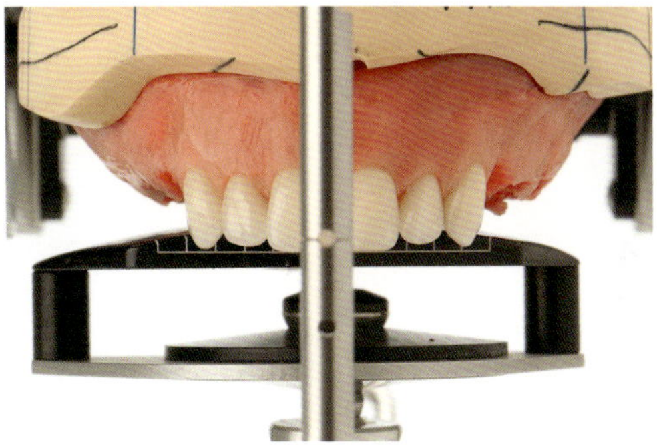

The laterals are set 0.5mm vertically higher than the centrals, since there is no anatomical landmark for set up

Fig 29 Maxillary and mandibular central and canine set up.

12 Denture teeth set up for the easy clinical case

The dental technicians have been setting the denture teeth by relying on their experience and intuition. However since the recent development of BPS technique to analyze the master casts anatomically allows the dental technician to set up the denture teeth more accurately.[62,63] Then what is the denture tooth set up technique by using BPS anatomical landmarks as a reference? In this section, the overview of this technique will be introduced by treating " The easy clinical case".

(1)Standard tooth set up (Maxillary anterior teeth) for the ideal ridge condition case

The cervical area of the maxillary central incisors are positioned in line with the center of the incisive papilla anteroposteriorly for the ideal ridge condition case. Incisal denture tooth's hight of contour is supposed to be positioned 7mm (for a male) and 9mm (for a female) from the center of the incisive papilla (Fig 29).

The maxillary canine's hight of contour is supposed to be positioned 9mm anteriorly from the the first large palatine rugae[60]. Since there is no anatomical landmark for setting of the maxillary lateral incisors, the canines should be set up first and the lateral incisors set up should follow. If there is a big space between the central incisor and canine, the bigger size lateral incisor should be chosen and set up. On the other hand, if there is a narrower space, the lateral incisor can be set by slightly rotated or can be set pallatally.

(2) How to use 3D tooth setting templates?

The tooth setting devices allow more esthetically symmetric denture tooth set up than the tooth set up is done by the technician's intuition or the eye measurement. By using BPS system's 2D or 3D template, anterior teeth's horizontal line should be determined. If the model mounting was done without facilitating the face bow, the symmetrical denture tooth set up can be accomplished efficiently by using 2D template that has been incorporated with the curve of Spee and the curve of Wilson.

If the models are mounted with the UTS face bow (BPS system), the models cannot be situated in the center of the articulator, since the human face is not completely symmetrical. In this case, the 3D template allows tooth set up efficiently.

(3) Setting the mandibular canines (Fig 30)

After the maxillary anterior teeth are set up for the ideal alveolar ridge case, the both side's canines should be set up on the crossing points between the alveolar crest line and the posterior tooth setup line. Adjust the position of canine so that its labial prominence is in line with the anterior arch medially and with the posterior arch distally. The cusp tips of mandibular canine is positioned near the inter proximal contact between the maxillary canine and lateral incisor on each side.

(4) Setting the mandibular posterior teeth (Fig 30)

For the mandibular posterior tooth set up with the ideal alveolar ridge case, the teeth should be set up along the line between canine and outside of retromolar pad and aligned the central grooves of the posterior teeth on this line. The order of the teeth set up should be starting from the first premolar and followed with second premolar, first molar and second molar. The normal type denture teeth were selected for this case. Once maxillary and mandibular first premolar position is determined, following tooth set up becomes effortless. Finally, the denture teeth should be set up anterior to the Pound line in order to keep the enough space for the tongue activity.

If the ridge sagittal angle is more than 22.5 degree, the denture teeth should not

Full balanced occlusion (one tooth to two teeth occlusion for premolar setup one tooth to one tooth occlusion for molar setup)

Posterior teeth buccal and lingual cusps should touch the anteroposterior curvature of the template

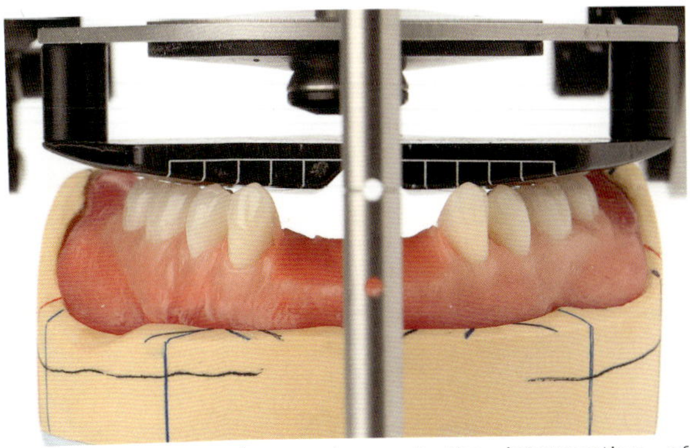

Set the mandibular canines at the intersection of transverse line for the anterior ridge and that for posterior set up. The cusp tip of the canine is positioned near the inter proximal contact between the maxillary canine and lateral incisor on each side. Denture tooth's labial prominence is in line with the anterior arch mesially and with the posterior arch distally

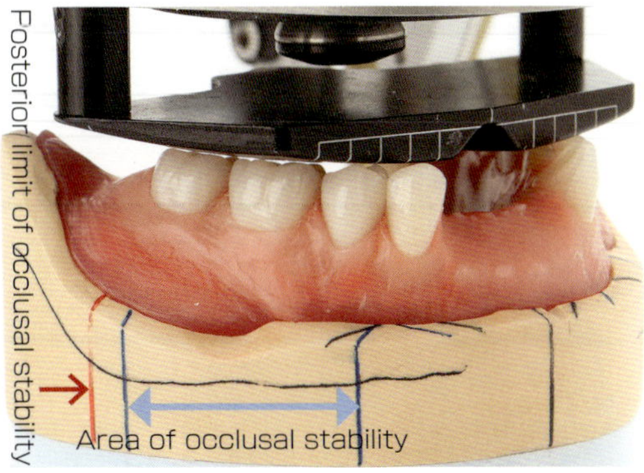

Once mandibular canine set up is done, first premolar-second premolar-first molar-second molar are set up in this order. In this case, anteroposterior length is short, therefore, only second premolar is set in this order. Buccal and lingual cusps should contact with the curvature of the template

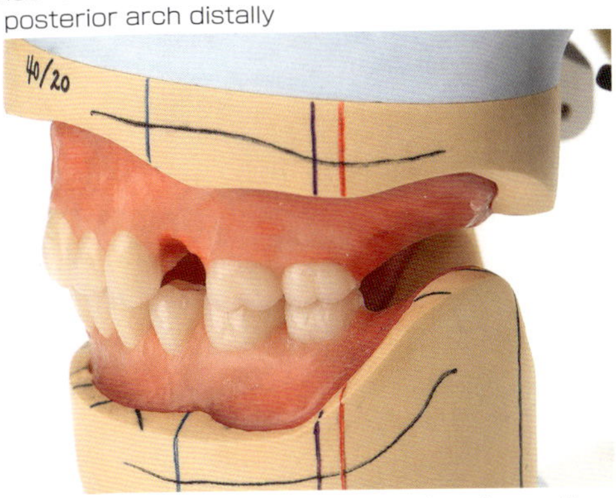

Once mandibular molar set up is completed, maxillary molar set up will follow. Generally, the order of the set up should be maxillary first molar-first premolar-second premolar-second molar. In this case, since first premolar was eliminated, teeth set up was done by the order of first molar, second molar, second premolar

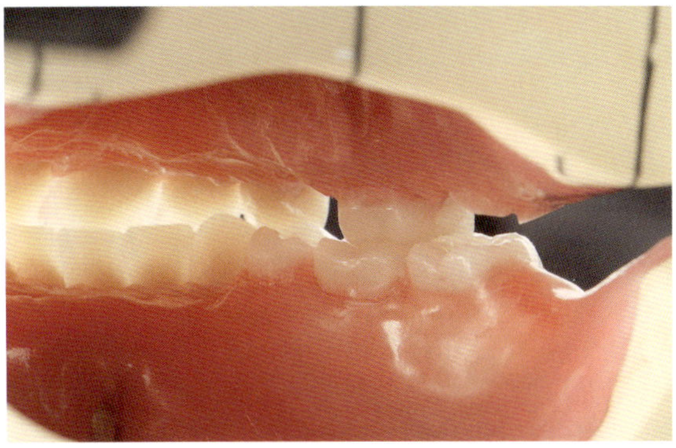

Maxillary first molar lingual cusp is occluding to mandibular first molar central fossae. In this case, maxillary and mandibular buccal cusps are occluding since full balanced occlusion is applied

Fig 30 The method of applying an appropriate occlusion in the simple case. There is no too much difference between one tooth to two teeth occlusion and one tooth to one tooth occlusion or full balanced occlusion and lingualized occlusion.

be set up on the area. If the patient masticates on this area, the denture may slide anteriorly then this may cause the denture drop out.

(5)Setting the maxillary molar teeth(Fig 30)

For this case, one tooth to two teeth (cusp to ridge) occlusion is facilitated in the maxillary first premolar's setup and one tooth to one tooth (cusp to fossa) is fascilitated in the maxillary first and second molar's setup. The occlusal stability zone should be taken into the consideration during the final check up facilitation, especially considering occlusal adjustment after remounting. Most of the post denture

Mandibular 6 anterior tooth set up

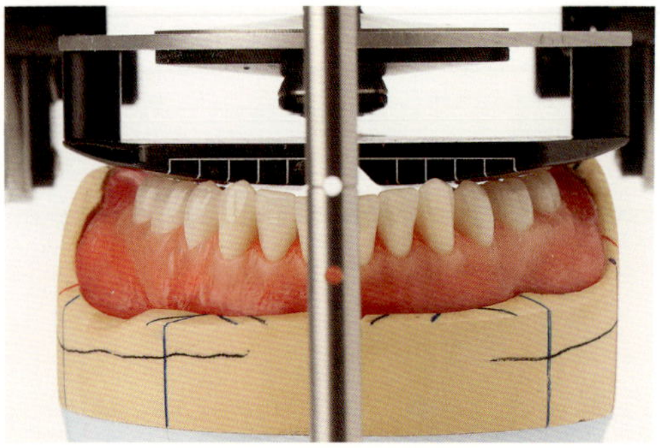

In order to create natural appearance, slight anterior tooth rotation and crowding were applied on the 6 anterior tooth set up

Fig 31 Mandibular 6 anterior set up is completed at last order.

insertion issues such as sore spots or ill fitting will occur to the mandibular denture for the ideal ridge condition case of the maxillary arch. Therefore, tooth set up should be focused on the mandibular denture stability.

(6) Characteristic mandibular anterior tooth set up

Mandibular 4 anterior teeth are set up in the space that is left. Distinctive characterization has been seen by slight crowding has been applied (Fig 31).

(7) Creating an ideal occlusion for the easy case. (Fig 30)

For the easy case, teeth occlusal contact can be one tooth to two teeth contact or one tooth to one tooth contact. Also full balanced occlusion or lingualized occlusion cannot make a big difference to the patient's satisfaction[38].

The denture is the prosthesis that moves frequently on top of the elastic alveolar ridge tissue[83]. This feature is completely different from the fixed prosthesis such as crowns & bridges. The patient feels comfortable with the minimum movement of the denture; therefore, it is necessary to minimize the denture movement during function.

Bi-lateral balanced occlusion ; bilateral molars are sliding together during right and left lateral movement, is created on the articulator reduces the denture movement during function. Also anteroposterior balanced occlusion ; anterior teeth and posterior teeth will slide together during the protrusive movement, also creates the denture stability during the function. Therefore, even though lingualized occlusion has been chosen as the tooth set up method, those two functional movement characterizations should be applied intraorally and on the articulator in order to provide the denture stability during function.

Maxillary posterior tooth set up matching to the ridge crest line(green)

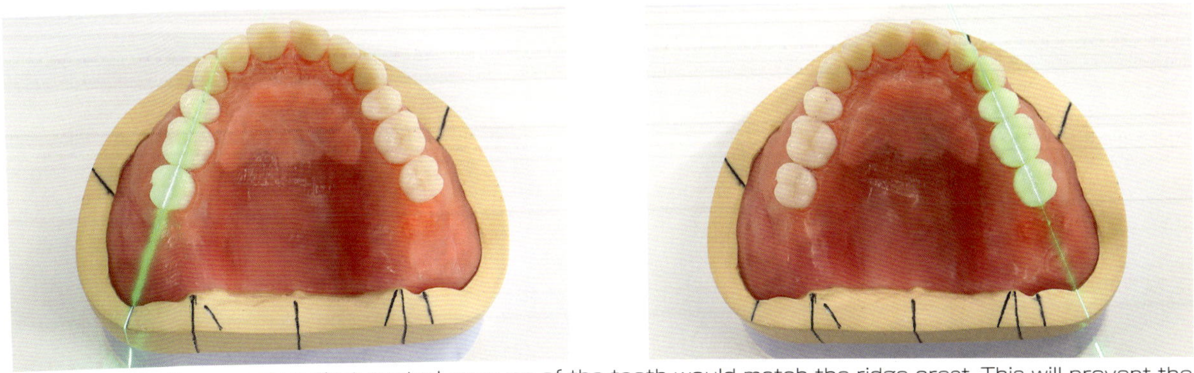

Maxillary : Teeth are set up that central grooves of the teeth would match the ridge crest. This will prevent the denture movement during function

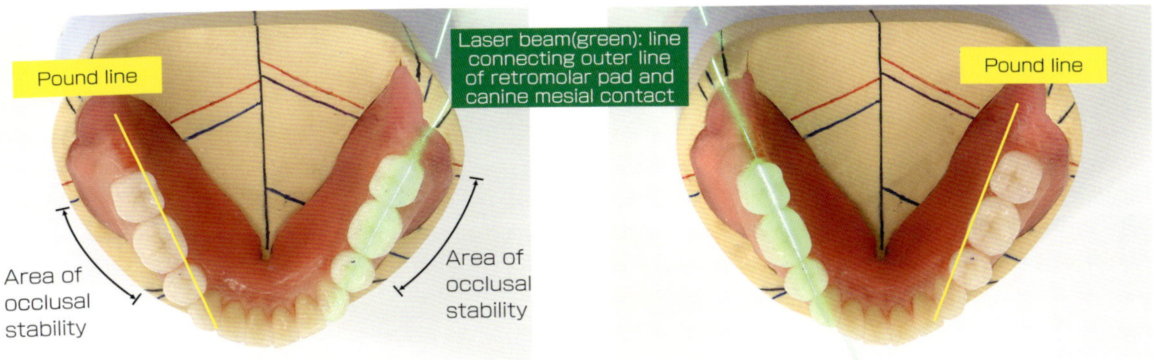

Mandible : It is important to pay attention that posterior lingual cusps are not set up lingually beyond the line connecting inner line of retromolar pad and canine mesial contact. Moreover, since posterior teeth are set up within the area of occlusal stability, the denture movement will be minimized during function

Fig 32 Occlusal view of denture tooth set up. Maxillary posterior tooth set up matching to the ridge crest line.

(8) Occlusal view of the denture tooth set up

Fundamental denture tooth set up has been introduced until now. However, there are so many case varieties ; therefore, the denture tooth set up should be modified according to the case with the emphasis of the maxillary denture stability and the mandibular denture suction (Fig 32, 34).

(9) Suction effective wax up method and application of polished denture surface characterization

Denture surface wax up characterization has a lot of influences for maxillary and mandibular dentures suction and patient's conformability during the function[64]. The denture polished surface characterization will be discussed in this section (Fig 37).

The method of wax up and application of denture polished surface to obtain denture suction

The method of buccal and lingual contour go the polished surface

①Maxillary first premolar teeth length should be adjusted transitionally according to adjacent teeth in order to apply esthetic and function (It is not root exposure). There is a cervical height discrepancy between canine and premolar since there is a deference of the root length. In order to overcome this issue, wax up is done to lengthen the premolar tooth length so transition area becomes more esthetic.

②Interproximal papilla anatomy is applied by considering esthetic, cleansability and appearance.

③S shape on the mandibular lingual surface (bluegreen) is applied to ensure the rest portion of the tongue, anterior tongue position and tongue positional stability. Denture seal is completed by having buccal mucosa on the buccal polished denture surface. Also by creating enough lingual space with the denture, this prevents for the tongue to retrude, therefore, denture lingual seal is completed.

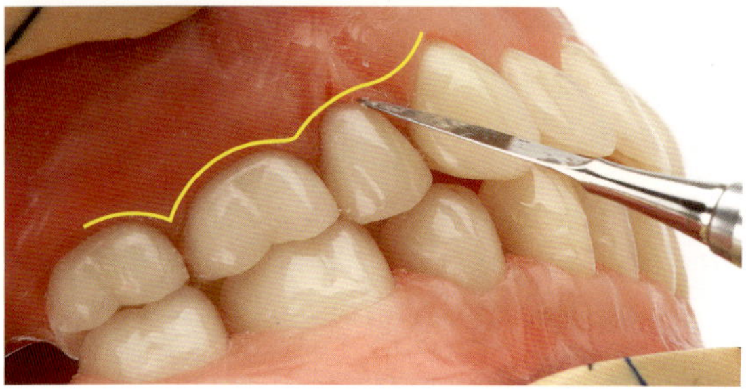

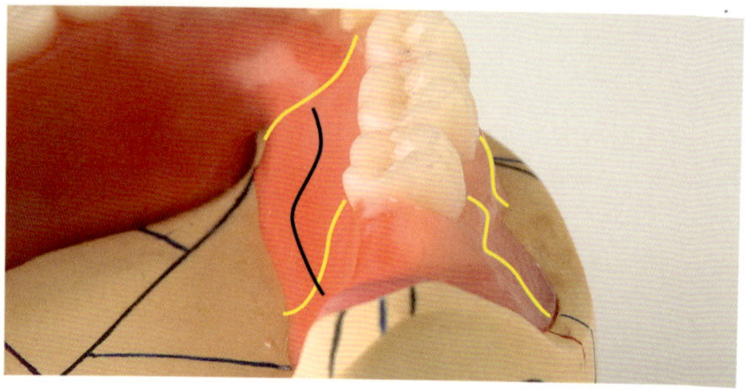

The method of buccal contour on the polished surface

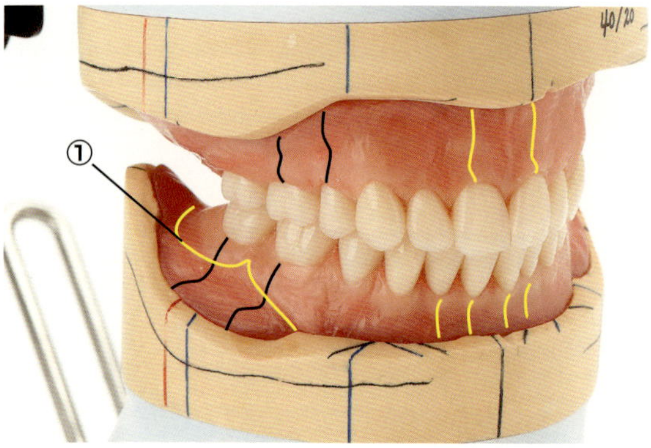

Lately, 3D digital scanning method is increasingly popular since it allows to obtain accurate impression and to produce the accurate denture with highly polished surface. This is so-called CAD/CAM denture. However this technique is not so popular in Japan. Therefore, in the regular lab, the best way to produce highly polished surface is to fabricate the core of the impression. (Fig 23,26) As it shows on the left Fig A, the line from buccal frenum, posterior teeth area and to the retromolar pad should be drawn at first and then polished surface contour should be created.
Polished buccal surface area of mandibular anterior teeth should have slight concavity that will create a lip support.

The method of lingual contour on the polished surface

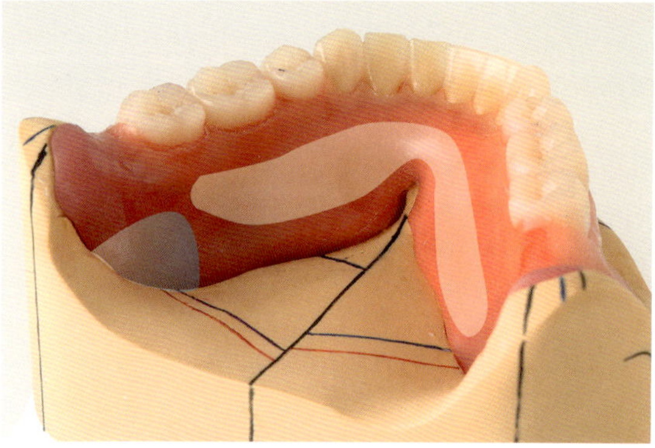

The method of lingual contour on the polished surface :
The gentle concavity on the posterior lingual surface for the base of the tongue to support the denture polished surface should be created.
This concavity allows the tongue to stabilize the denture; therefore, this feature will help to provide more denture suction.

Fig 33 The method of wax up and application of denture polished surface to obtain denture suction.

Completion of denture tooth set up

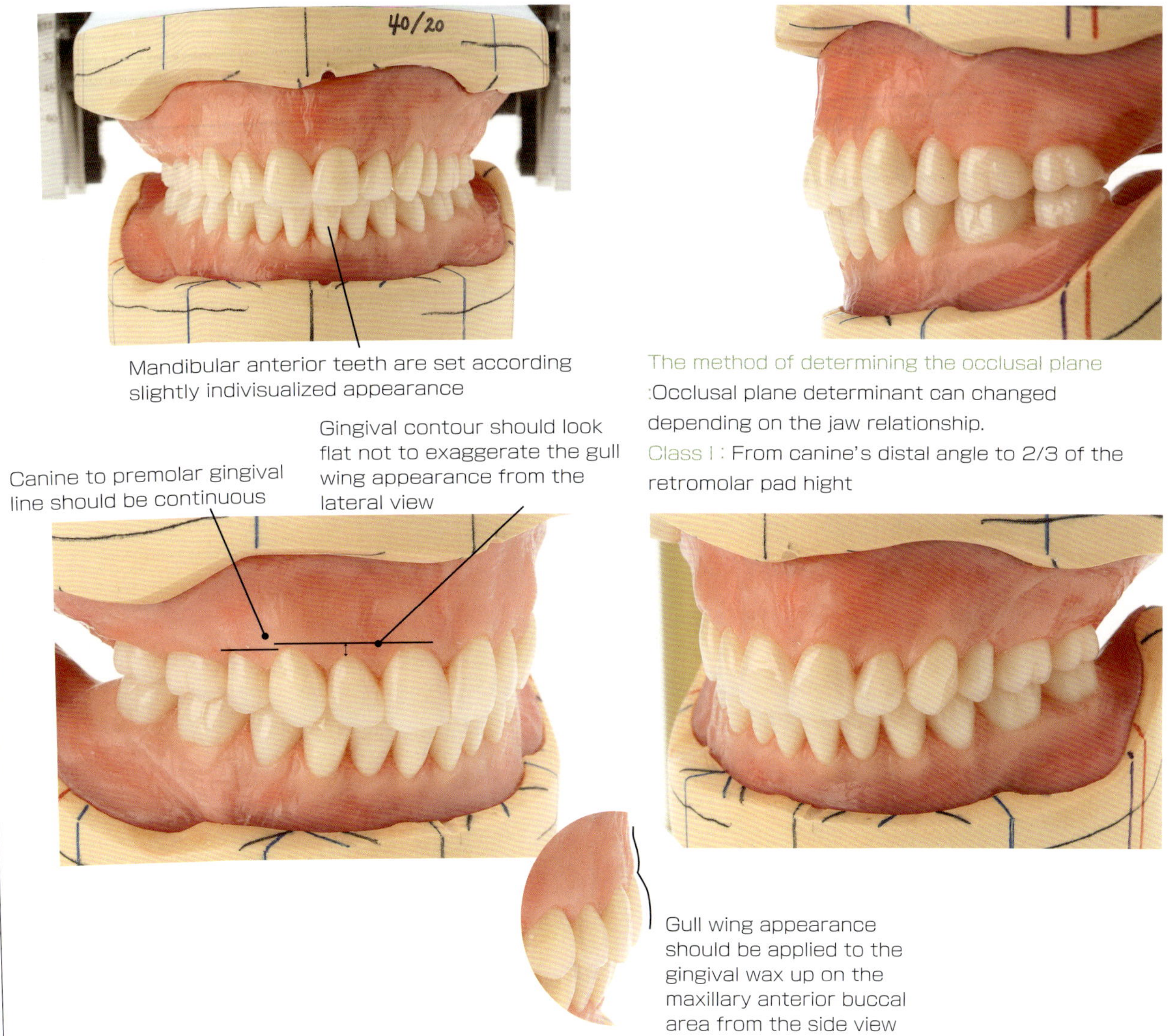

Fig 34 Completion of denture tooth set up. SR-Phonaeres (Ivoclar Vivadent) 6 anterior teeth are manufactured with the strong feature of buccal contour. Once the cervical area is covered with wax, food impaction can be well prevented for the elderly population who lost the normal lip function.

In this case, tooth set up minor adjustment was done with the following order : mandibular second premolars-maxillary second premolars-mandibular first molars-mandibular second molars-maxillary first molars-maxillary second molars. Regarding to the canine set up, if the template is placed according to the distal angle of mandibular canine, maxillary molars appear to be set buccally with the lingualized occlusion denture teeth; therefore, maxillary molars should have setting adjustment according to the maxillary second premolar location.

(10) Completion of denture tooth set up and resin polymerization

The stabilizing test during the wax try in and the method of curing resin will be discussed in Part 5 ClassII-2 case.

13 Denture coloring using SR Nexco (Fig 35)

The patient would like to present him/herself well and attractive. The denture coloring improves their esthetic and it helps branding the denture value. In this book, the special coloring technique after processing the denture by using SR Nexco

Completion of denture teeth set up ①

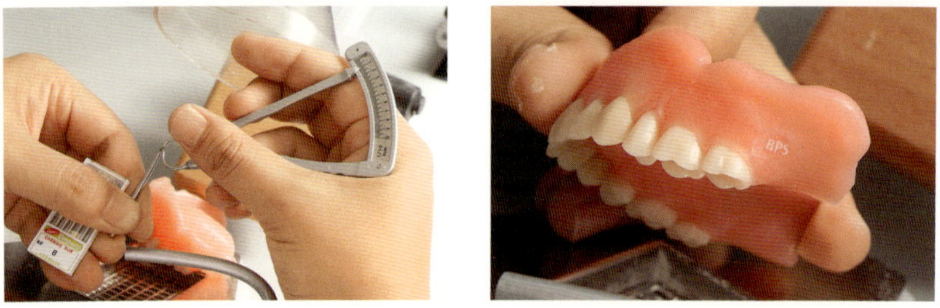

Step1 : The clearance(1～1.5mm) for Nexco (ivoclar vivadent) : laboratory light cure composite should be created. Carbide bur #8 (Emesco) diameter 1mm should be used. It is important not to grind the area 5mm away from the denture border since this area is very important for the denture suction

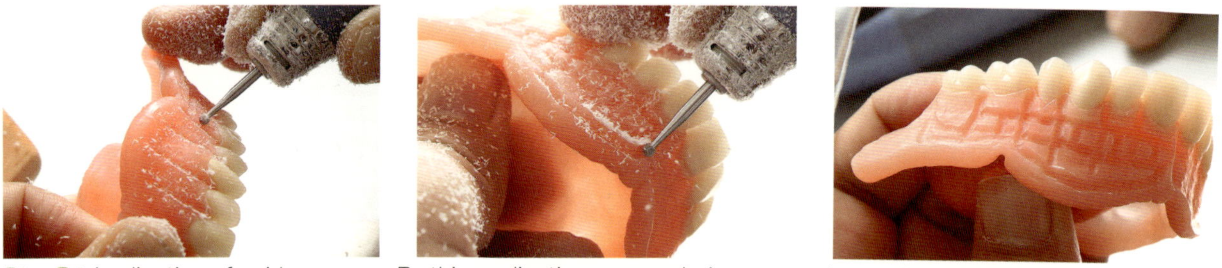

Step2 : Application of guide grooves. By this application, even coloring composite application is possible

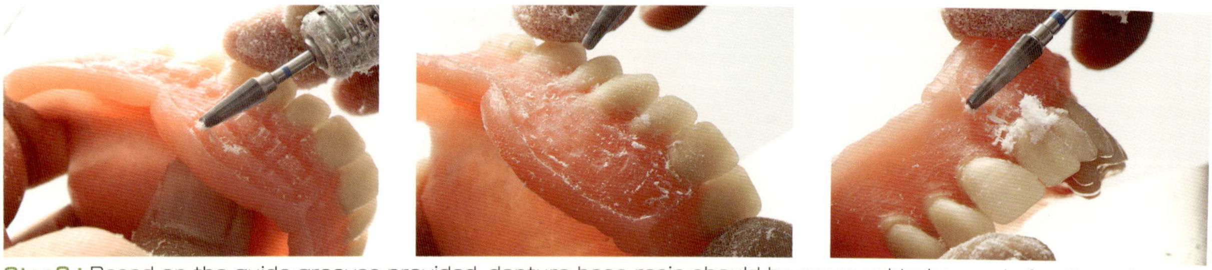

Step3 : Based on the guide grooves provided, denture base resin should be removed to be ready for the coloring composite application

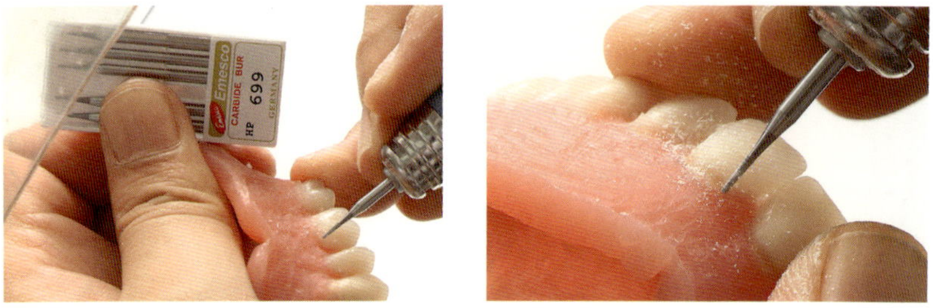

Step4 : Cervical area and papilla area denture base resin should be carefully removed with using Carbide bur HP699 (Emesco)

Fig 35a The sequence of denture coloring ①.

(Ivoclar Vivadent) will be explained with Class I(Part 4,Class II-1<Part 5>) and Class II-1 (Part 6) cases. The other coloring technique in the flask by using Candulor denture coloring kit (Candulor, Rinkai) will be explained with Class III (Part 7) case.

Step5 : Contact point area denture base resin should be carefully removed with Shofu fissure carbide HP (Shofu)

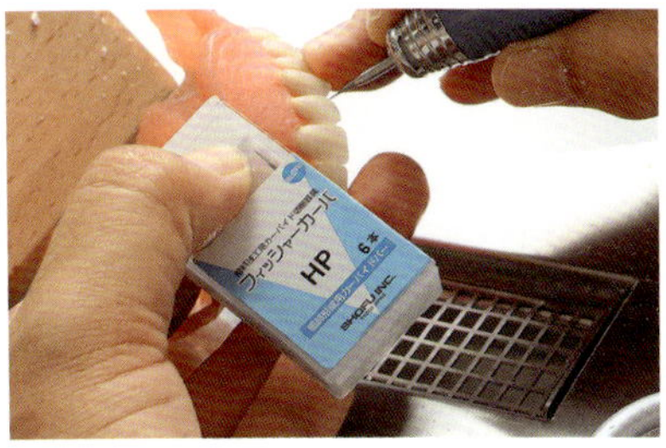

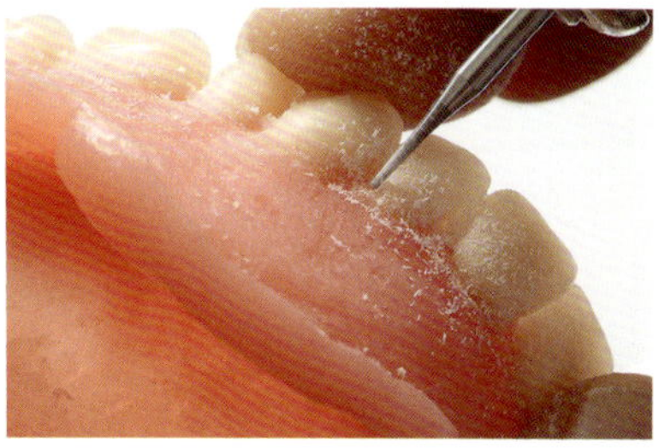

Step6 : Alumina sandblast treatment is done (0.2MPa)

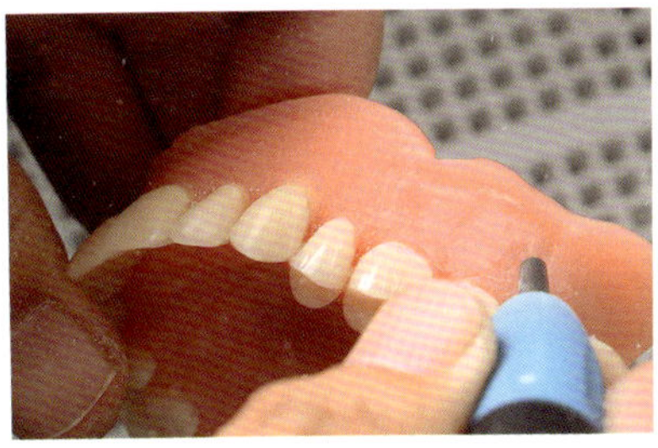

Step7 : Clean denture in the ultrasonic cleaner. This removes alumina from the denture surface. After then the denture should be cleaned with the steam cleaner

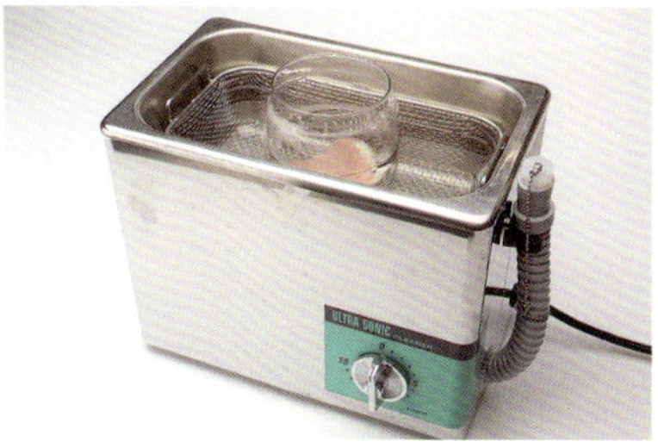

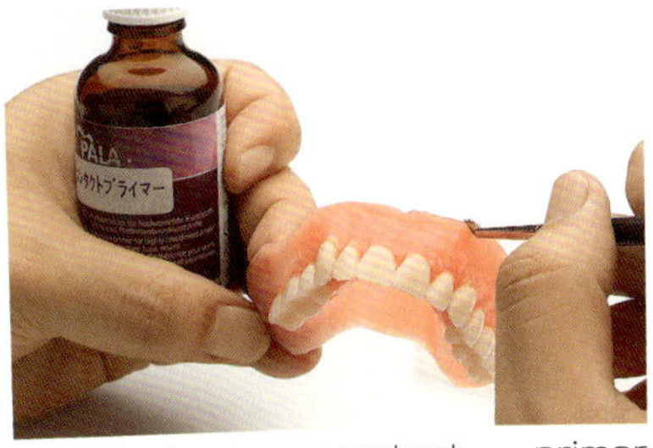

Step8 : Apply contact primer (Kulzer). This melts the denture resin surface, consequently the bond with Signum connector becomes stronger. (Attention : This should be applied to 1/3 of cervical area of denture teeth and denture base to avoid peeling during polishing. Wait for complete dryness)

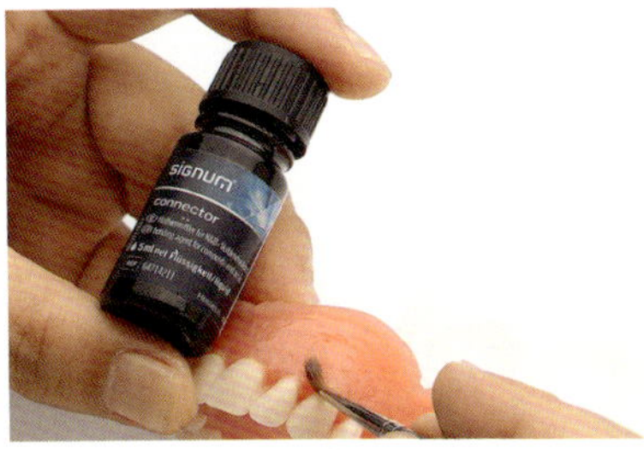

Step9 : Primer : Signum connector (Kulzer) is applied. (Attention : It is important to make sure that this wouldn't stay too much on the papilla area)

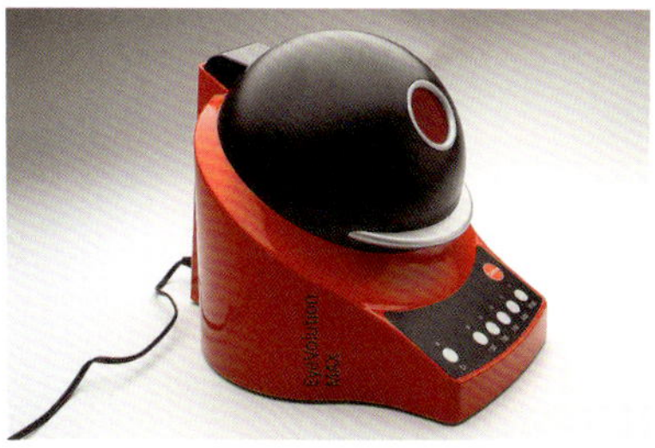

Step10 : After completing Step 8,9, the denture is light cured for 180 seconds in the Evolution Max: LED light cure machine (Dreve). This machine doesn't create too much heat; therefore, the denture deformation can be prevented

The sequence of denture coloring ②

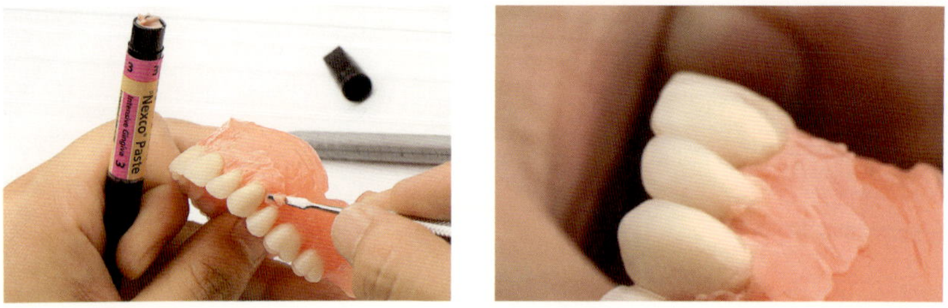

Step11 : Root contour area composite is applied with Nexco Intensive Gingiva #3 (Attention : Pay attention to the Canine eminence)

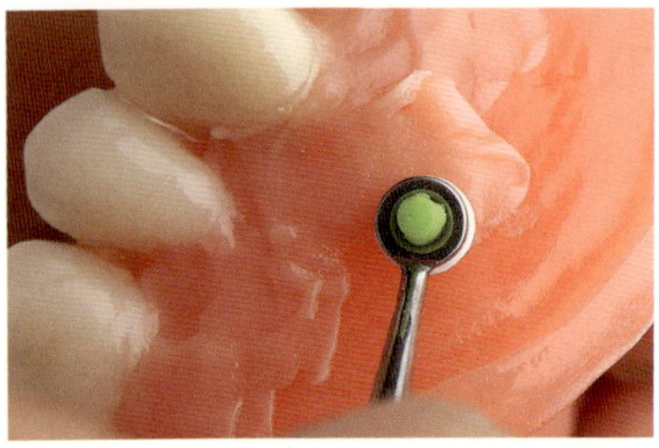

Step12 : Nexco should be compressed and eliminate bubbles by using OptraSculpt Pad (Ivoclar)

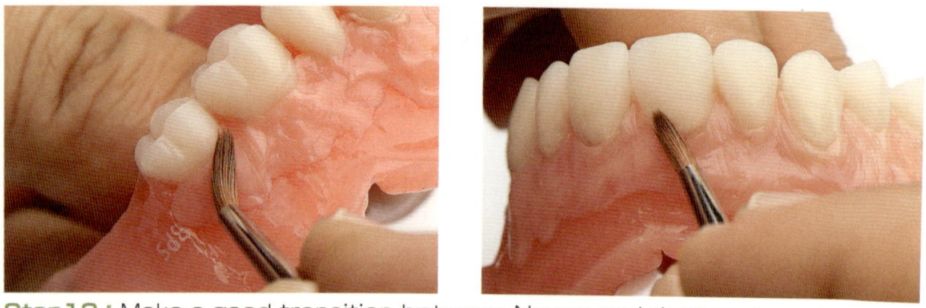

Step13 : Make a good transition between Nexco and denture base by using pile brush No.1 (Shofu) (Attention : Do not use composite primer liquid. This may cause degrading material and Nexco peeling off)

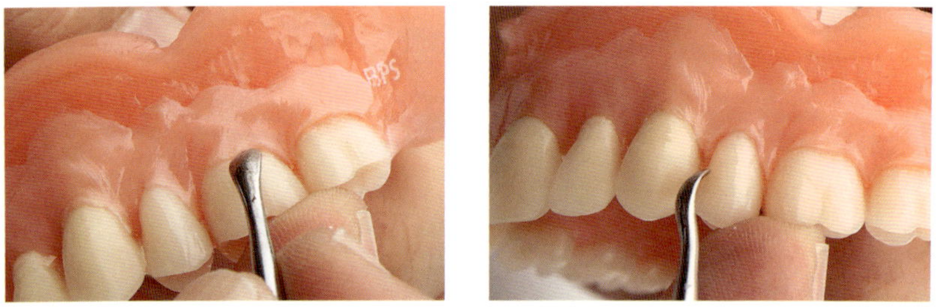

Step14 : Remove excess material from the cervical area with spoon shape instrument

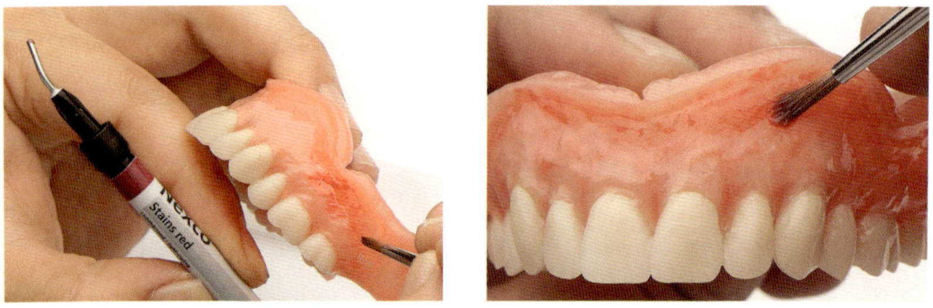

Step15 : Create alveolar mucosa esthetic with Nexco stain red

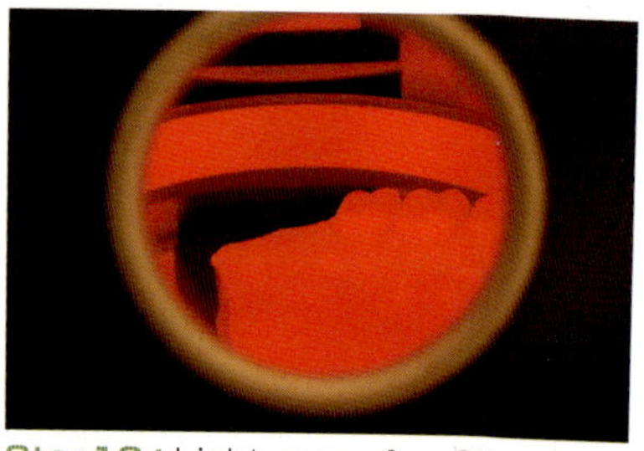

Step16 : Light cure for 60 sec in Evolution Max light cure machine

Fig 35b The sequence of denture coloring ②.

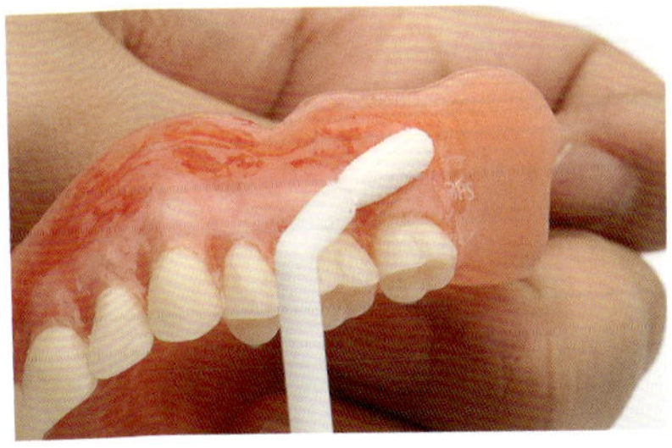

Step17 : Residue monomer after light curing should be removed with disposable sponge (Ivoclar Vivadent) (Attention : Residue monomer will cause a negative effect on the material)

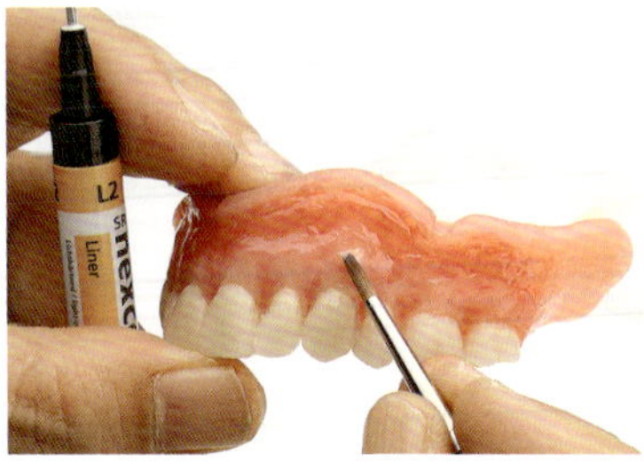

Step18 : Reproduction and esthetic enhancement of root contour should be achieved with Nexco Liner 2

Step19 : First layer and second layer should be painted seamlessly with pile brush No.1 (Attention : Do not use other composite primer. This may cause degrading material and peeling Nexco)

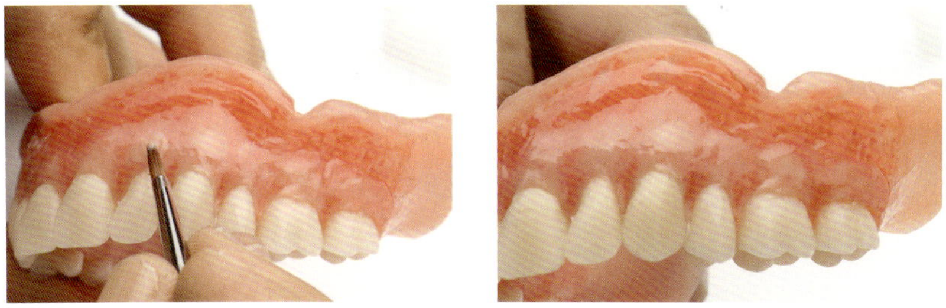

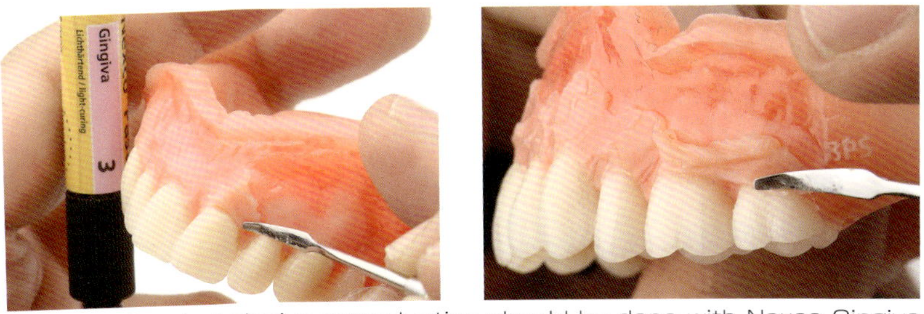

Step20 : Cervical gingiva reproduction should be done with Nexco Gingiva #3 (Applied on top of Nexco Intensive Gingiva(first layer))

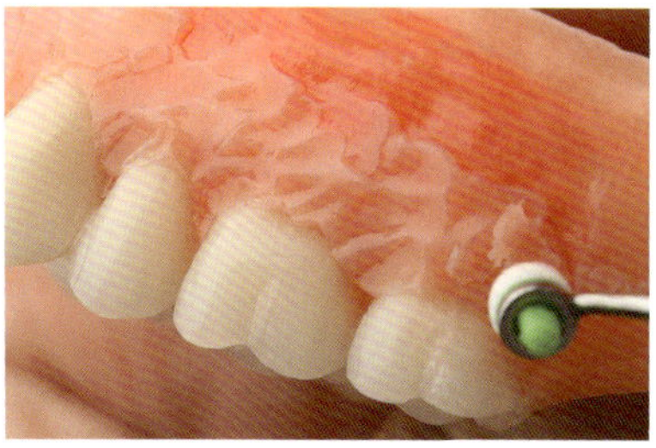

Step21 : Nexco gingiva #3 should be compressed and eliminate bubbles by using OptraSculpt Pad (Ivoclar)

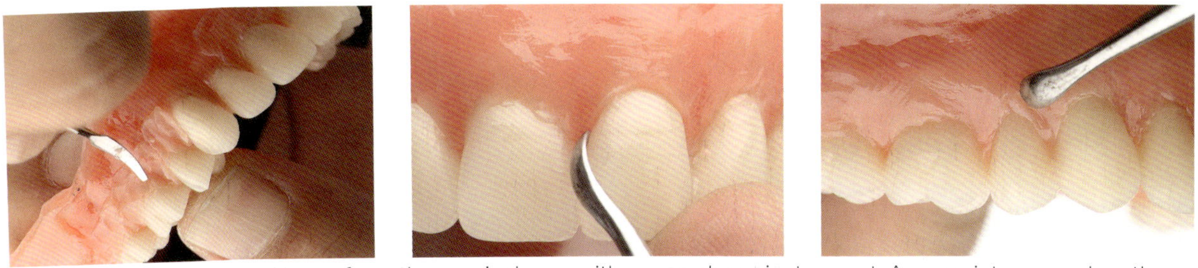

Step22 : Remove excess Nexco from the cervical area with spoon shape instrument. Appropriate crown length should be reproduced

The sequence of denture coloring ③

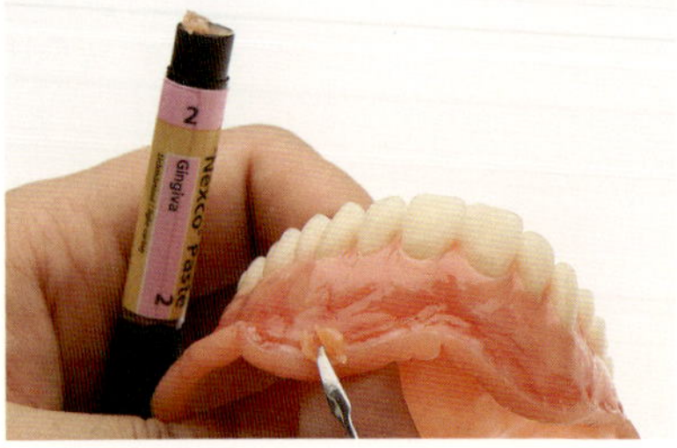
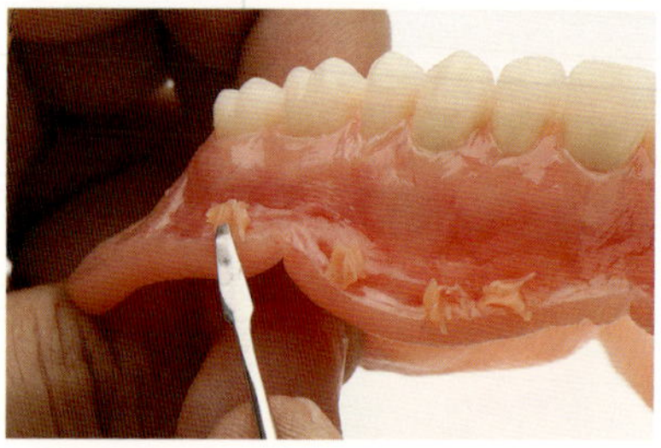

Step23 : Nexco Gingiva 2 is randomly applied to alveolar mucosal transition

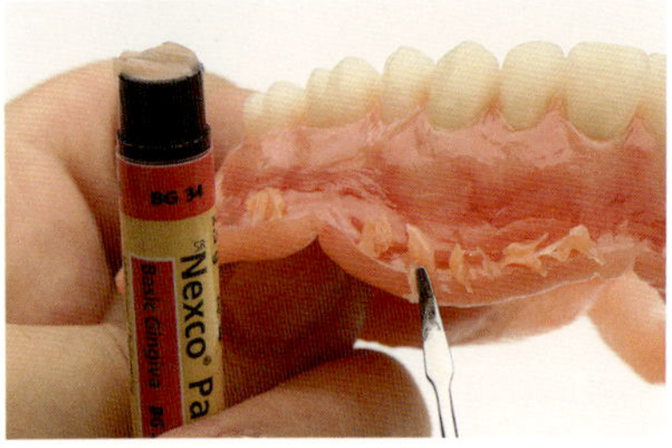
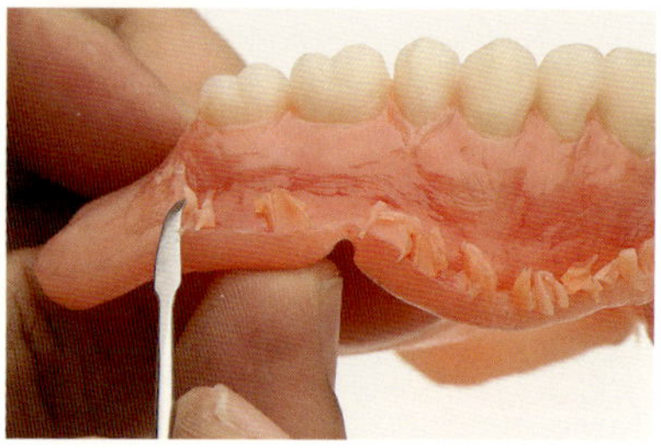

Step24 : Nexco Basic gingiva 34 is randomly applied to alveolar mucosal transition

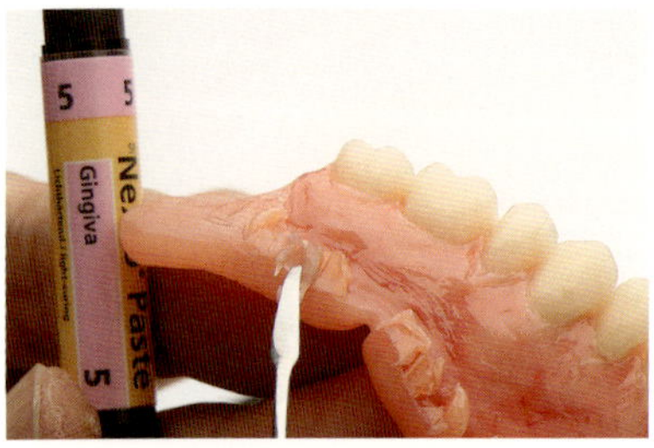
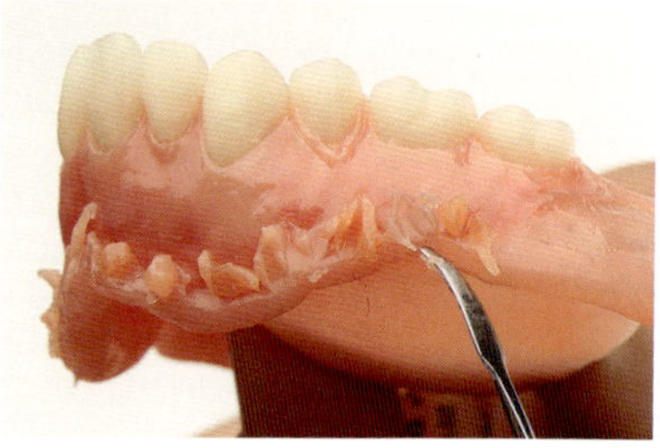
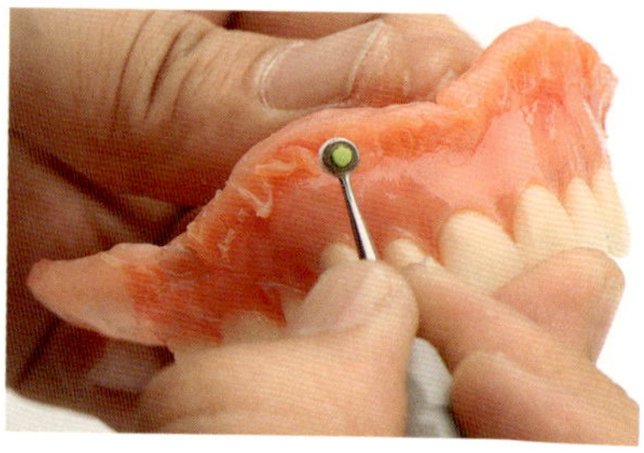
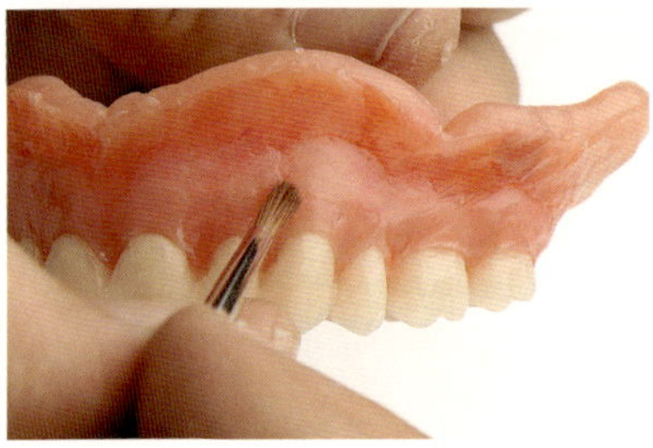

Step25 : Nexco gingiva 5 can be applied to molar area alveolar mucosa transition as an accent

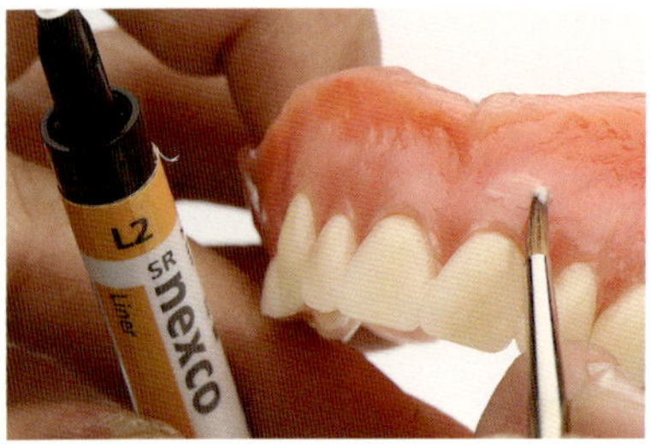

Step26 : Final application adjustment (Color adjustment)
①If the gingival color is darker :Nexco Liner 2 should be added on the cervical area

Fig 35c The sequence of denture coloring ③.

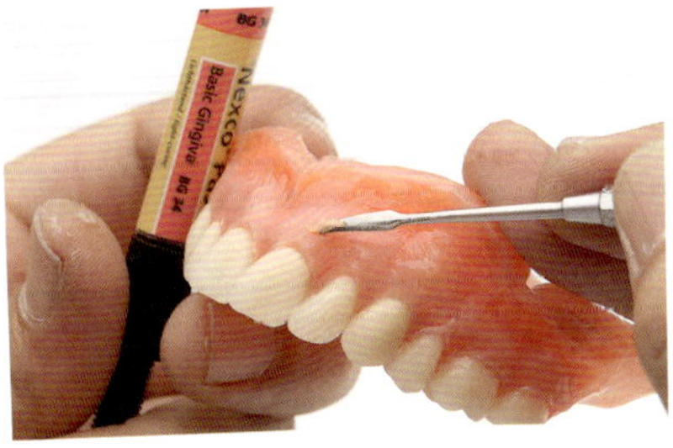

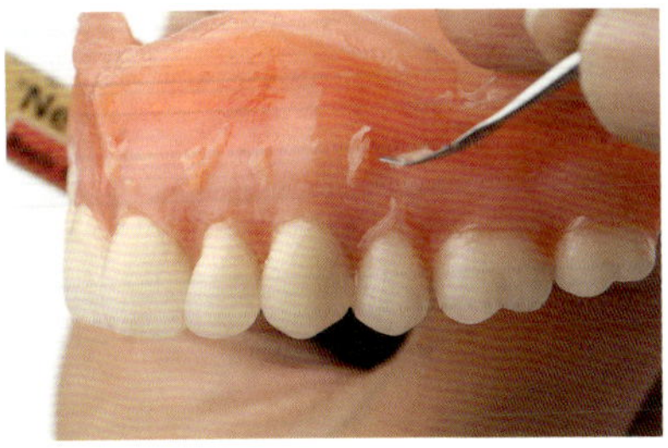

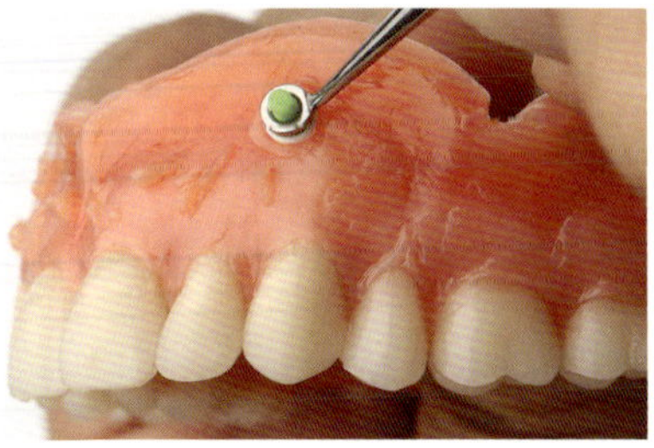

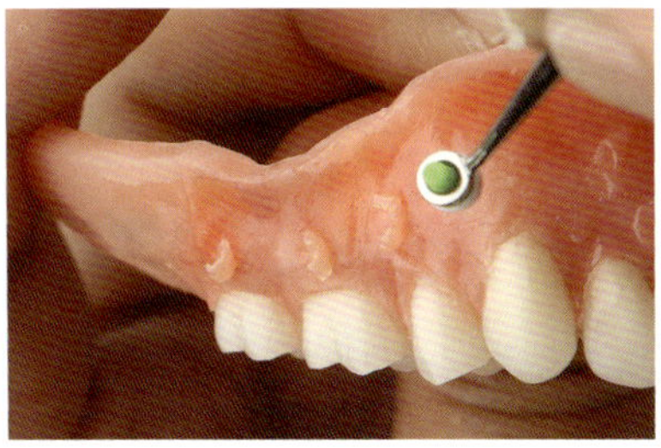

Step27 : Final application adjustment (Color adjustment)
②If the gingival color is lighter : Nexco stain red should be applied to give value and gradation

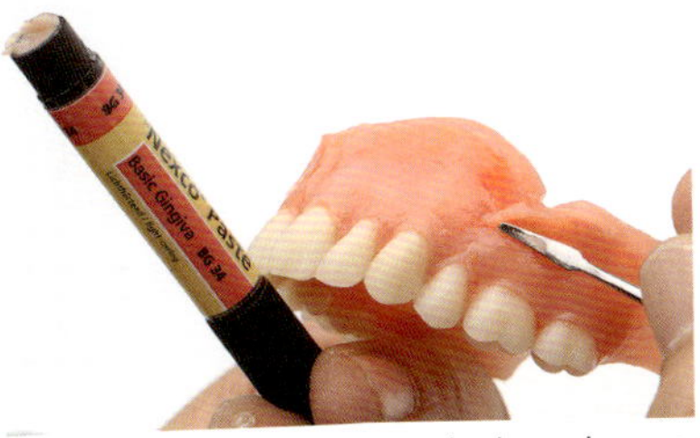

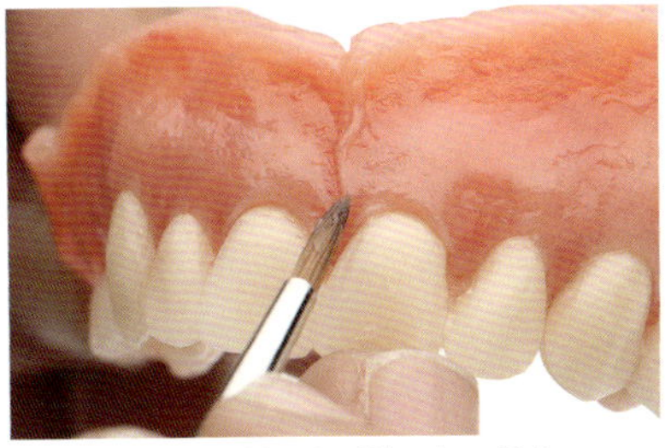

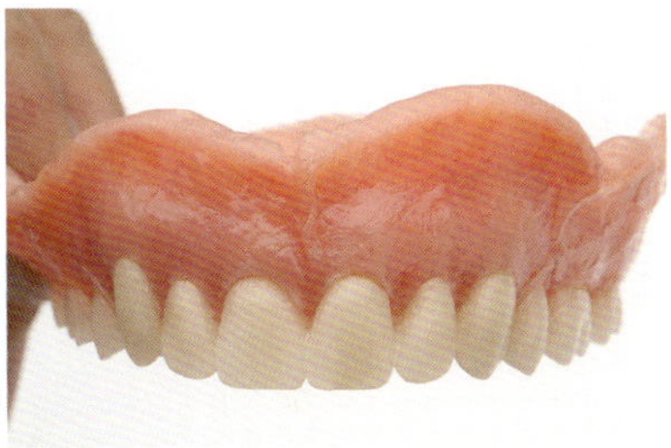

Step28 : Frenum morphology is created with Nexco Basic Gingiva 34

Step29 : Light cure for 60 sec in Evolution Max light cure machine.
Step30 : Vacuum light polymerization for 12 minutes with Visio Beta Vario (3M ESPE)

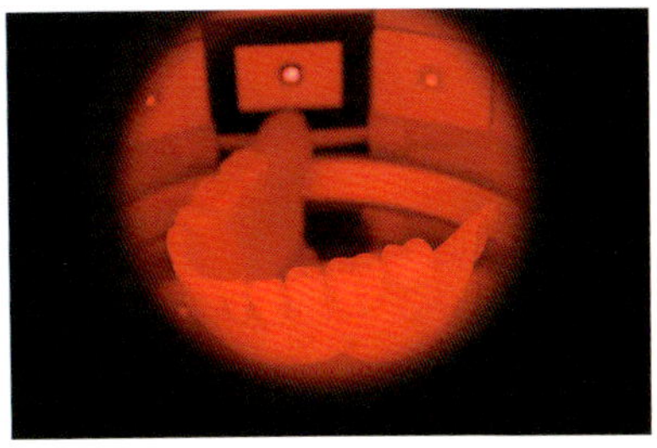

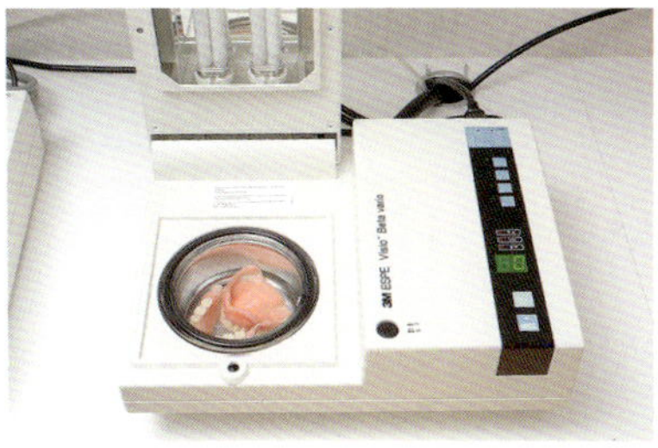

Step31 : Excess composite around cervical area and papillary area should be trimmed with EMESCO carbide bur HP699
Step32 : Surface texture and polished surface morphology are created with Meisinger HM77MF 023HP (Meisinger/GC)

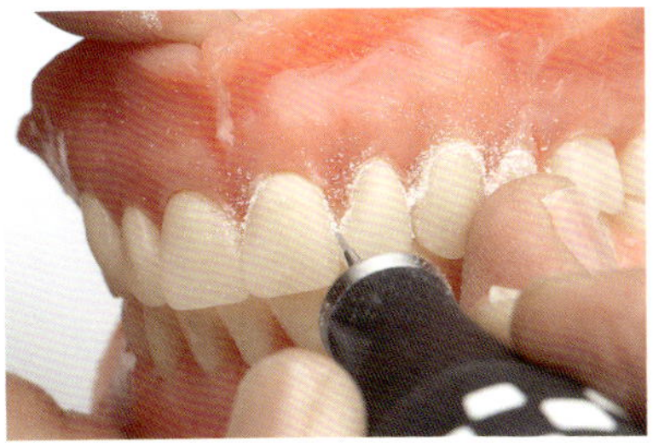

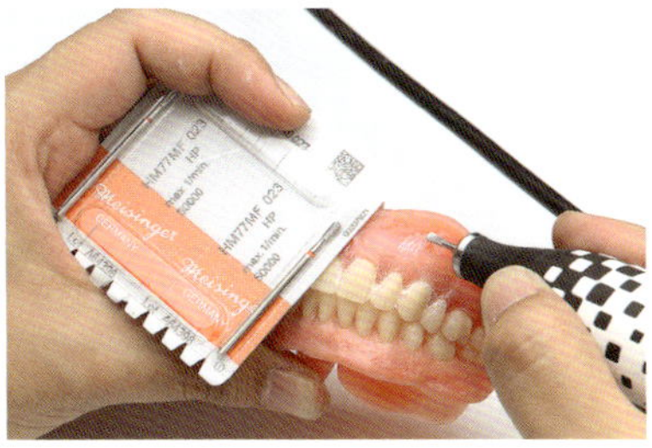

Finalized complete denture

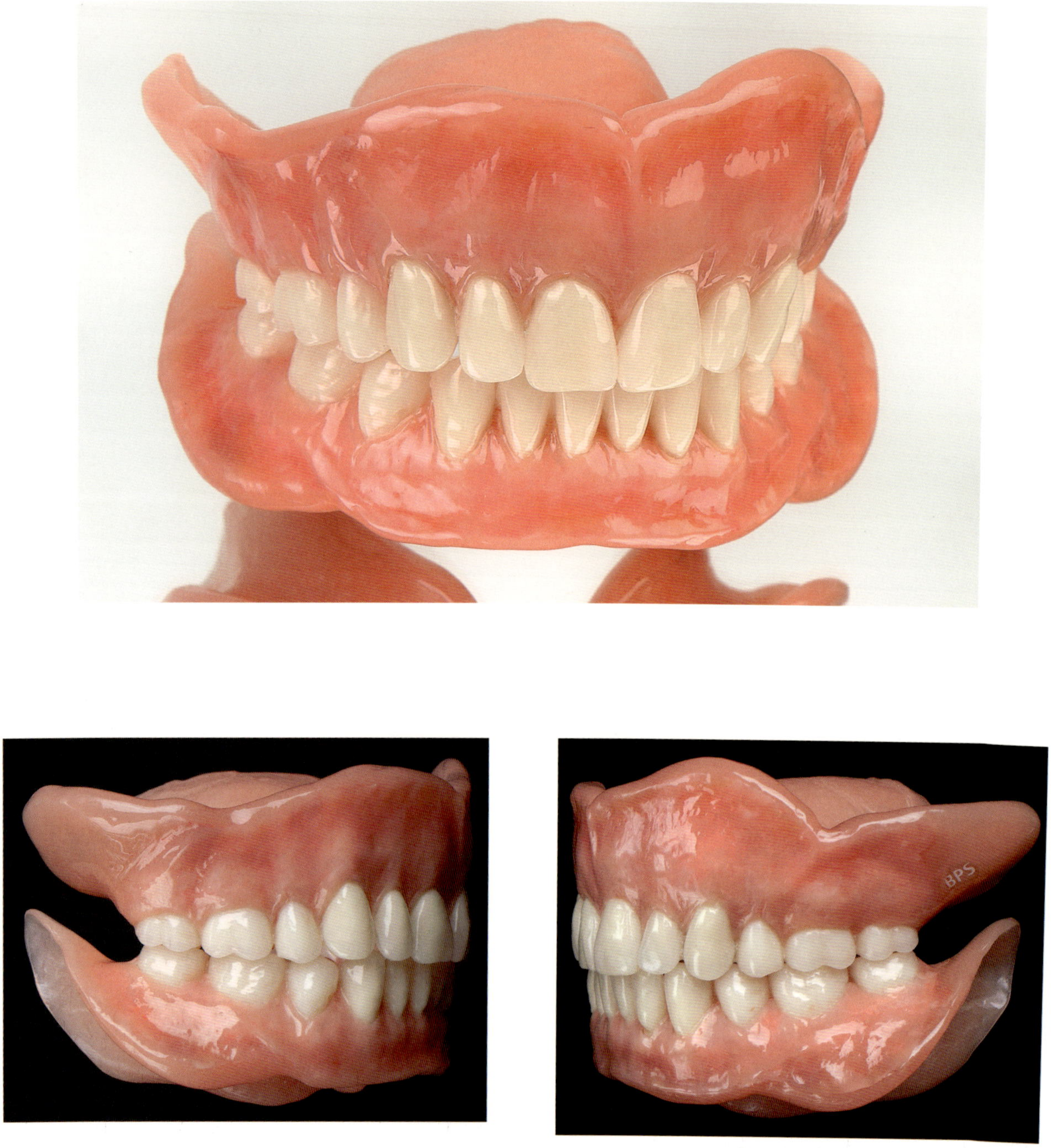

Fig 36 Finalized complete denture.

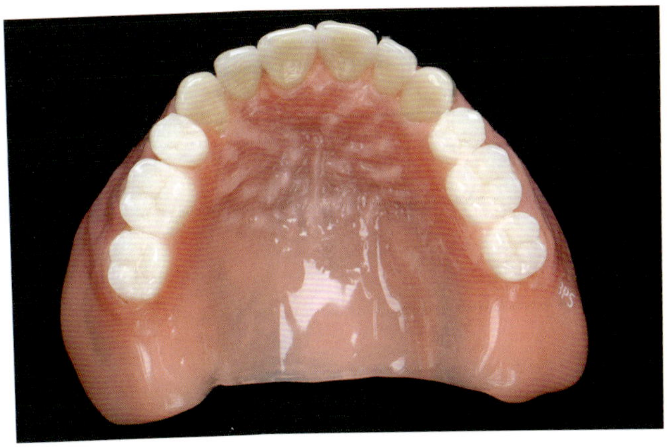

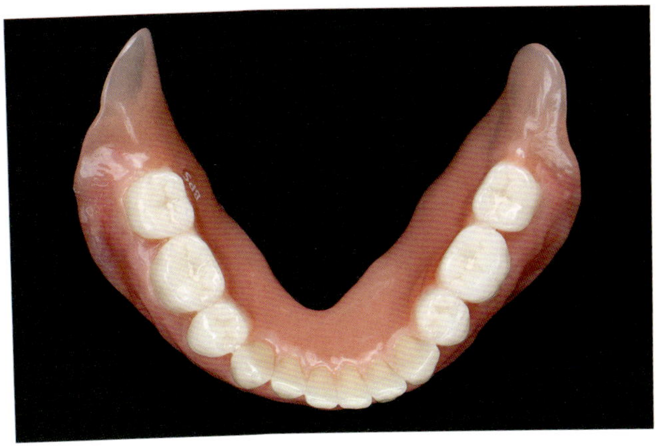

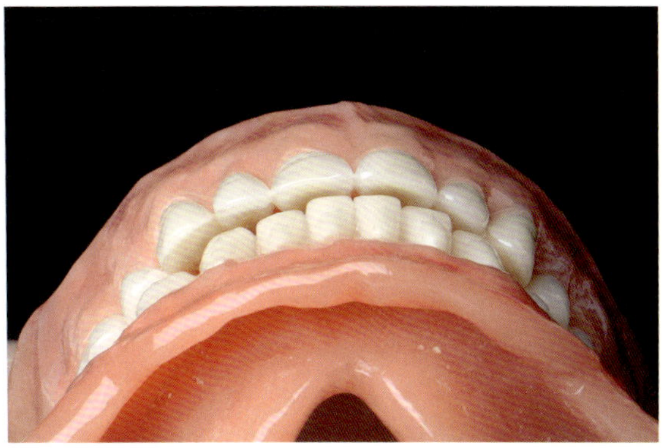

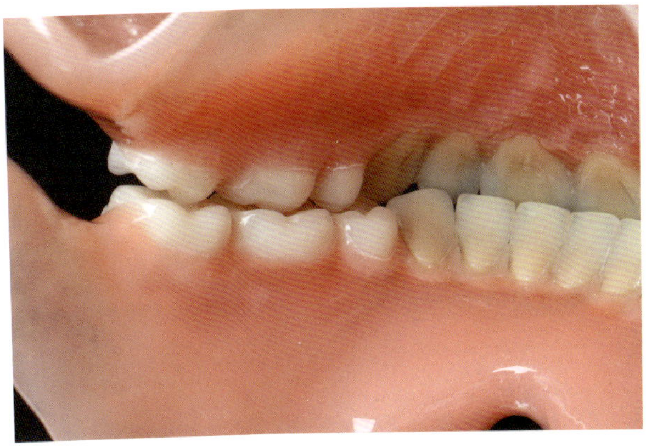

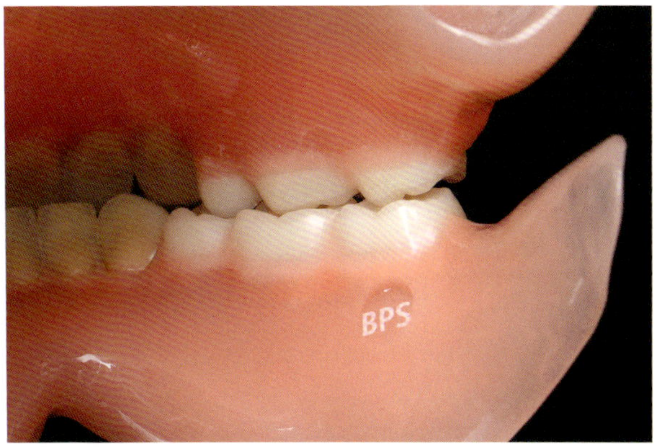
BPS

Fundamental complete denture esthetic

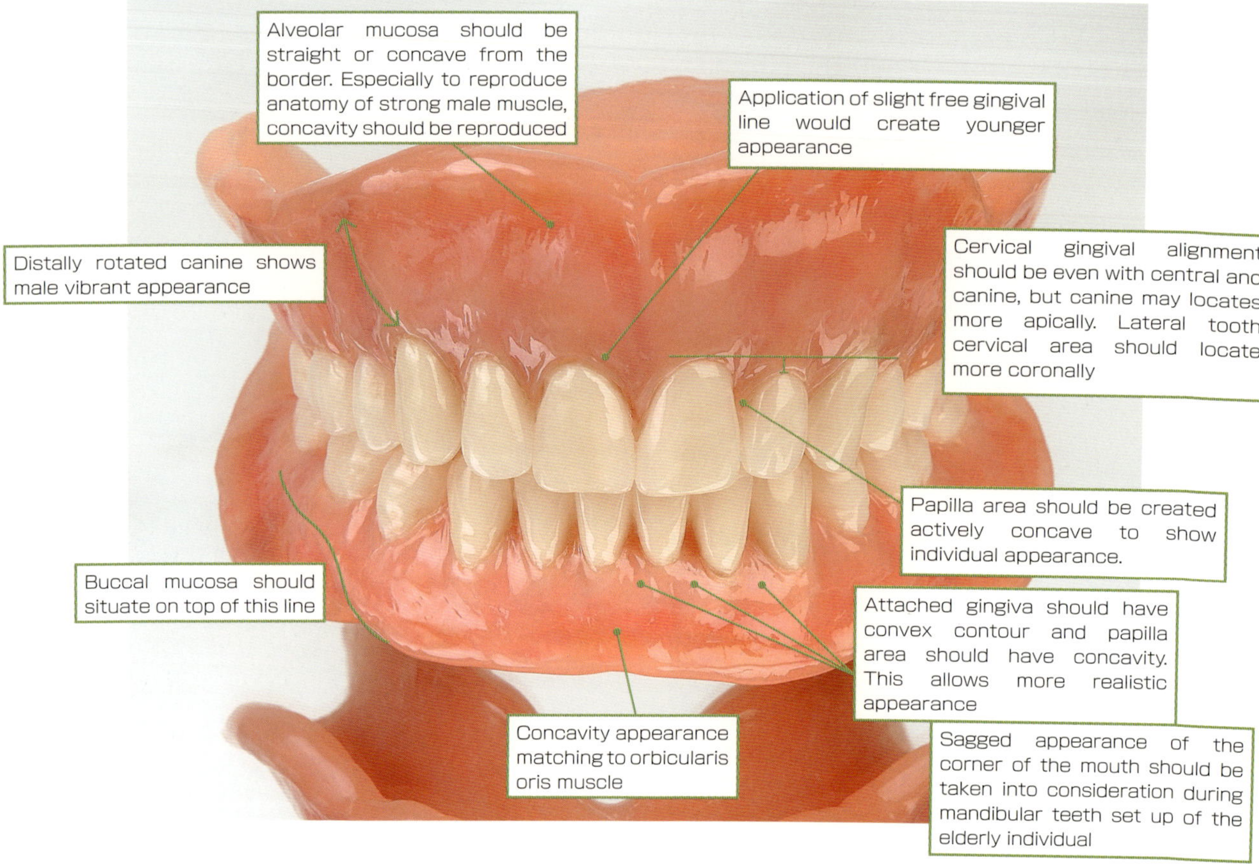

Fig 37 Fundamental complete denture esthetic. Interdental papilla area should be concave to create more individual appearance so the denture doesn't look like a denture. There are 2-3% of the patients in the authors clinic request to have slightly crowding teeth setting. In this case, since the maxillary left incisal mesial corner is slightly overlapped with the maxillary right incisal distal corner, the maxillary left incisal cervical area is located slightly apical to the maxillary right incisal cervical area. The root position influences the gingival appearance. The cervical area of maxillary left lateral incisor locates more apically compared to that of the maxillary right lateral incisor. The appearance of this area should be adjusted according to the individual esthetic in conjunction with the lip. Gingival esthetic appearance should be well paid attention with the case that requires unique teeth set up or the lip has more concavity.

14 Summary

Clinical denture fabrication steps of the Class I jaw relationship with the normal ideal alveolar ridge condition and the laboratory denture fabrication steps by the dental technician have been described in this chapter.

The purpose of this chapter is to learn the denture fabrication basics and establish the fundamental ideas for denture fabrication. The author would like to emphasize the importance to learn and master the basic and fundamental concepts and this knowledge will eventually enhance the ability to treat the difficult cases in the future.

Part 5

Clinical case 2
Maxillary/Mandibular difficult case : Class II -division 2
with maxillary flabby ridge & extensive mandibular ridge resorption

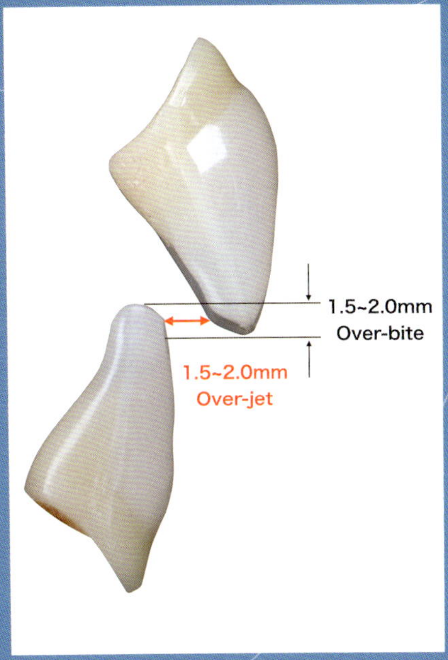

Dental Technician:
Kenji Iwaki

1 The goal of the treatment

Fabrication process of maxillary and mandibular complete dentures for Class II-division 2 malocclusion is presented in this chapter. The treatment approach for maxillary anterior flabby ridge as well as impression technique and denture tooth set up for mandible with extensive ridge resorption can be learned through this clinical case.

It is important to set the treatment goal, which is simple and achievable. Regarding the management of maxillary flabby tissue, stimulants causing inflammation of flabby ridge needs to be controlled by establishing bilateral posterior occlusion and eliminating the tendency of chewing with anterior teeth. Inflammation will be gradually resolved by maintaining the bilateral posterior occlusion. Quality of Life is improved by managing resorbed mandibular ridge establishing mandibular suction-effective denture through accurate clinical performance and precise fabrication process.

2 Initial condition at the first visit

The patient is 77 years old female. Chief complaints were dislodgment of the maxillary denture, unstable mandibular denture and accompanying soreness of the ridge.

1) Maxilla

Ridge size is relatively small and inflammatory flabby ridge is found between right and left second premolar area. Torus is appreciated at mid palatal anterior region (The optional impression technique for flabby gum and maintenance to control inflammation are required).

2) Mandible

Severe ridge resorption is appreciated and the mental foramen is palpable at the crest of the ridge at second premolar region (Precise impression technique is required).

The retromolar pad is likely distorted even under the impression with gentle pressure using frame cut back tray, since the anterior portion of the retromolar pad consists of mainly soft mucosa glands without firm fibrous tissue. Large amount of changes in the shape of the retromolar pad during opened and closed

Fig1a, b Patient is 77 years old female. Occlusal classification is Class II-2, severe flabby ridge is observed between areas of maxillary second molars. Protruded bone is observed posterior to the flabby ridge.

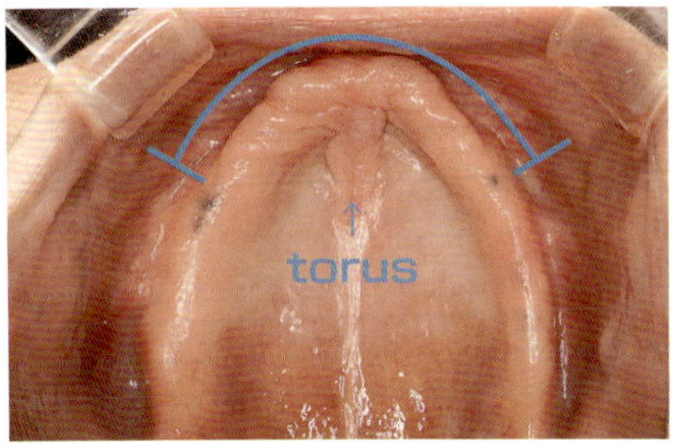

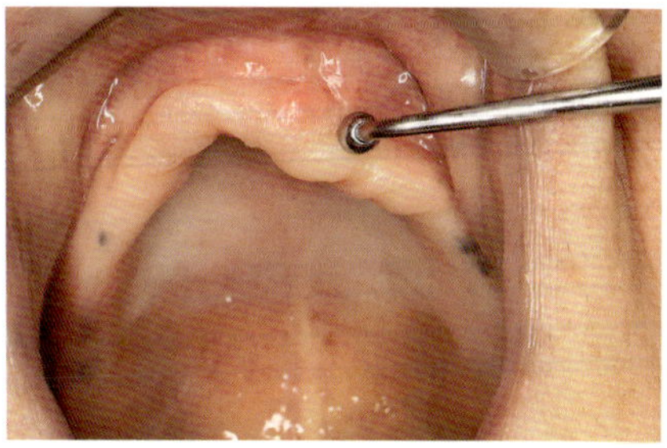

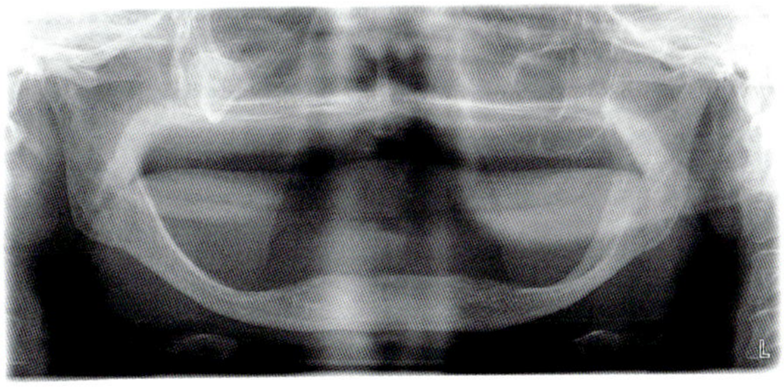

Fig1c Panoramic x-ray. Extensive mandibular ridge resorption is appreciated.

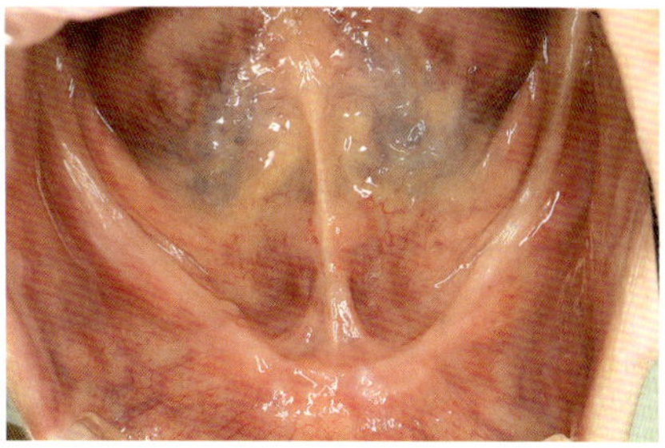

Fig1d Extensive retraction of the tongue upon opening the mouth.

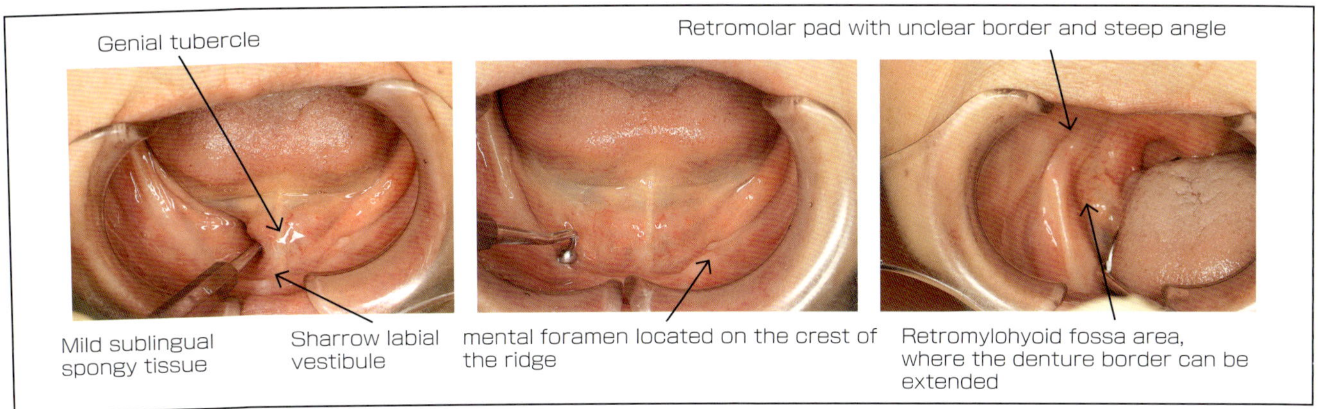

Fig1e Condition of the mandible with various kinds of problems.

motion was found. Further, the retromolar pad that is steeply inclined forward due to extensive resorption of the ridge (Process of improving adaptation of the custom tray in the retromolar pad region is required before taking final impression).

Vestibule is rather narrow in the anterior area due to attachment of mentalis to the ridge crest (The optional impression technique in order for the denture border of anterior region to be thickened and gain additional lip support is required).

To make matters worse, the tongue retraction at opened position and the genial tubercle posterior to the anterior region are appreciated (The optional technique to seal lingual denture border while the tongue is retracted is required).

The sufficient space where the denture border can be extended is present in the retromylohyoide fossa.

There is 8mm discrepancy between patient's habitual occlusal position of the existing denture and the mandibular posterior guided position, but no functional

Chair side evaluation

Examination items for mandibular complete denture

Suction inhibiting factor	Right: Good	Right: Fair	Right: Poor	Left: Good	Left: Fair	Left: Poor
1. Ridge form			☑			☑
2. Spongy tissue in sublingual fold region		☑			☑	
3. Space for denture extension in retromylohyoid fossa region	☑			☑		
4. Pear-like shaped retromolar pad			☑			☑

Retromolar pad (one risk is ☑ as Fair, ☑ as Poor, if more than two risks are marked)

	Right	Left
1. The presence of firm fibrous tissue in anterior half	(Yes slightly No✓)	(Yes slightly No✓)
2. Size	(Large Moderate✓ Small)	(Large Moderate✓ Small)
3. Tilt angle	(Shallow Moderate Steep✓)	(Shallow Moderate Steep✓)
4. Change during open and close movement	(Small Moderate Large✓)	(Small Moderate Large✓)

5. Tongue retraction upon opening mouth	☐ Normal (less than 2cm)	☐ Further retraction (2～4cm)	☑ Even further retraction (more than 4cm)
6. Jaw relationship	☐ Class I	☑ Class II	☐ Class III
7. Mandibular jaw position	☐ Guided position and habitual occlusal position coincide or within 2mm of discrepancy	☑ More than 2mm of discrepancy	☐ More than mm of discrepancy and unstable tapping point
8. Temporomandibular joint function	☑ Normal	☐ Disfunction	☐ Severe disfunction with pain

Special Note :
Wearing time of the denture, (Maxillary) Flabby tissue, Tori (Mandibular) Flabby tissue, Genial tubercle shallow labial vestibule in mandibular anterior region, etc

→ Maxilla: flabby ridge in anterior and premolar region and torus on anterior aspect of palate.
Mandibular: Lingual genial tubercle, shallow labial vestibule, mental foramen is located on the ridge crest.

The special impression technique for flabby ridge and the maintenance to control inflammation is required (P107-111)
The technique to maintain the thickness at the mandibular anterior denture border is required (P115-116)
The technique to seal the mandibular lingual genial tubercle is required (P111-114)

Precise impression is required (P117-121)

Seal of the sublingual fold needs to be reinforced / Optional sublingual sealing impression technique is required(P111-124)

Fit of the custom tray at the retromolar pad area needs to be improved before the final impression (P105, Fig33)

The technique to seal the lingual denture border needs to be utilized when the tongue is retruded (P111-124).

Denture teeth have to be set up so that esthetics, function and stability are maintained (P128-140)

The mandibular position after delivery of the new denture could be displaced due to elevated VOD and improvement of mandibular horizontal position (relining could be indicated)

Table 1 Suction (Seal) is broken if there is even one area of air leak. Obtaining suction is difficult if more than 2 anatomical inhibiting factors of 1~5 are marked (there are 2 factors checked in unfavorable and 1 check in severe tongue retraction in this case). However, suction can be obtained in many cases by employing some optional sealing technique. The measure to overcome the inhibiting factor is discussed later.

Laboratory side evaluation

Examination items for mandibular complete denture

Suction inhibiting factor	Right Good	Right Fair	Right Poor	Left Good	Left Fair	Left Poor
1. Ridge form			☑			☑
2. Spongy tissue in sublingual fold region		☑			☑	
3. Space for denture extension in retromylohyoid fossa region	☑			☑		
4. Pear-like shaped retromolar pad			☑			☑

Retromolar pad (one risk is ☑ as Fair, ☑ as Poor, if more than two risks are marked)

	Right	Left
1. The presence of firm fibrous tissue in anterior half	(Yes slightly No✓)	(Yes slightly No✓)
2. Size	(Large Moderate✓ Small)	(Large Moderate✓ Small)
3. Tilt angle	(Shallow Moderate Steep✓)	(Shallow Moderate Steep✓)
4. Change during open and close movement	(Small Moderate Large✓)	(Small Moderate Large✓)

5. Tongue retraction upon opening mouth	☐ Normal (less than 2cm)	☐ Further retraction (2～4cm)	☑ Even further retraction (more than 4cm)
6. Jaw relationship	☐ Class I	☑ Class II	☐ Class III
7. Mandibular jaw position	☐ Guided position and habitual occlusal position coincide or within 2mm of discrepancy	☑ More than 2mm of discrepancy	☐ More than mm of discrepancy and unstable tapping point
8. Temporomandibular joint function	☑ Normal	☐ Disfunction	☐ Severe disfunction with pain

Special Note:
Wearing time of the denture, (Maxillary) Flabby tissue, Tori (Mandibular) Flabby tissue, Genial tubercle shallow labial vestibule in mandibular anterior region, etc

→ Maxilla: flabby ridge in anterior and premolar region and torus on anterior aspect of palate.
Mandibular: Lingual genial tubercle, shallow labial vestibule, mental foramen is located on the ridge crest.

Fabrication of the special custom tray for the flabby ridge or case specific denture tooth set up and adjustment are required (P94-96).
Slight thickness of the denture border should be provided at the labial region
Laboratory idea should be provided to be able to seal at the genial tubercle with the denture base

Well fit custom tray is required (P98, Fig22)

Enough thickness of the denture border needs to be provided at the sublingual fold region (P92-99)

The tray must thinly cover the whole retromolar pad (P98, Fig22)

Enough thickness of the denture border should be provided at the sublingual fold region (P92-99)

Special tooth setup technique to achieve high esthetic and function is required not to affect maxillary and mandibular denture stabiity

Laboratory work should be rendered taking the possibility of changing denture teeth or relining into consideration

Table 2 Various dental laboratory techniques, which are shown in this table, are required to fabricate the maxillary denture, which does not fall, and the mandibular denture, which does not rise up, under the tough condition described above.

problem was found in the temporomandibular joint.

Jaw relationship is Class II Division 2 according to the photo of the patient when she was still dentate (Denture tooth set up technique to facilitate denture stability fulfilling esthetics and function is required).

Various types of suction inhibiting factors are found in the difficult case. Appropriate optional techniques need to be utilized for successful denture treatment.

3) Everything starts from Intra-oral Examination

The outcome of mandibular complete denture suction-effect diagnosis sheet is shown in Table 1 and 2. Diagnosis should be shared between the dentist and the dental technician. Collaboration between the dentist and the dental technician sharing the result of diagnosis and the common treatment goal is imperative to accomplish good result even in the difficult denture case.

4) Consultation

The approach and the explanation to the patient would be different among dentists depending on their experience and skill for Suction-effective complete denture fabrication or the character of the dentist. The author keeps it in mind to talk in a matter-of-fact approach as follows according to the diagnosis.

[The maxillary denture can be made so that it would not fall down during opening your mouth in spite of the maxillary flabby gum. On the other hand, the condition of your mandible is considerably unfavorable and suction-effect rate would be only up to 60% with my experience and skill. However, the mandibular denture can be fabricated so that it would not lift up during opening your mouth with 90% of success chance even with the weak suction-effect. In any case, if you are not satisfied with the denture, I would recommend transition to the implant over denture. What would you think about it?]

After patient's consent, the treatment is started.

3 Maxillary preliminary impression

(1) 3 types of maxillary preliminary impression technique

Three different types of maxillary impression techniques for general case, flabby ridge case and palatal torus case, are discussed in this section.

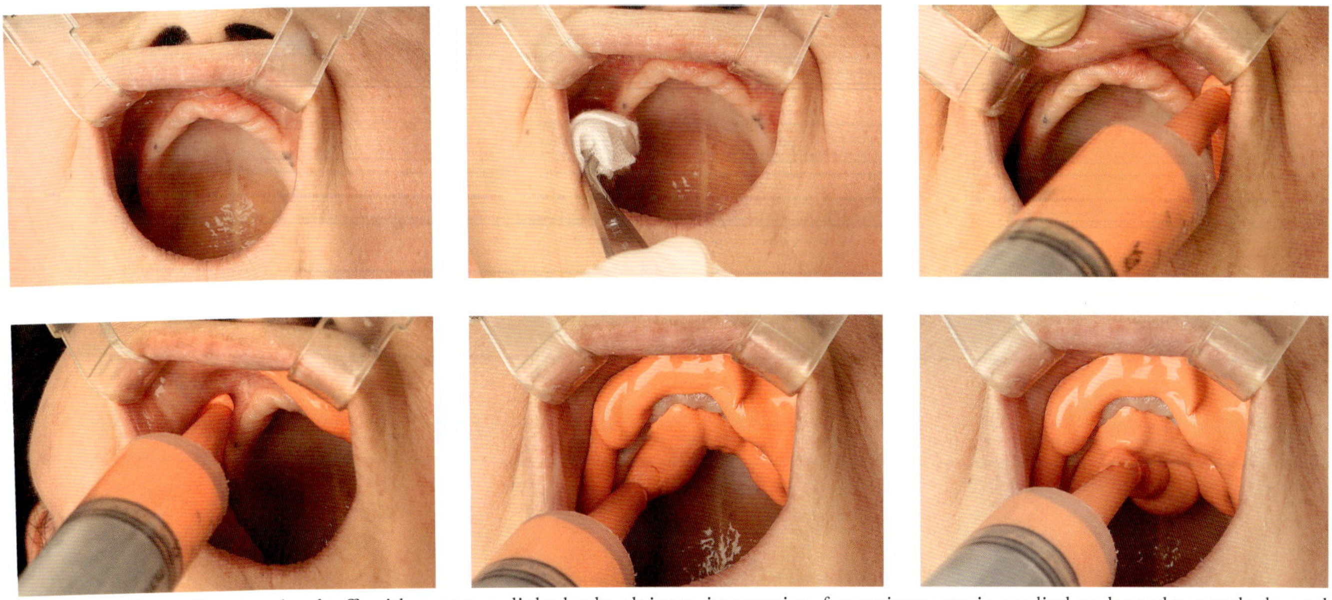

Fig2a~f After saliva is wiped off with a gauze, light body alginate impression for syringe use is applied to hamular notch, buccal side of maxillary tuberosity up to labial frenum areas on one side. Upon reaching midline, the impression material is applied to the other side in the same manner starting from the maxillary tuberosity and moving toward to the midline. The impression material should be applied over the labial frenum to avoid air trap. Next, the impression material is applied to undercut area posterior to the anterior flabby ridge and midpalatal area to avoid air trap.

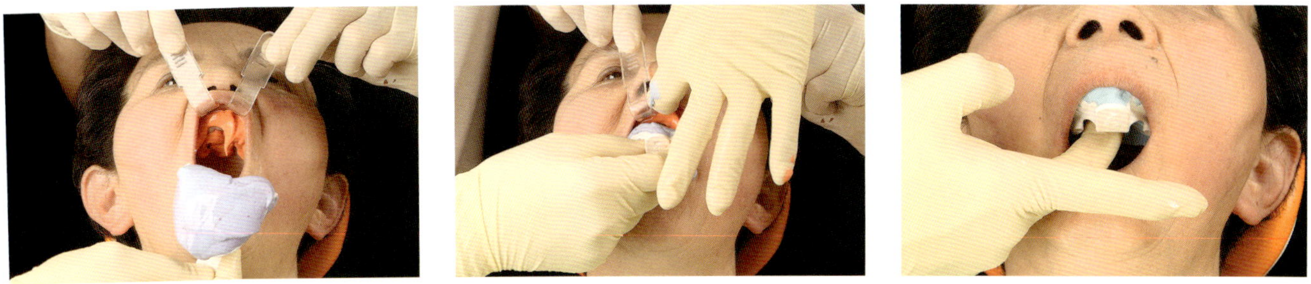

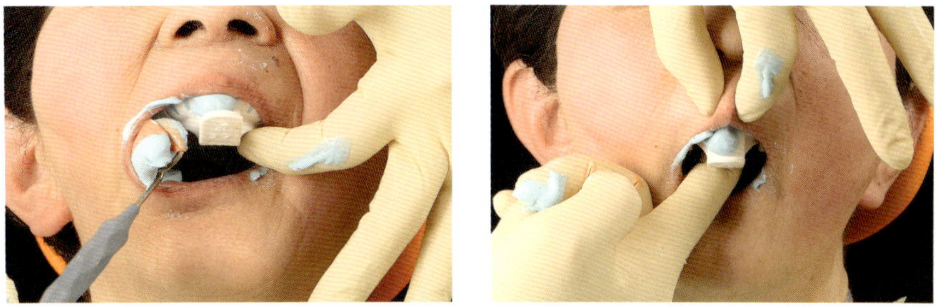

Fig2g~k The tray, loaded with heavy body alginate impression material is inserted in the mouth. The tray is pressed against the mucosa by rotational movement from anterior to posterior direction. Excess material is scooped up with the mirror to prevent gag reflex. Impression material flows deep into the flange by pinching the upper lip.

1) General technique

General maxillary preliminary impression technique is shown in fig 2 and the left column of Fig3. Light-body alginate impression material is squirted to the hamular notch, mucobuccal fold, and labial frenum area for both sides. Lastly, squirt to the palatal vault as shown in photos. The tray molded with heavy-body alginate impression material is inserted from anterior to posterior direction with upright

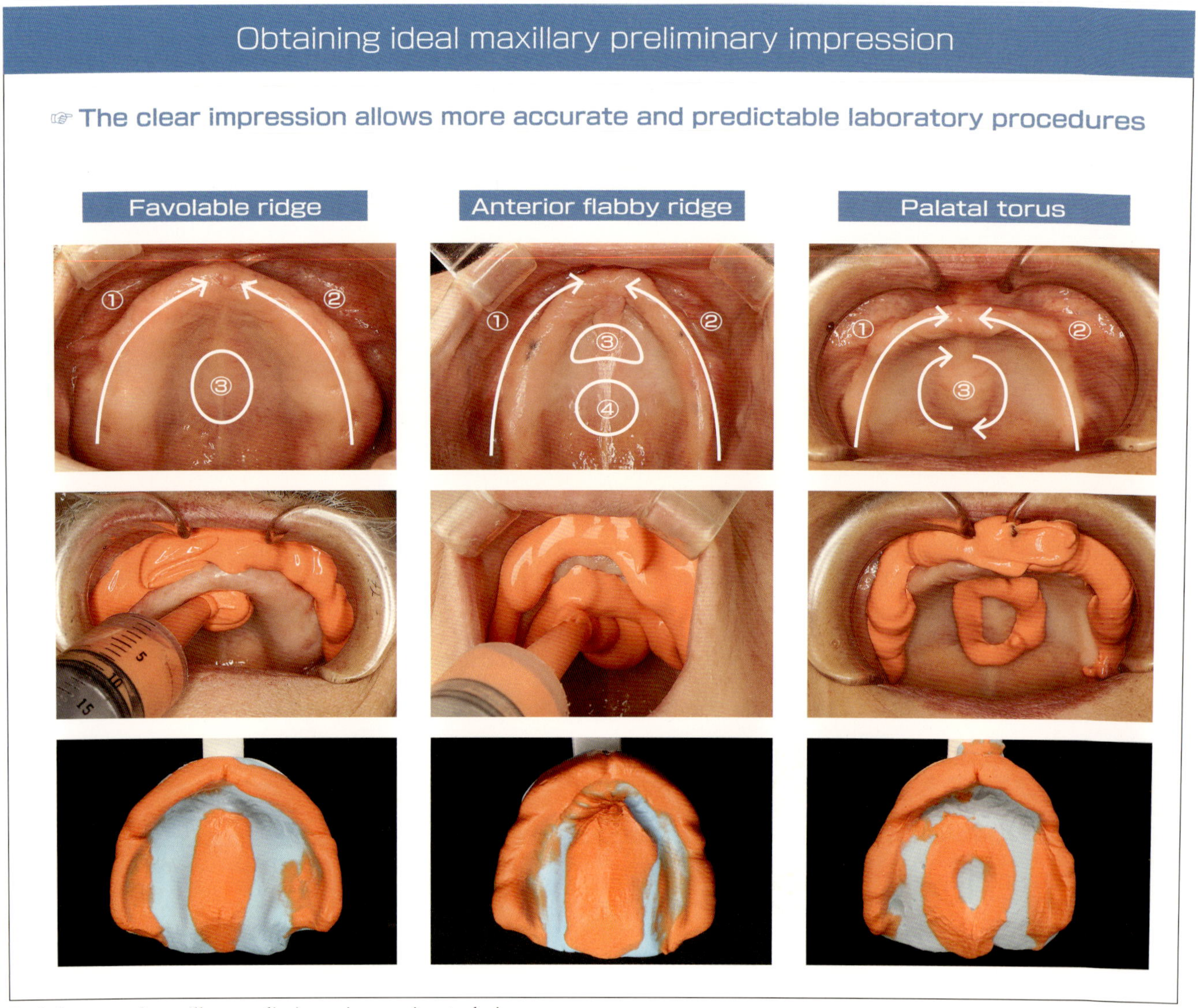

Fig3 3 types of maxillary preliminary impression techniques.

rotational maneuver.

2) The impression technique for the case with flabby ridge

the preliminary impression technique for the case with maxillary anterior flabby ridge is shown in the middle column of Fig 3. Light-body alginate impression is squirted to the hamular notch, mucobuccal fold and labial frenum area first and then to posterior part of anterior flabby ridge in order to prevent air trap in posterior undercut area of flabby ridge. Palatal vault area is squirted lastly, and then the tray molded with heavy-body alginate impression material is inserted from the anterior to posterior direction with upright rotational maneuver.

3) The impression technique for the case with the palatal torus

The preliminary impression technique for the case with the palatal torus is

Determination of posterior border of the custom tray

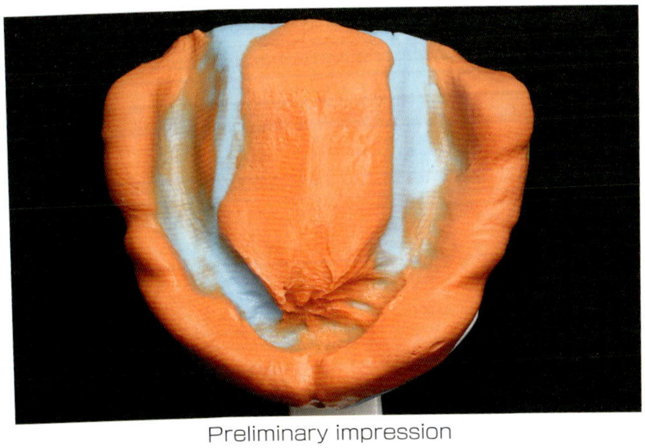

Preliminary impression

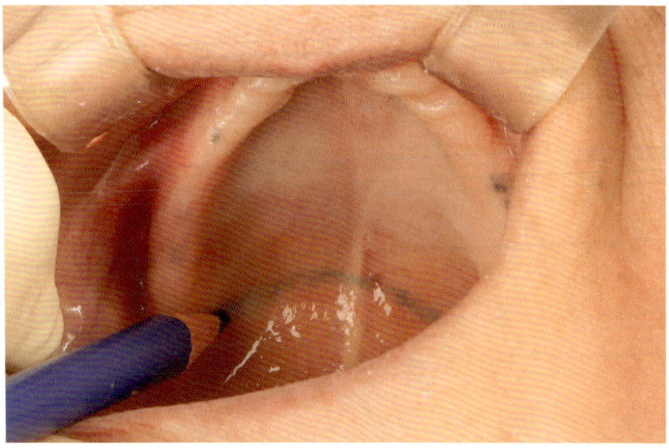

Soft palate is raised and vibrates when the patient says "Ah" (A-line Method) or the area, immediately posterior to hard palate, drops when the patient is asked to breathe through the nose, which is pinched by the operator (Nose Blow Effect). Border between hard and soft palate is identified and marked by the pen

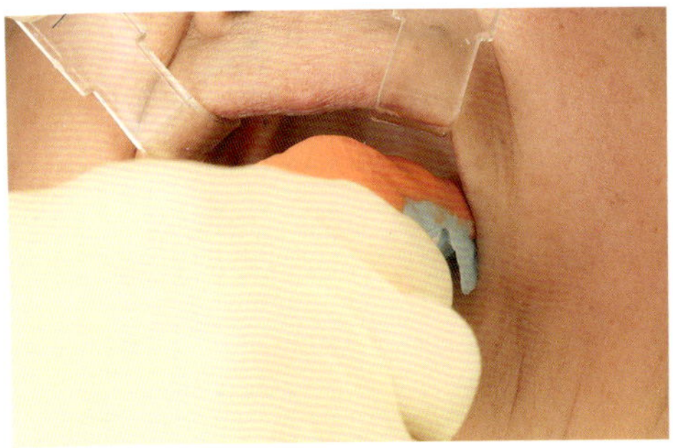

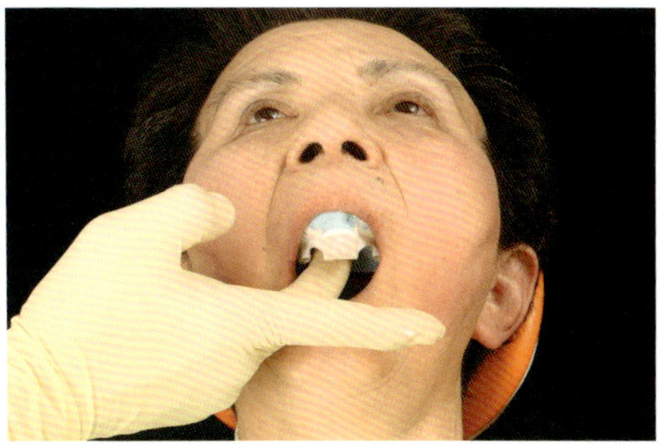

The preliminary impression is put back in the mouth and pressed against the mucosa and the line is printed on the impression

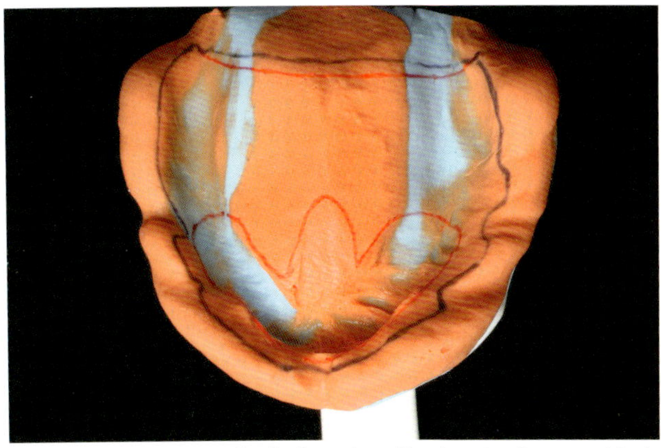

Outline of the custom tray is designed on the impression considering the movement of the frenum or condition of the flabby ridge by observing intra orally. This line is printed on the model once the stone is poured

Fig4 Determination method of the posterior border of the custom tray.

The measures when the FCB tray is located rather low due to extensive ridge resorption

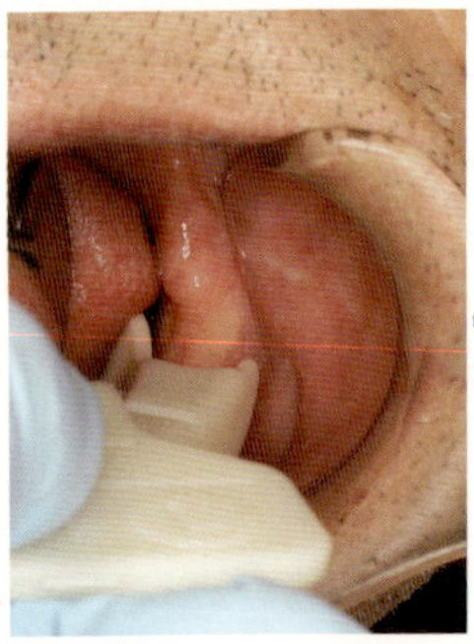

The tray is located low position. The retromolar pad is located way above

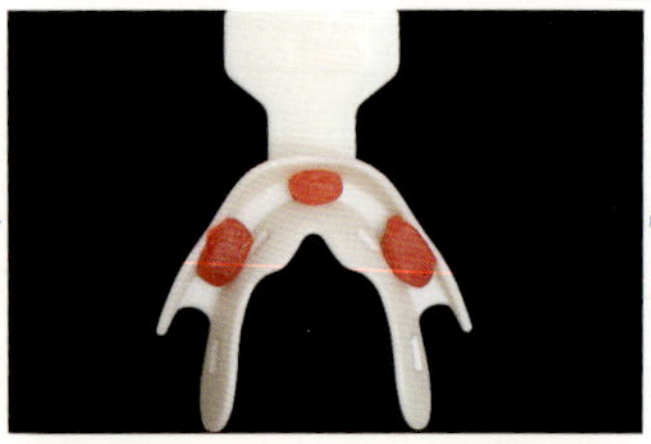

Hight of the tray is improved by placing soft wax on 3 projections of internal surface of the tray

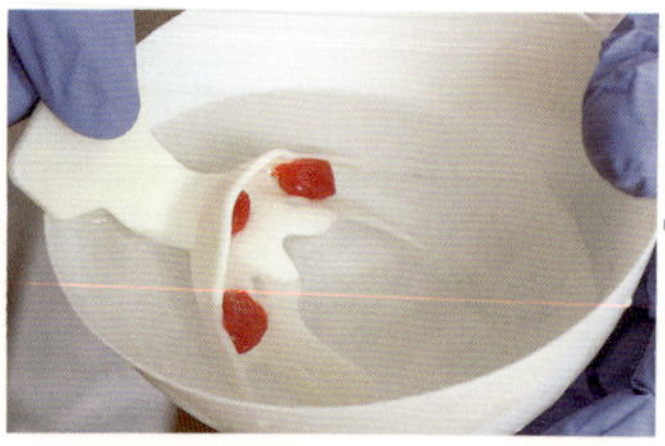

The wax is softened with warm water and it is pressed in the mouth to adjust the hight

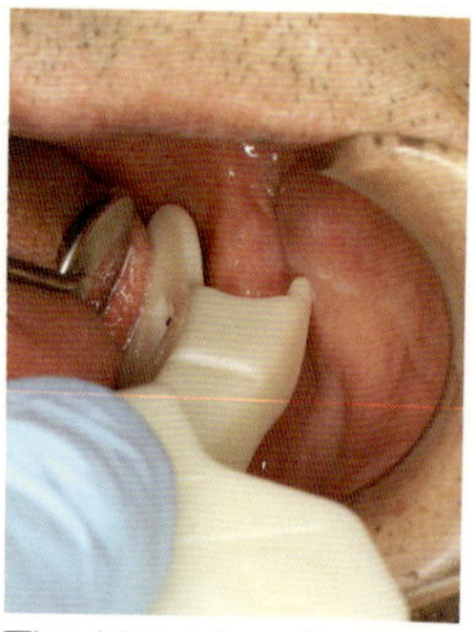

The hight is adjusted to the level of retro molar pad

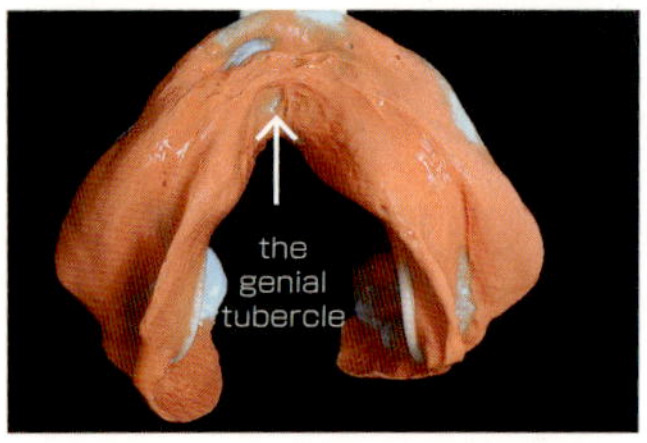

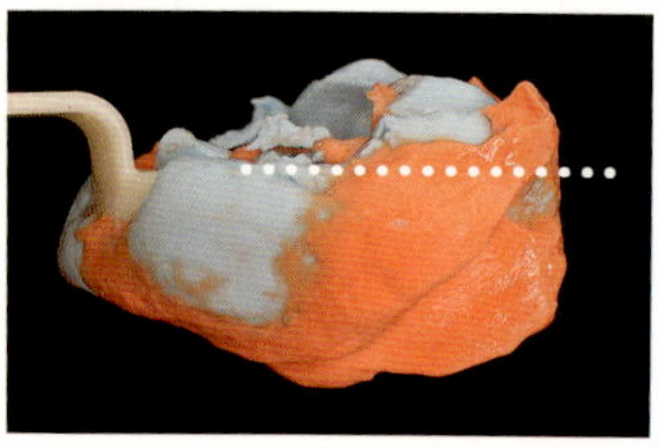

It is ideal to adjust the hight of the tray equal to the level of retromolar pad

Fig 5 The tray would be located way below the level of the retromolar pad in the case with extensive ridge resorption. Unsupported impression material would be distorted easily by the weight of the stone. The hight of the tray is adjusted to the level of the retromolar pad by placing wax to the 3 projections on the internal surface of the tray.

shown in the right column of Fig 3. After light-body alginate impression material is squirted to mucobuccal fold and labial frenum area, periphery area of the palatal torus is loaded to prevent air trap. The tray filled with heavy-body alginate impression material is inserted as other techniques.

(2) Posterior border of the maxillary custom tray

Excess material is trimmed away with scissors or a knife extraorally.

Vibrating area is identified by Ah-line technique. Nose-Blow Effect method can be utilized as well by asking the patient to blow air through the nose, which is pinched by the dentist, to identified the border since the soft palate drops down. The tay border, which is slightly extended posteriorly from the border line in the soft plate, is marked directly in the mouth by the pen. This line is printed on the impression once it is placed back in the mouth and pressed as ti is shown in the photo. The line on the impression is repainted with the pen, which is transferred to the model (Fig 4).

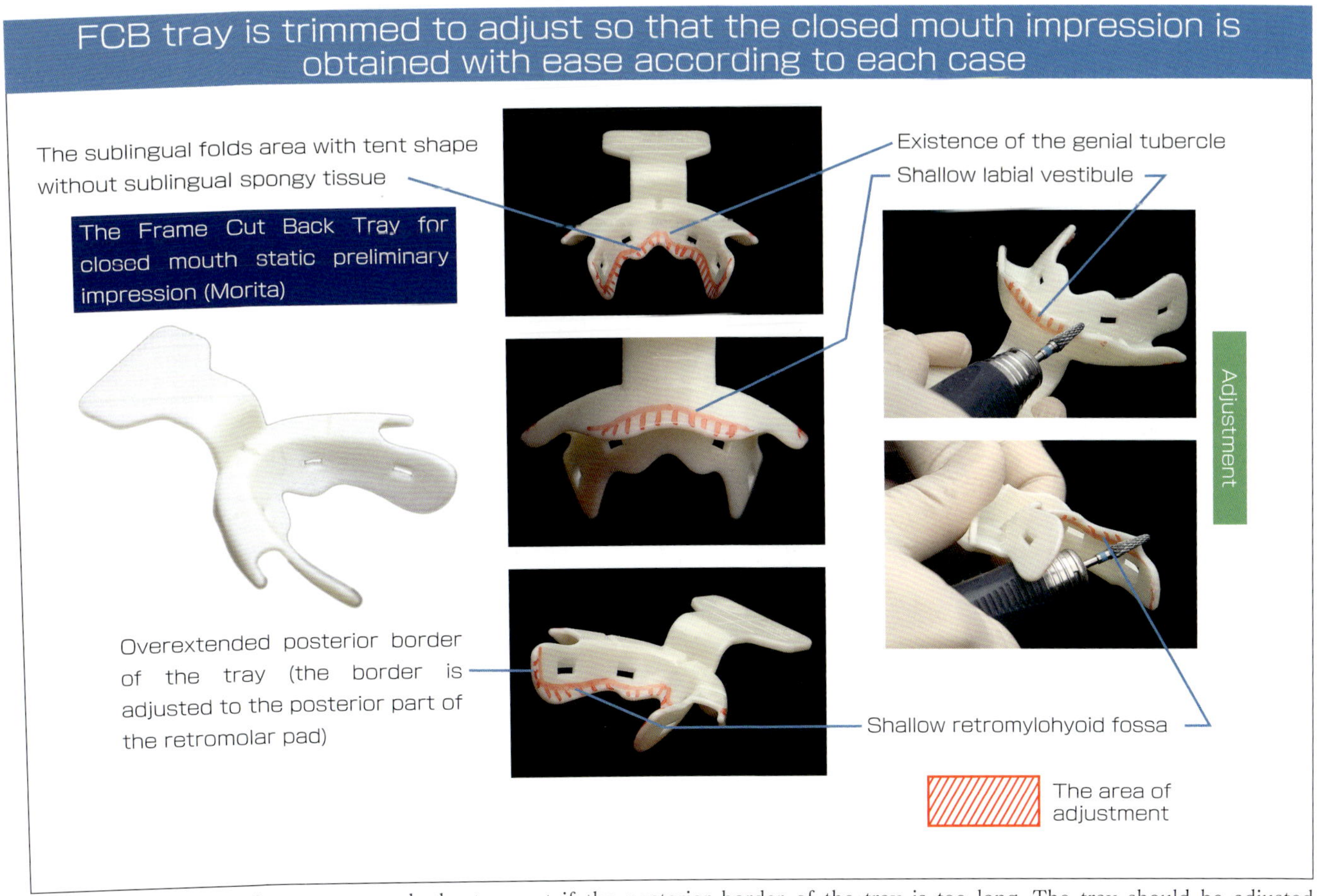

Fig 6 The patient tends to try to push the tray out if the posterior border of the tray is too long. The tray should be adjusted accordingly so that it would not touch the genial tubercle and would not interfere with the attachment of the mentalis, which is close to the ridge crest due to severe ridge resorption in this case for smooth closed-mouth impression.

4 Mandibular preliminary impression and the Frame Cut Back Tray (FCB Tray)

The impression process with Frame Cut Back Tray for difficult cases is almost the same as other general cases.

The shape of FCB tray often is not appropriate for preliminary impression as it is for certain cases such as extensive ridge resorption, shallow mucobuccal fold or shallow retromylohyoid fossa and often requires modification. Examples of modification of FCB tray for various clinical conditions to take an ideal preliminary impression are presented in this section.

Posterior border length of the tray is first adjusted to the position of the posterior boarder of the retromolar pad to correspond with the posterior end of the retromolar pad.

Otherwise, too much length of the posterior border of FCB tray may induce gag reflex.

Solution to prevent the thin impression on labial aspect with the FCB tray in the case of shallow labial vestibule

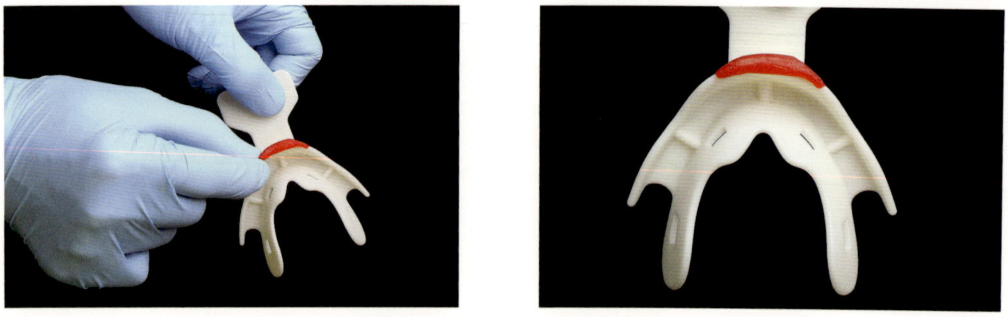

Fig 7 The labial aspect of the impression tends to become rather thin with the patient who has tendency of pushing the tray up strongly with the lower lip or shallow labial vestibule. The soft wax is applied to the anterior border of the tray to obtain thick enough preliminary impression.

(1) The case with extensive ridge resorption

In extensive ridge resorption case, the tray sometimes fits much lower than the level of the retromolar pad. The impression of the retromolar pad area, taken with this condition, deforms when the stone is poured because of the lack of support for sufficient amount of alginate impression material. In such a case, soft wax is added on three protrusions in the internal surface of the tray and the hight is adjusted intraorally to be equal to the height of the retromolar pad before taking impression (Fig5). The depth of lingual side of the tray is adjusted so that the patient is able to hold the handle of the tray comfortably when the mouth is closed (Fig 6).

(2) The case with the shallow and narrow lavial vestibule

Labial border of the tray is trimmed so that impression is taken at naturally mouth closed condition for shallow vestibule case (Fig 6). Certain types of patients such as discussed in this section or Class III, have tendency of lifting up the tray with their tensed lower lip as a result, labial border of the impression tends to become thinner. Preliminary impression with enough thickness can be obtained by adding soft wax to anterior border area of the tray (Fig 7).

(3) The case with the genial tubercle

The bony protrusion at the lingual side of severely resorbed mandibular anterior ridge is called the genial tubercle. The corresponding area of the tray should be relieved (Fig 6).

Steps of the preliminary impression 1

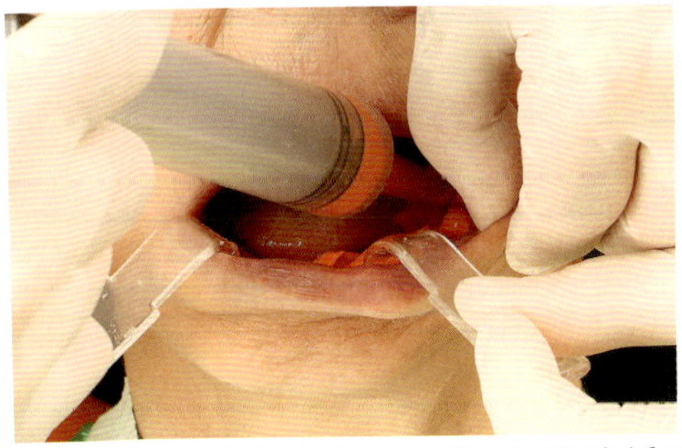

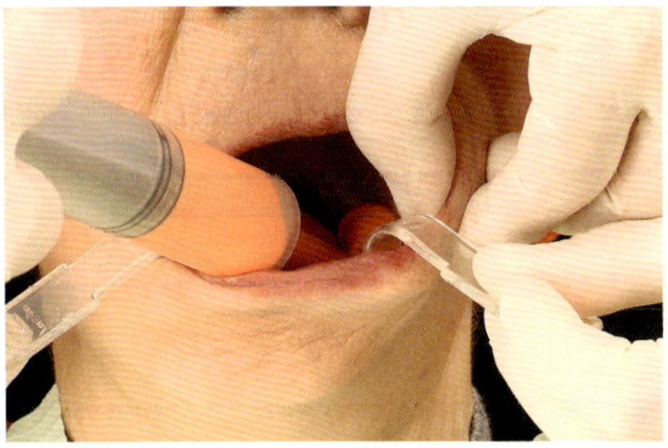

Step1 : Light body alginate impression material for syringe use is squirted in the order of the lingual side of left retromolar pad → mid lingual → right retromolar pad → buccal shelf → labial side of anterior region → left buccal shelf → left molar pad. It has to finish over the start point on the retromolar pad continuously

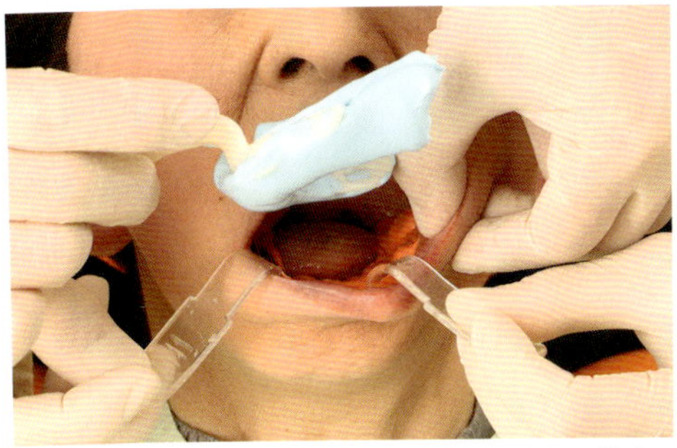

Step2 : Next, the position, where the tray will be placed, is checked by pulling the patient' s lower lip anteriorly in left and diagonal direction using left fingers (It is the most important step in this procedure to visualize the location to place the tray clearly for the edentulous patient). The handle of the FCB tray is held firmly. The tray is inserted with rotating motion (buccal aspect of the tray interferes with the corner of the mouth if it is tried to insert the tray straight)

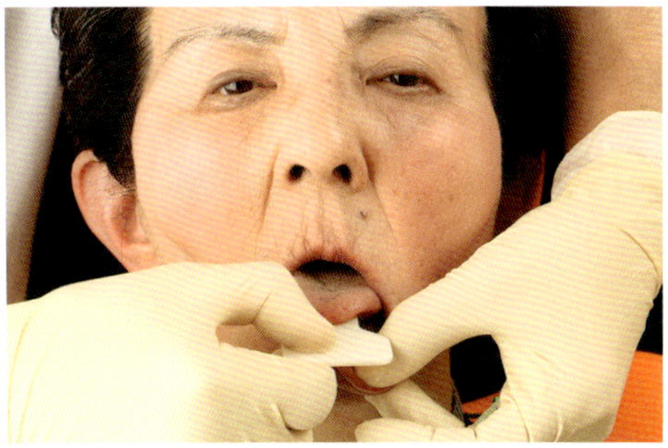

Step3 : Patient is asked to stick the tongue out after the tray is inserted (it raises soft spongy tissue, at sublingual fold area and retromylohyoid fossa area, above the tray preventing them to be caught under the tray)

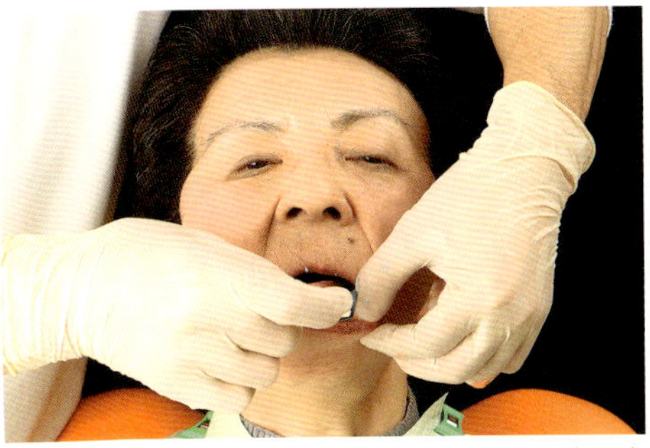

Step4 : Patient is asked to move the tongue back to the relaxed position and rest in that position for 5~7 seconds (it takes longer than 5 seconds for the tongue to be relaxed)

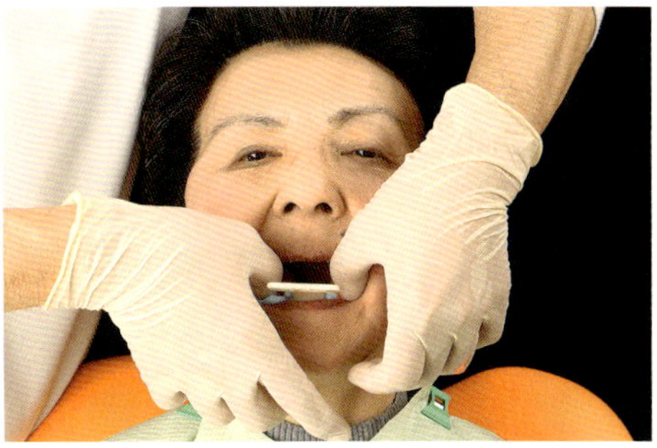

Step5 : The operator lightly presses down the tray at the molar region with both thumbs (strong force is not required to press down since there is no frame to cover the upper part of the retromolar pad with FCB tray)

Fig 8a The purpose of the preliminary impression is to take the alginate impression at mandibular rest position without distorting the retromolar pad using a FCB tray, which is designed not to have the frame covering upper part of the retromolar pad and buccal shelf.

Steps of the preliminary impression 2

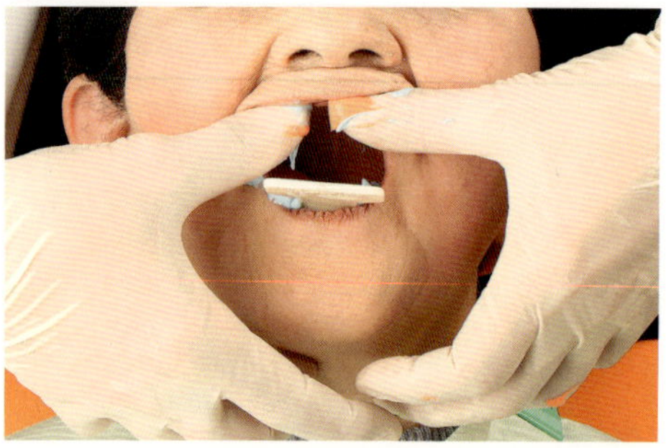

Step6 : Then, the upper lip is lifted up and the patient is asked to close the mouth slowly down to the mandibular rest position and hold the handle of the tray in the patient's mouth (attention must be paid not to close excessively, since it could let the maxillary tuberosity press the retromolar pad causing distortion)

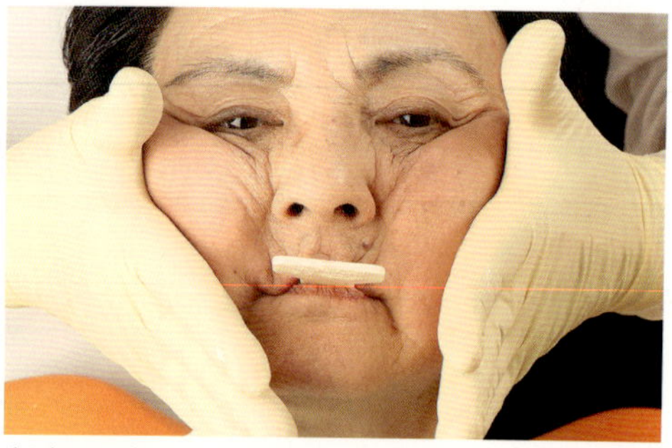

At last, the operator massages the cheek of the patient using the palm (the technique to prevent accumulation of the impression material within the cheeks)

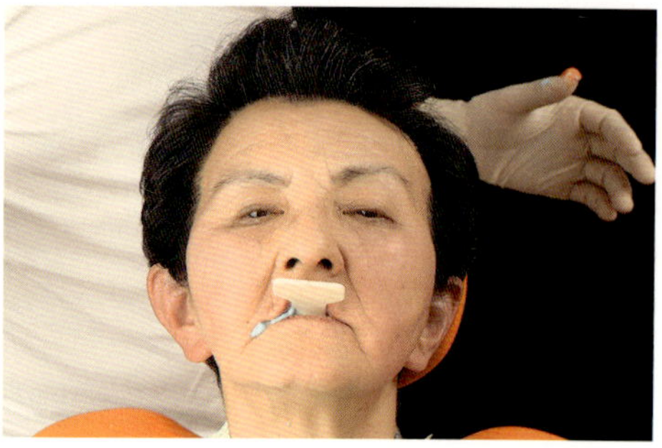

Wait for setting of the impression material at the rest position

Fig 8b Steps of the preliminary impression (continued from the previous page).

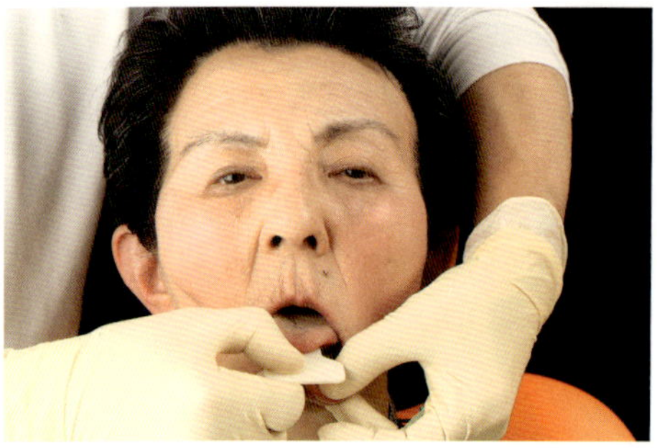

Fig 9 Standing position of the operator: the operator stands diagonally behind the patient on the right side while impression procedure. The patient chair should be tilted about 60°, at which the operator is able to perform the procedure with ease.

(4) The case with the shallow retromylohyoid fossa

The tray is adjusted according to the depth of retromylohyoid fossa (Fig 6).

The Class II - division 2 case presented in this section is one of rare cases, which present with all conditions above.

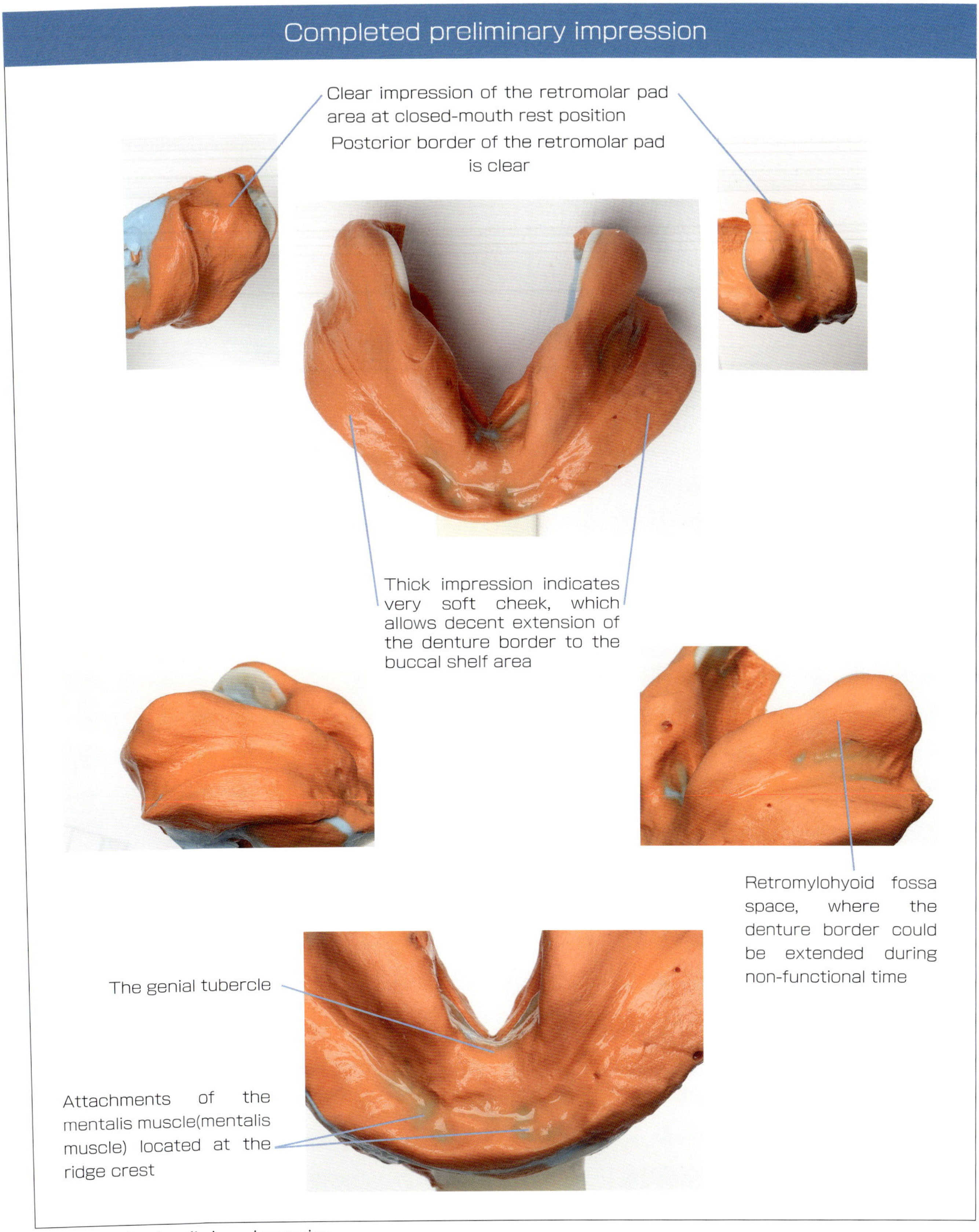

Fig 10 Completed preliminary impression.

Proper use of silicone putty and alginate (heavy body type) impression material

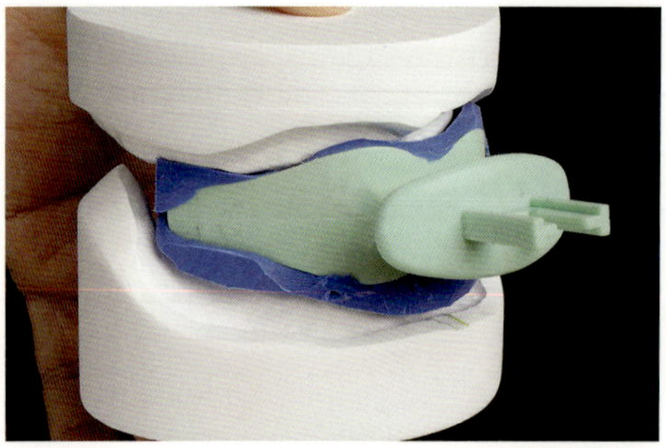

Easy-to-treat case : Laboratory procedure of fabrication of the models and mounting can be performed with enough time by using silicone putty for the case with the favorable ridge condition

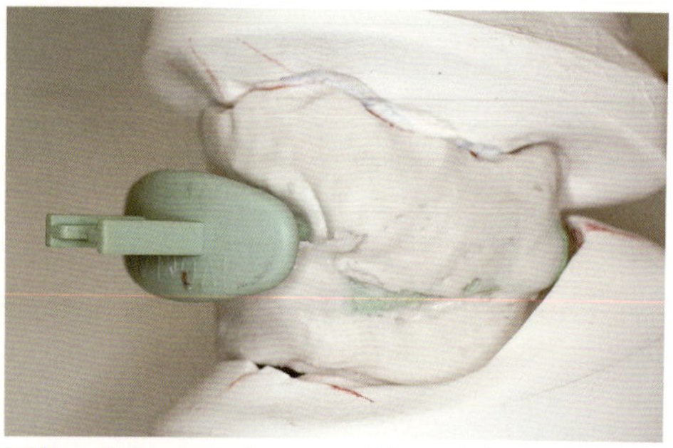

Difficult-to-treat case : The alginate (heavy body type) is used for flabby ridge case. Accu tray Gel from Ivoclar Vivadent does not distort for 24 hours in the humidity box. However, the alginate impression material from other brands require immediate work of modeling and mounting

Fig 11 Proper use of silicone putty and alginate (heavy body type) impression material.

Basic FCB Tray impression technique is carried out even for the difficultly case with severe ridge resorption (Fig 8, 9). Completed preliminary impression is shown in Fig 10.

5 Simplified bite registration technique using the Centric Tray (Professional technique)

Advanced bite registration technique for maxillary anterior flabby ridge or severely resorbed ridge is presented.

(1) The case with maxillary anterior flabby ridge (using heavy-body alginate impression material)

Maneuver of Centric Tray and the process in the difficult cases are same as the ones of general cases.

However, silicone putty used for general cases deforms flabby ridge due to its rigidity resulting in discrepancy between the preliminary model and the bite registration record.

It is recommended to use heavy-body alginate impression materials (AccuDent Tray Gel, Ivoclar Vivadent), or other alginate impression material mixed harder with less amount of water for mobile tissue such as flabby ridge (Fig 11). It is often difficult to capture mandibular ridge impression clearly if it is severely resorbed (Fig 12).

Flabby ridge impression technique (by heavy body type alginate) using the Centric tray

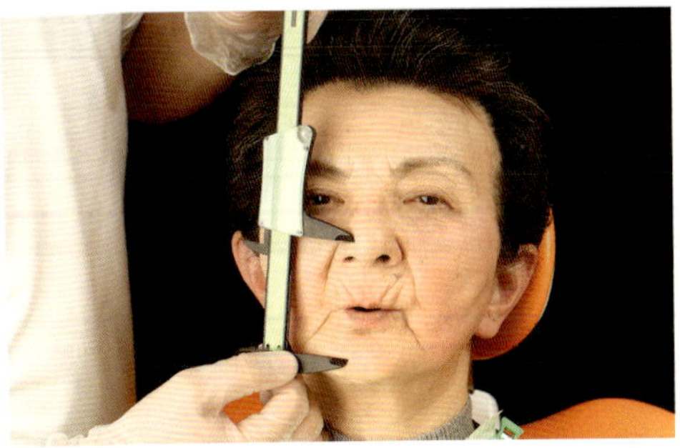

Step1 : VDO is measured and recorded using interocclusal rest space or Air-blow method

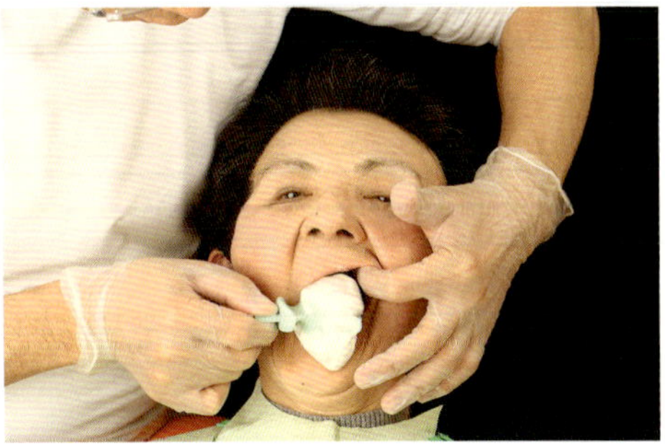

Step2 : Heavy body type alginate impression material is applied on both sides of the tray

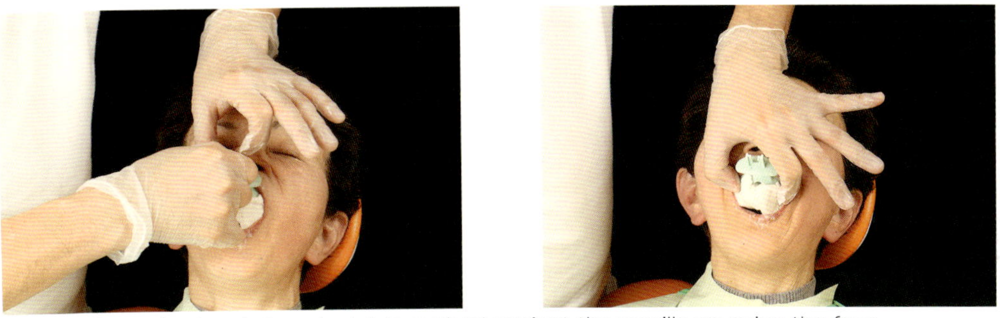

Step3 : Once the tray is inserted, it is pushed against the maxilla covering the face

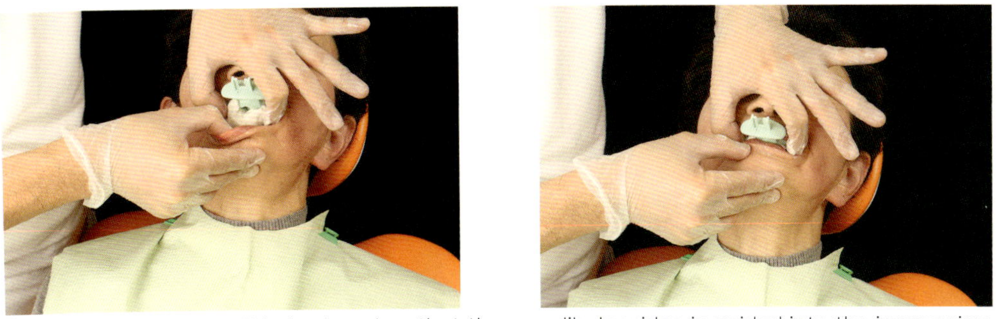

Step4 : Then the mandible is closed so that the mandibular ridge is guided into the impression material in retruded position by the guidance

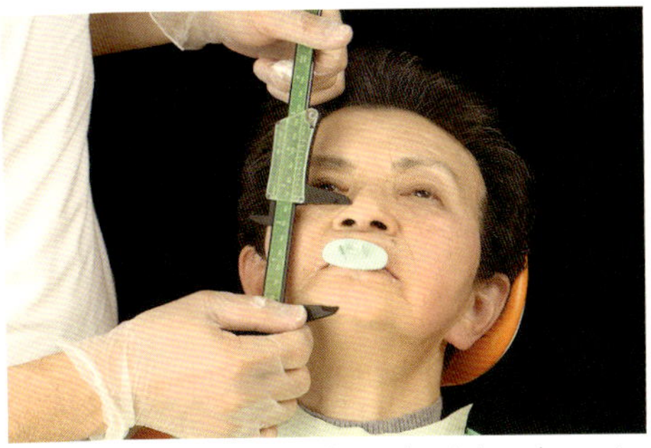

Step5 : The patient is asked to close to the level of the previously measured VDO

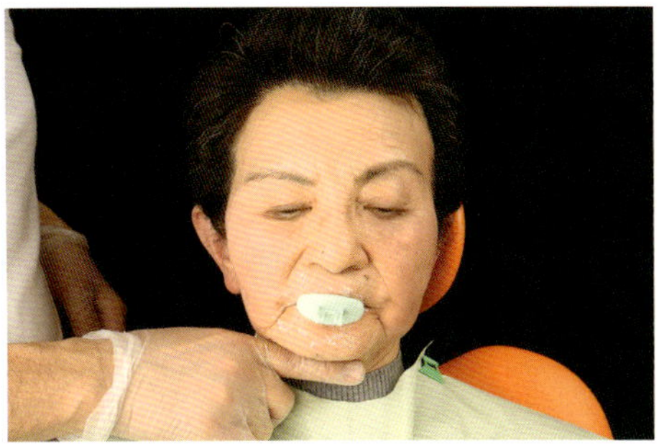

Step6 : The mandible is retruded by swallowing. The patient is asked to stay in this position while waiting for setting of the impression material

Fig 12 Flabby ridge impression technique using the Centric tray.

The technique to obtain clear bite registration record for severely resorbed ridge

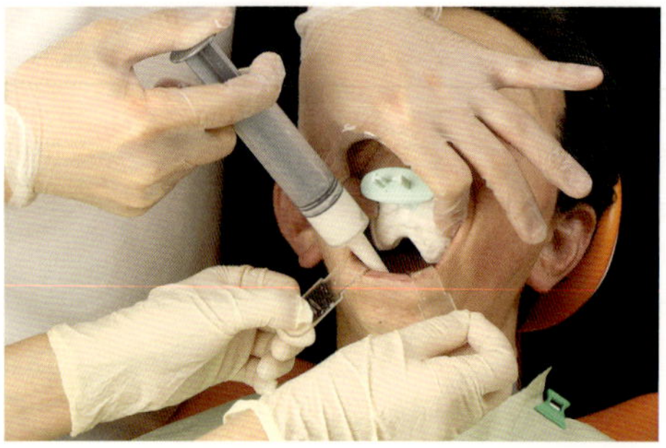

Step1 : The impression body is removed out of the mouth and the condition of it is checked. If the impression is found to be unclear, softly mixed same impression material, mixed with increased amount of water, is injected in the mouth using the syringe. The impression body is re-inserted in the mouth and the patient is asked to swallow. Clearer impression surface is obtained with this technique

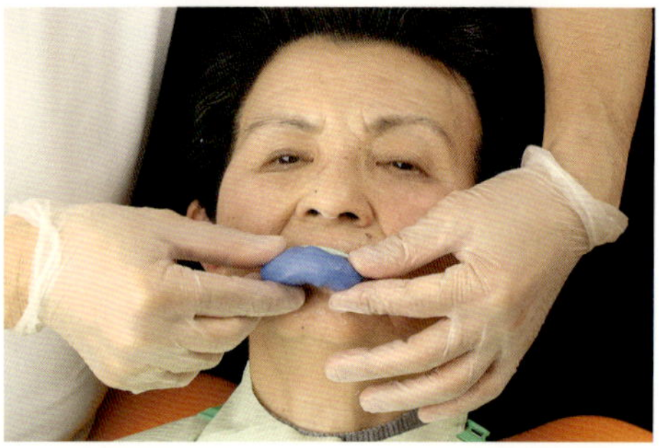

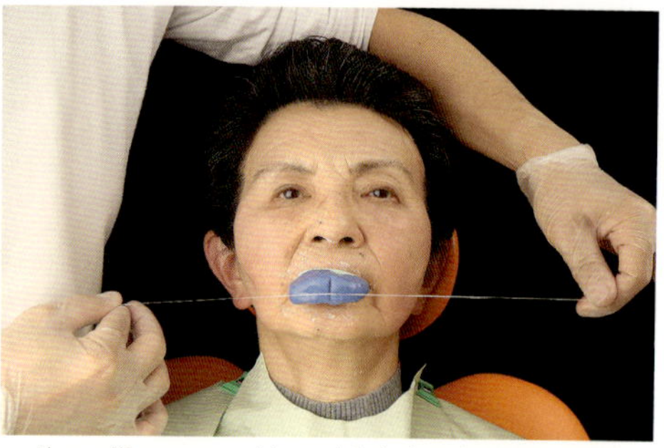

Step2 : Horizontal line and mid line are recorded on the silicone putty, which is placed on the handle after the impression material is hardened. These lines will be the guide for mounting on the articulator

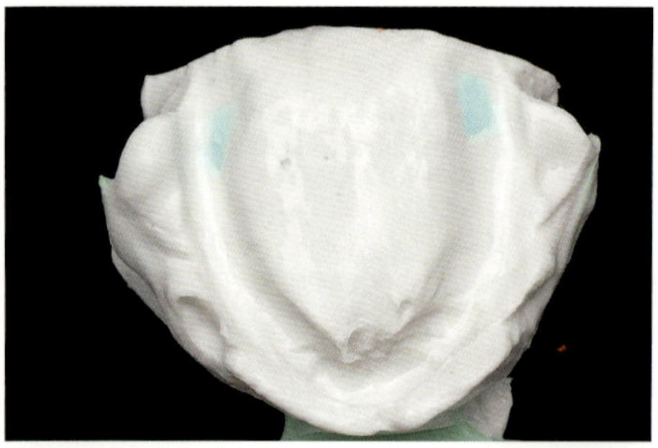

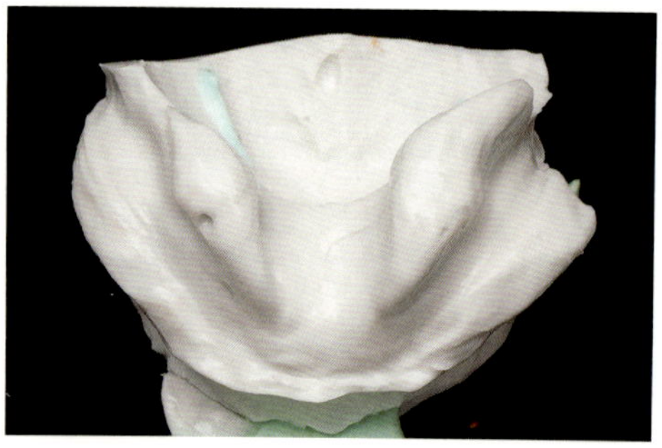

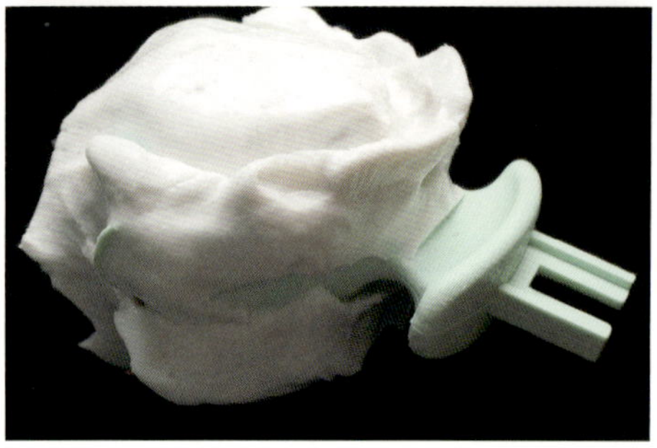

Step3 : Bite registration body using the Centric tray with maxillary and mandibular clear impression

Fig13 The technique to obtain clear bite registration record for severely resorbed ridge.

If the impression surface is not clear, it can be relined (The same impression material that is mixed softer with more water). The impression taken by the Centric Tray is placed back with to the mouth after adhesive is applied, and then the patient is asked to bite and swallow. Clear impression is obtained by applying appropriate pressure on the alveolar ridge mucosa (Fig 13).

Change in the occlusal vertical dimension due to addition of the impression material is not significant for fabrication of custom trays. Definitive occlusal vertical dimension will be determined before pin tracing (Gothic arch tracing) after the final impression.

(2) The cases with favorable maxillary ridge condition and severely resorbed mandibular ridge

It is recommended to use silicone putty for bite registration for this type of cases. In these cases, taking clear mandibular impression is difficult taking due to ridge resorption, the same process discussed in (1) is carried out using Monophase (silicone impression material with the middle viscosity between heavy-body and light-body In order to obtain clear mandibular impression).

(3) The Class III cases with severe mandibular ridge resorption and maxillary flabby ridge

The bite registration technique[45] taking impression of maxilla and mandible separately using the Centric Tray is discussed (Fig 14).

1) Support wings for partial denture are attached to the Centric Tray.
2) The base is formed in the middle with silicone putty so that proper pressure is applied toward the ridge[45].
3) After the silicone putty is set, additional silicone putty is placed on mandibular side in arch shape and it is inserted in the mouth with pressure to take impression of mandible.
4)After the silicone putty is set, adhesive for alginate impression material is applied on the maxillary side. The Centric Tray loaded with heavy-body alginate impression material, which is selected to avoid deformation of the flabby ridge, is inserted in patient's mouth. Patient is asked to bite down to the previously made occlusal vertical dimension and swallow.

(4) Severe Class II or III cases

Positioning of the Centric Tray using single step of double arch impression technique during bite registration for severe Class II or III cases are challenging. Patients often have complains with pain when the edge of the centric tray hits the

The technique to take impression of maxilla and mandible separately using the Centric Tray for Class III maxillary flabby ridge case (refer to Part 7)

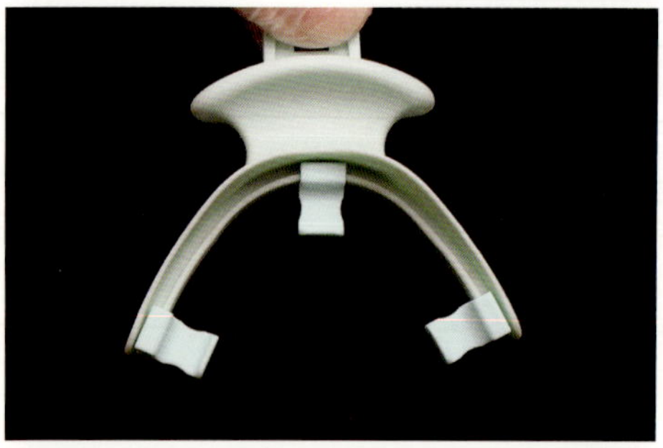

Step1 : The support wings for the partial denture are attached to the Centric Tray

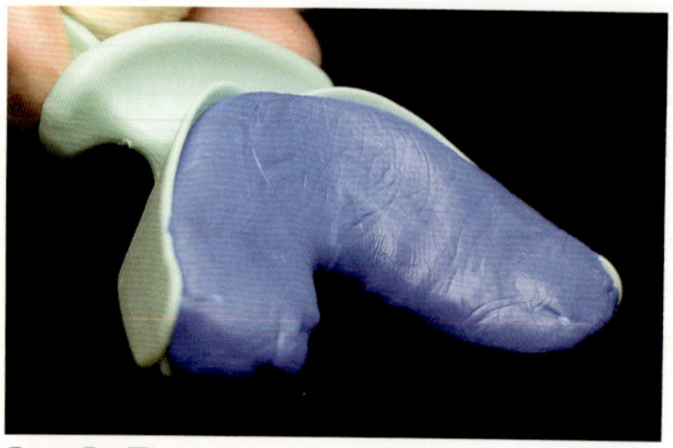

Step2 : The plate shape is formed in the middle with the silicone putty[45]

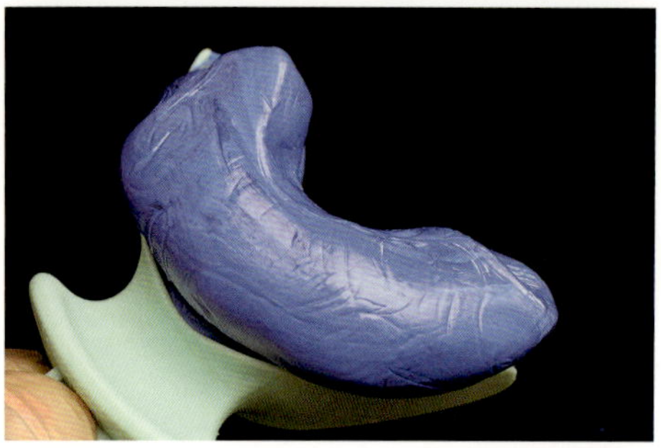

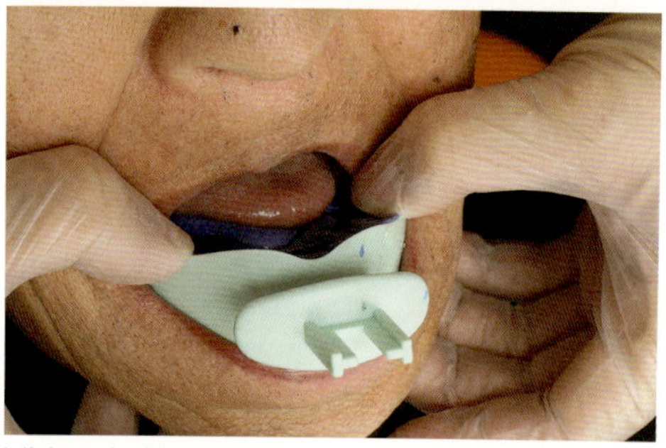

Step3 : Once the plate shape putty is hardened, additional silicone putty is placed on one side of the tray in arch shape. It is pressed on the mandibular ridge to take the impression of the mandible, with unfavorable ridge shape, first

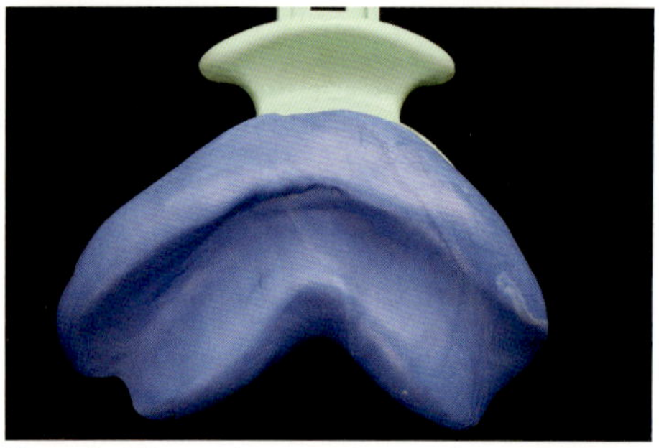

Step4 : Clear impression of mandibular ridge

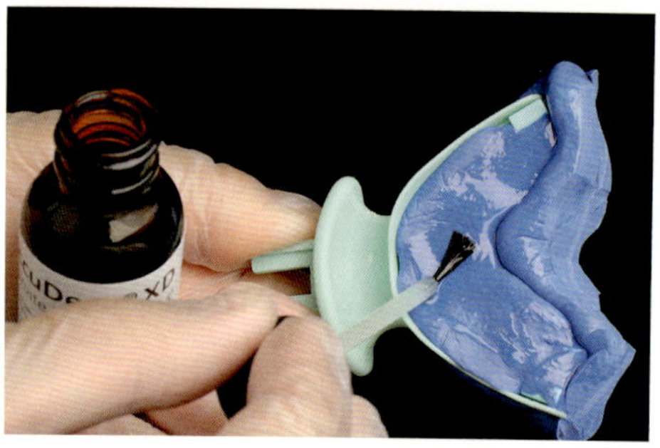

Step5 : Once it is hardened, adhesive for alginate impression is applied on the other side

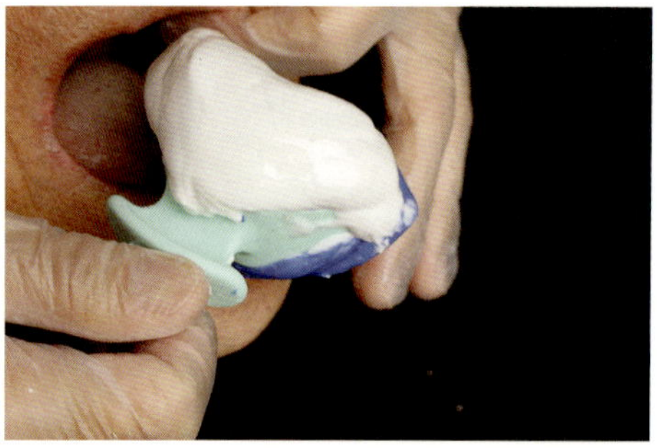

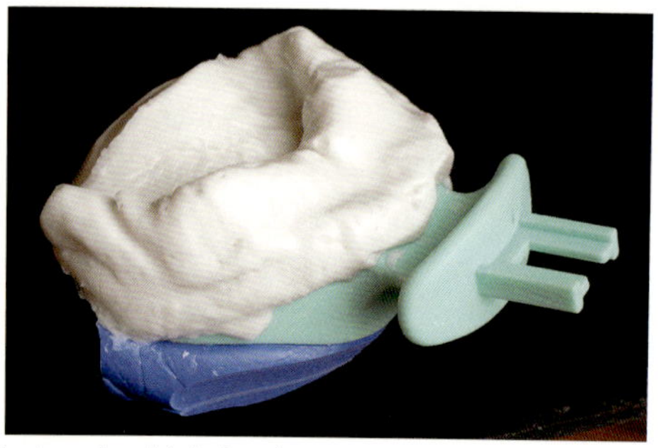

Step6 : The tray filled with the alginate (heavy body type), which is chosen to avoid distortion of the flabby ridge, is inserted in the mouth and the patient is guided to close the mouth to the proper VDO

Fig14 The technique to take impression of the maxilla and the mandible separately using the Centric Tray.

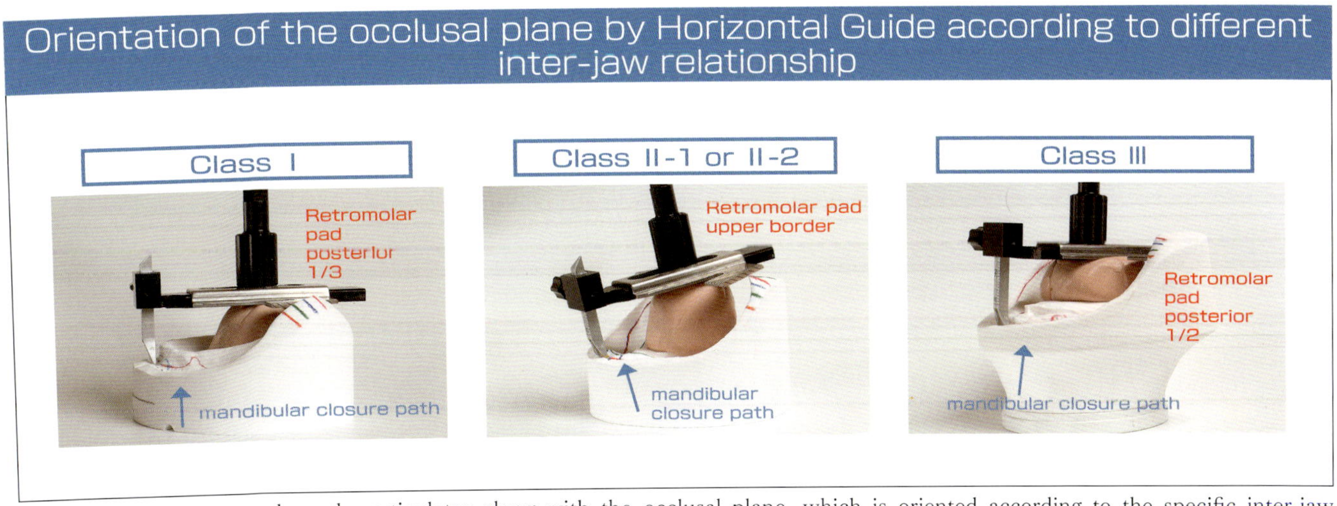

Fig15 Casts are mounted on the articulator along with the occlusal plane, which is oriented according to the specific inter-jaw relationship.

gums. Combination of the techniques described above allows obtaining proper maxillary and mandibular relationship even in difficult cases.

If the bite registration recorded by bite registration techniques I have introduced is questionable, conventional technique with the resin base and wax rim should be employed to mount the preliminary casts first and temporary bite records are taken. Subsequently, preliminary models are remounted. And next, the custom tray with the gnathometer M is fabricated for final impression and pin-tracing. Obtaining accurate bite registration record is critical, since occlusion is the key factor for successful suction-effect.

6 Mounting preliminary casts

Free hand mounting of preliminary casts to the articulator often creates errors such as tilted occlusal plane, malpositioned casts in all directions. The custom tray for closed mouth suction-effective functional impression, which is fabricated on the casts mounted incorrectly, results in the impression under uneven pressure causing problems later on. BPS recommends the Horizontal Guide to be utilized (Fig 15) to prevent these problems.

(1) Mounting preliminary casts using the Horizontal Guide

The Horizontal guide assists the casts to be mounted on center of the articulator. The wing of the Horizontal guide acts as the occlusal plane. This wing is slidable back and forth. Once the Horizontal Guide is set to the hight of posterior 1/3 of the retromolar pad, the wing is supposed to be equivalent to the Camper line.

In some cases, the level of right and left retromolar pads are not equal. Occlusal plane is sometimes set wrongly slanted if the Horizontal Guide is not used properly. In order to correct this discepancy, silicone putty is attached, which is removable, on the handle of the Centric Tray and mark the horizontal and mid line when the bite registration is taken. Proper occlusal plane is set by the guide of this record. This technique is useful as well to mount the casts in the middle of the articulator when the Horizontal Guide is not available.

Occlusal plane is set by the wing of the Horizontal Guide guided by the retromolar pad, which is higher level, if the level of right and left retromolar pads are not equal.

(2) Determination of the occlusal plane by the Horizontal Guide in cases of Class I, II and III

The occlusal plane of Class I is about parallel to Caper line, Class II is toward upper edge of the retromolar pad and Class III is toward the middle of the retromolar pad. This difference is due to the difference in the angle of [maxillary occlusal plane] in responce to the forces applied on it by the direction of chewing pattern of each jaw relationship (Fig 15). The custom tray for closed mouth impression technique is fabricated in next step. There are two methods of fabricating it with the Gnathometer M and with the wax rim (Fig 16).

7 Design and fabrication of the custom tray (Professional)

(1) Outline of the maxillary custom tray

The incisal papilla of severe ridge resorption or flabby ridge is not good anatomical land mark because it is often located off center. In such a case, the mid palatine raphe, mid point of fovea palatinae or right and left maxillary tuberosity is used as posterior mid reference point.

The tray border in molar area is drawn 2mm above the deepest point of mucobuccal fold avoiding frenum in general case. The tray border is drawn 1mm above or deepest point of the mucobuccal fold in both posterior and anterior region for the difficult case with severe ridge resorption. As the defect becomes more extensive, the border of custom tray should be designed to be thicker in order to restore the lost tissue with the denture. Border of the custom tray is

Orientation of the occlusal plane and mounting of the casts by Horizontal Guide

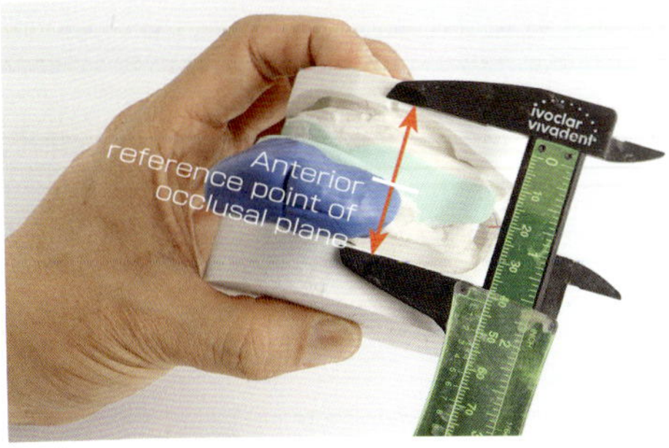

Step1 : Depth of the deepest point of the border by marking with the bur on the cast next to the labial frenum is recorded

Clay or the model block is used to stabilize the Horizontal Guide since the posterior portion tends to be unstable

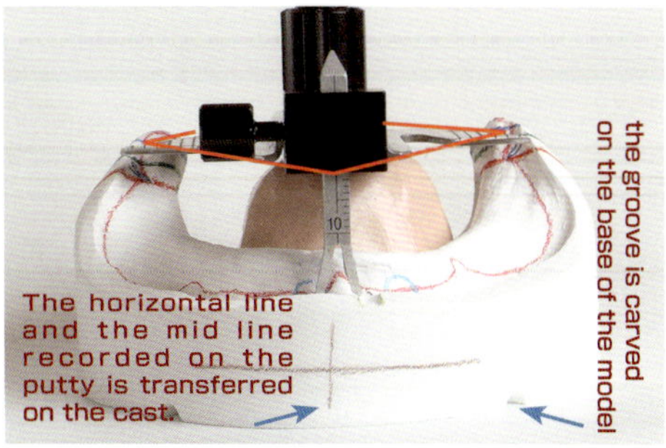

Step2 : The retromolar pad is the posterior reference point of the occlusal plane. The possible error in setting of the occlusal plane, which is generated by the difference in hight of right and left retromolar pads, is corrected with the horizontal line and mid line transferred from the putty

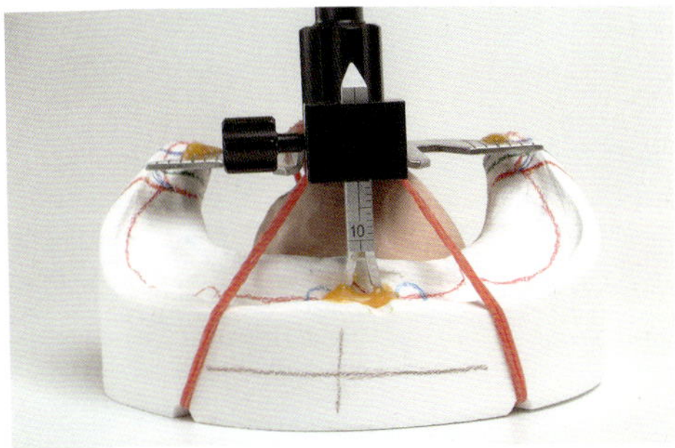

Step3 : The model and the Horizontal Guide are fixed by the rubber band, which is engaged in the grooves carved on the base of the model

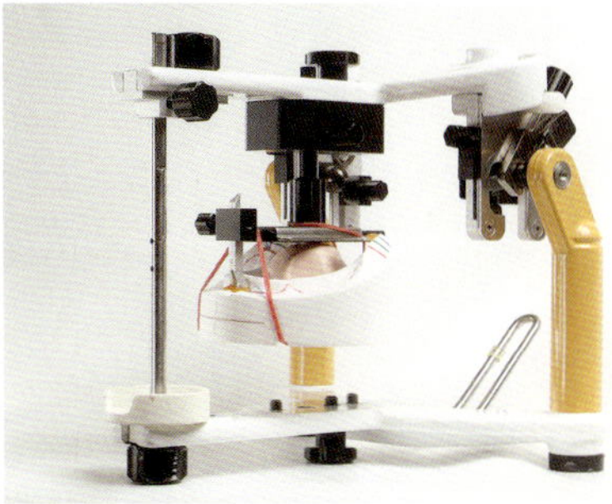

Step4 : The Mounting Carrier is attached firmly to the Stratos articulator. The mandibular cast is mounted by inserting the fixing pin of the Horizontal Guide fully in the carrier and the screw is tightened. Then the maxillary cast is mounted by inserting the Centric Tray Bite between the maxillary and the mandibular models

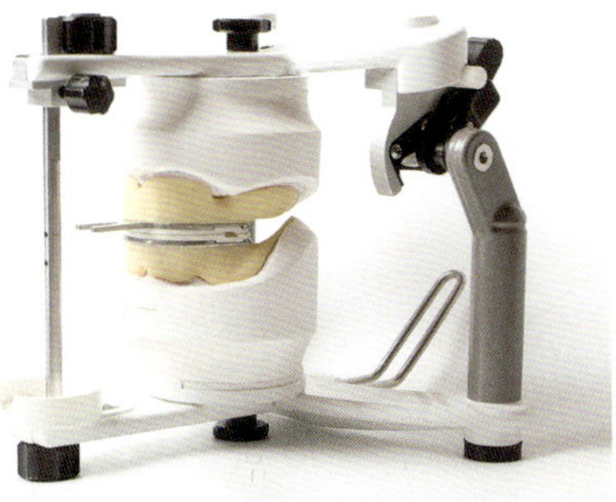

Completed custom trays for the closed mouth impression technique in combination with the Gnathometer M

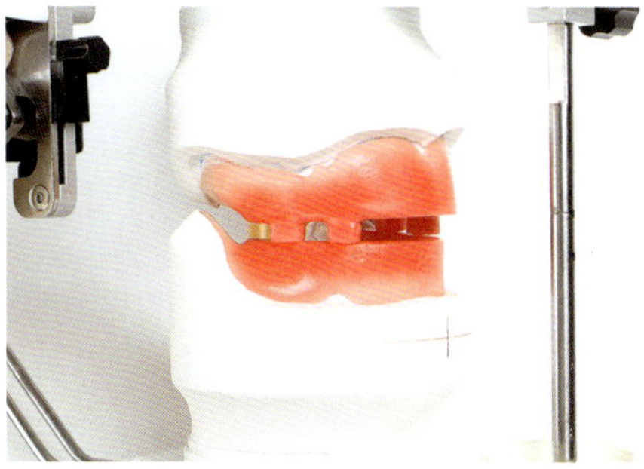

Completed custom trays for the closed mouth impression technique in combination with the wax rim

Fig16 Orientation of the occlusal plane and mounting of the casts by Horizontal Guide.

The design of the custom tray for the case with maxillary ridge resorption

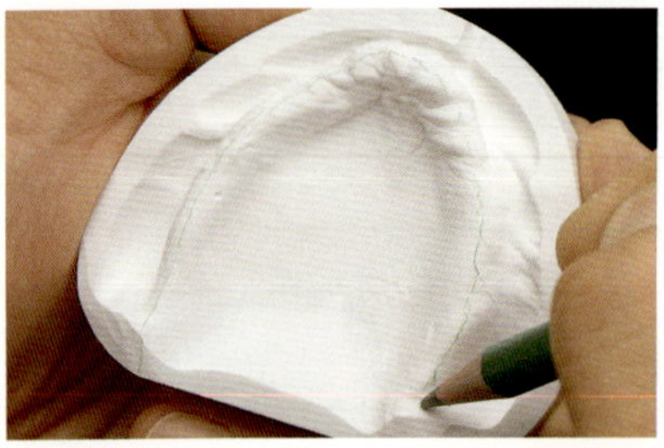

Step1 : The ridge crest line is marked

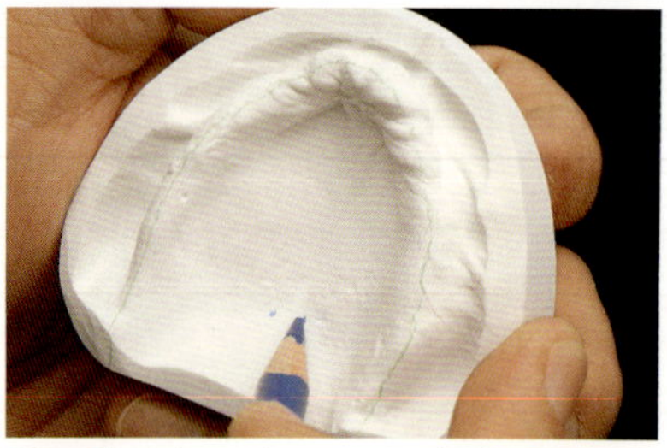

Step2 : The fovea palatinae are marked

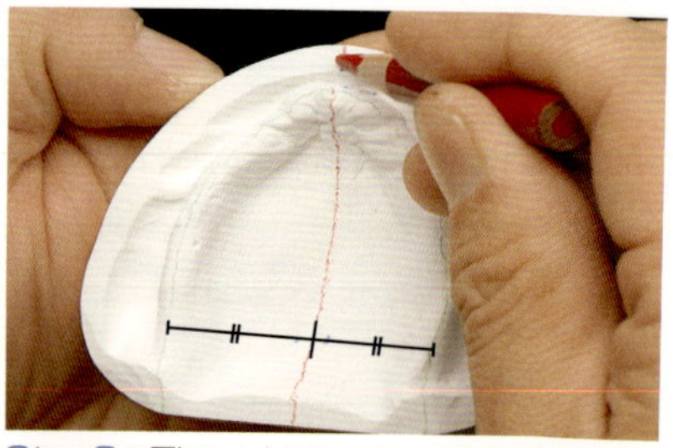

Step3 : The mid line is marked

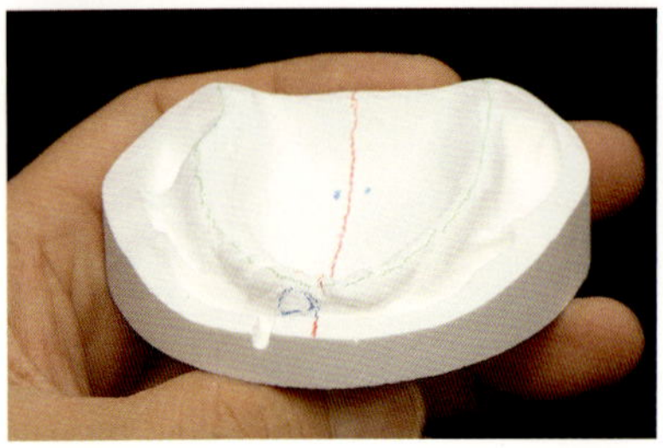

Step4 : Abnormal location of the incisive papilla away from the mid line

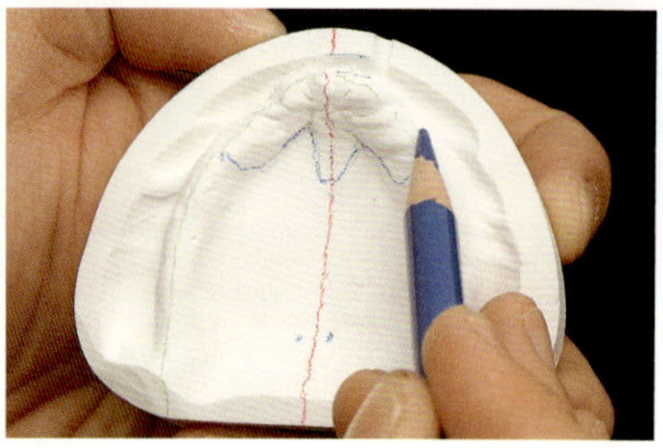

Step5 : Flabby ridge, where wax relief is required, is marked

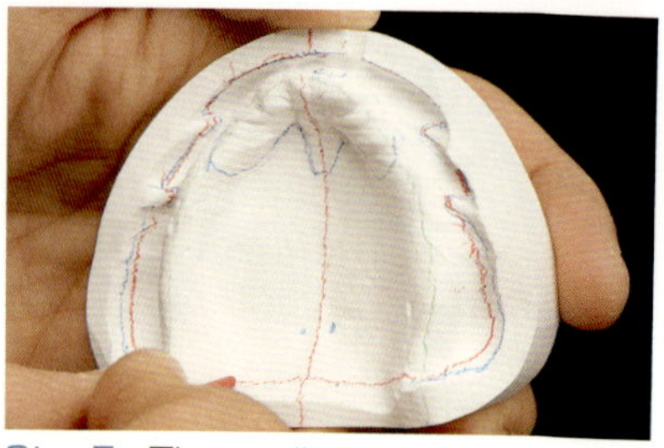

Step5 : The outline is drawn at the deepest part of the mucobuccal fold in the anterior region and 1 mm above the deepest part at posterior region in this case

Fig17 The design of the custom tray for the case with maxillary ridge desorption.

designed thicker as a result (Fig 17).

(2) The maxillary custom tray designed for treatment of inflammatory flabby ridge

Inflammatory flabby ridge in maxillary anterior region is the result of persistent pressure of the denture from habitual anterior biting pattern. In this condition, the maxillary and mandible dentures rotate in up-forward direction during articulation[65, 66]. Posterior palatal seal will break and maxillary denture will fall as a result. The mandibular anterior teeth push the maxillary anterior teeth up and forward during articlation[65,66]. Finally in this section, it will be limited to discuss management of maxillary flabby ridge. even though the case described in Kelly Combination Syndrome[67], maxillary single denture against the mandible with only anterior teeth left, is the most typical case of the flabby ridge.

First, it is important to minimize the occlusal pressure on maxillary anterior ridge as small as possible. Widest possible posterior stress bearing area including hard palate is utilized for that purpose. The middle of the hard palate, which usually is

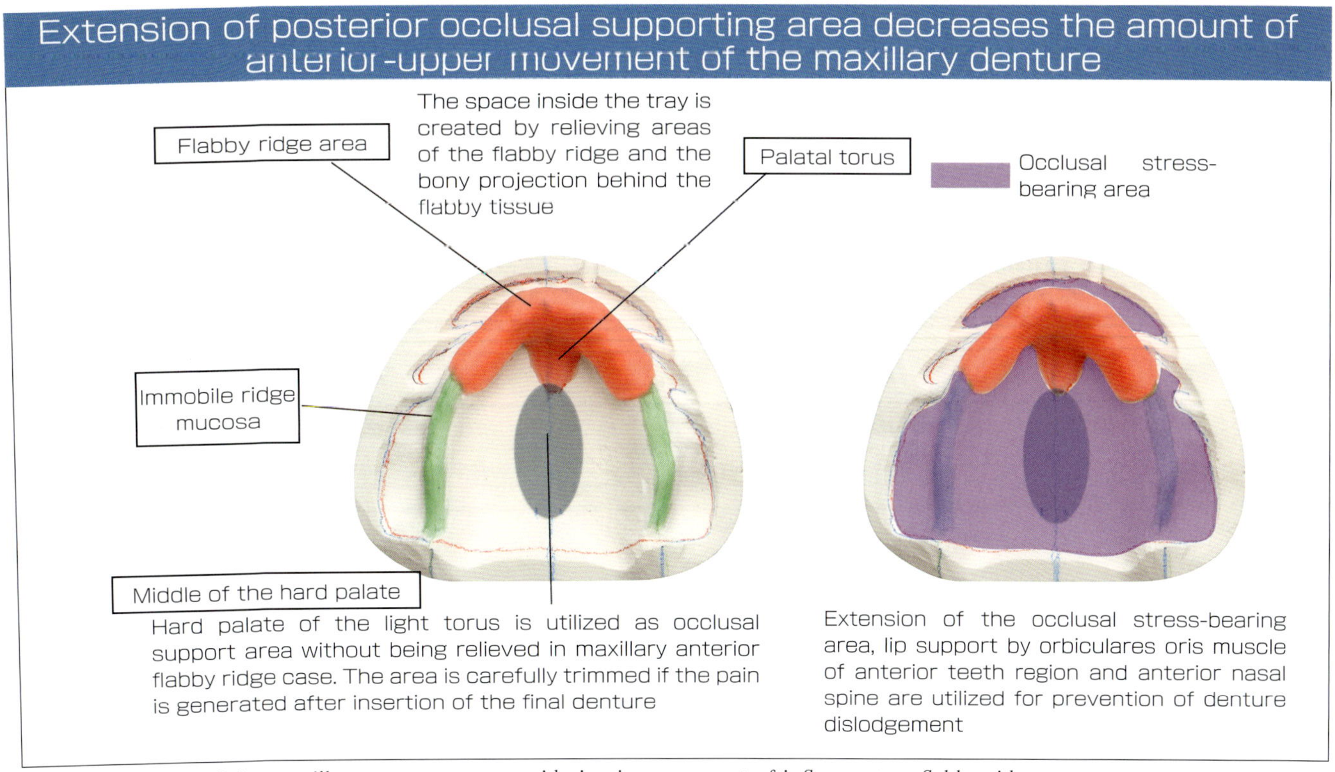

Fig18 The design of the maxillary custom tray considering improvement of inflammatory flabby ridge.

relieved with wax due to poor displacability before fabrication of the custom tray, is not relieved for fabrication of the custom tray for this case to utilize this area as stress bearing area.

Upper-forward shift of the denture is minimized by providing enough thickness to anterior border of the custom tray. Thickly formed anterior border is supported by orbicularis oris muscle and prevents upper-forward shift of the denture as anterior nasal spine acts as the stopper (Fig 18, 19).

1.5 ~ 2.0 mm of anterior clearrance is provided to avoid maxillary and mandibular anterior denture tooth contact and occlusion is adjusted periodically. Excessive force on the flabby ridge is controlled by maintaining this condition. Inflammation of flabby ridge subsides and edematous gingiva becomes more fibrous gingiva through this long-term treatment.

(3) Design of the custom tray for mandibular suction-effect denture

Fabrication of the custom tray, which starts from preliminary impression using the Frame Cut Back Tray, is the most important laboratory process for successful suction-effect of the mandibular complete denture. The quality of the custom tray

Modification of the maxillary custom tray for flabby ridge case

☞The better the condition of the ridge is, the thinner the tray border is fabricated. The more extensive the ridge resorption is, the thicker the tray border is fabricated. It is important to modify the thickness of the tray according to the condition of the residual ridge

Simple case | **Difficult-to-Treat case**

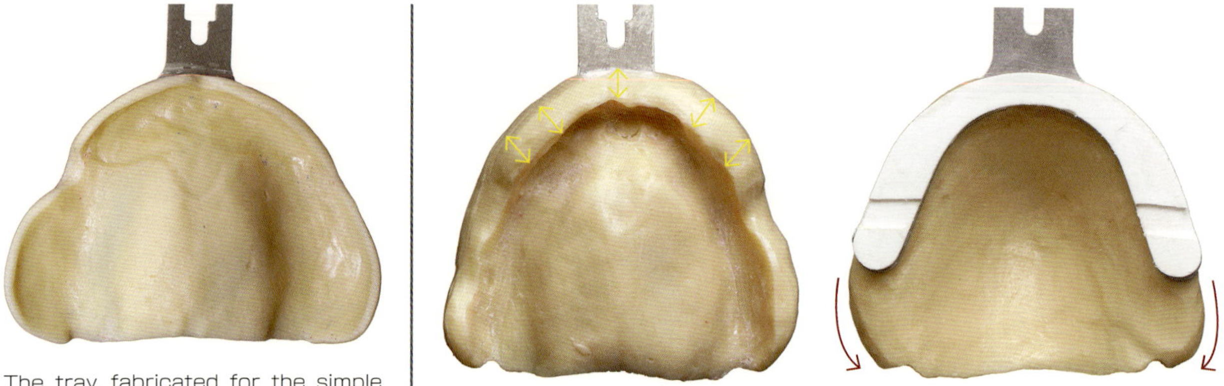

The tray, fabricated for the simple case in part 4

Upper-front movement of the denture is decreased by making the anterior region of the border thicker

The gentle curvature is formed toward the pterygomandibular raphe

Fig19 Modification of the maxillary custom tray for the flabby ridge case.

affects the quality of the final complete denture since the final impression is taken under the patient's functional movement using this tray[68-70] (Fig 20).

Drawing process of the custom tray border on the preliminary cast is almost identical between the general case with favorable ridge shape and the difficult case with unfavorable ridge shape. The only difference is the line of the anterior region on both labial and lingual aspect.

(4) Relief on the mandibular cast

The area of relief needs to be selected carefully in the case with unfavorable ridge shape. The denture does not tend to subside in the area with poor replaceability and tends to subside in the area with high replaceability. Better suction-effect is achieved by enabling the denture border all around to subside in the soft tissue by relieving the hard tissue (Fig 21).

The design of the custom tray of the mandibular ridge resorption case

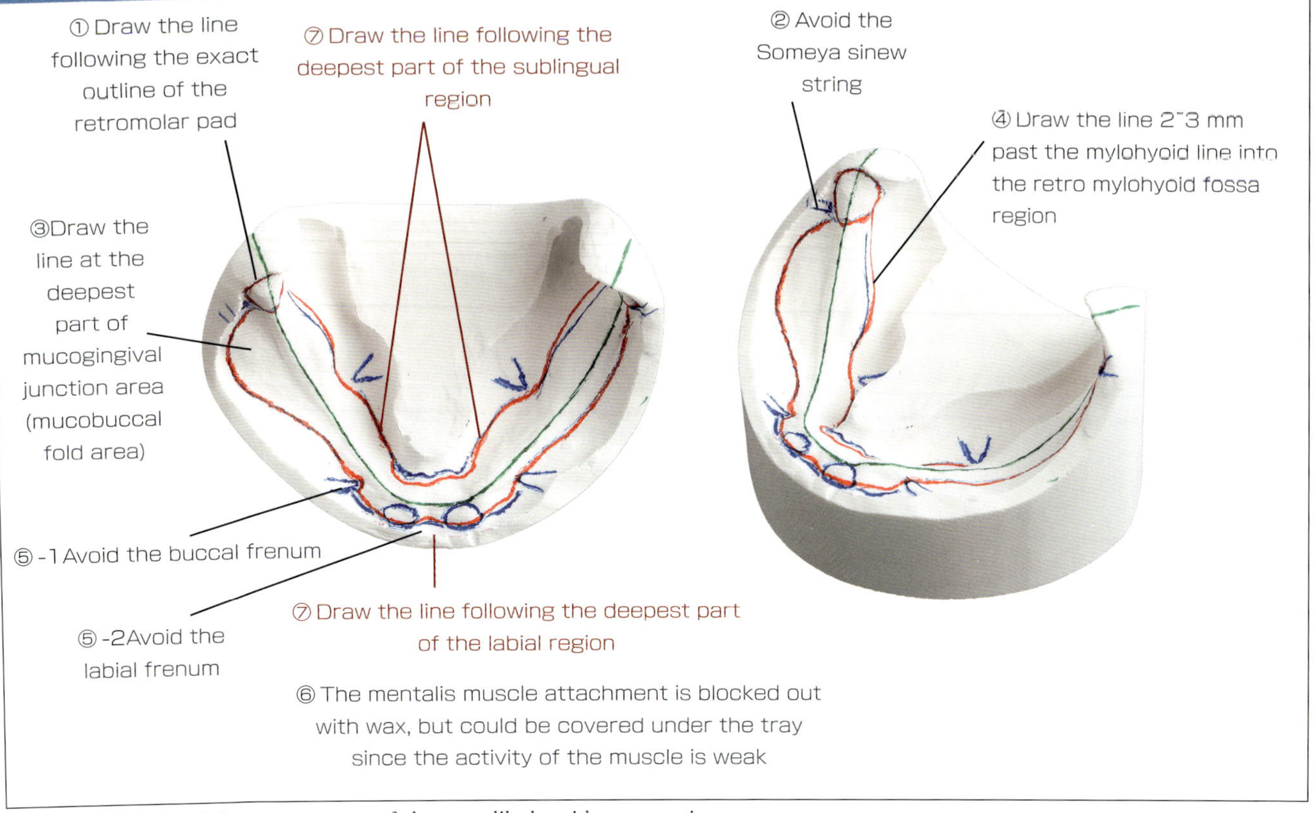

Fig20 The design of the custom tray of the mandibular ridge resorption case.

4 relieved areas by the wax

The alveolar crest area: The retromolar pad, which consists of soft glandular tissue without fibrous tissue in front part, as shown in this case is not relieved. The denture sinks down when occlusal force is applied with the circumferential denture border touching the soft tissue. The retromolar pad is completely sealed by the denture with the abundant replaceability

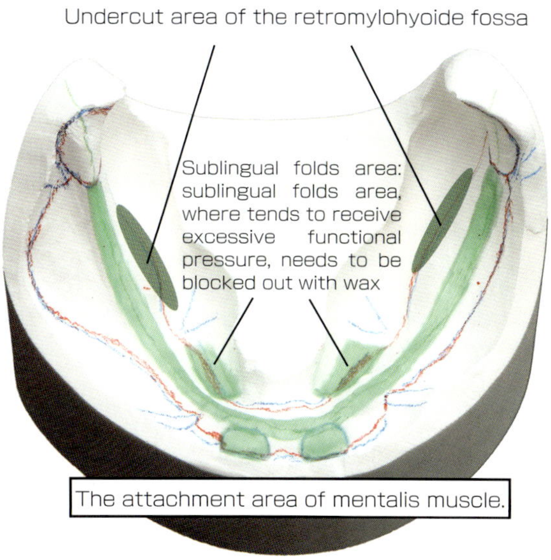

Fig21 4 relieved areas with wax.

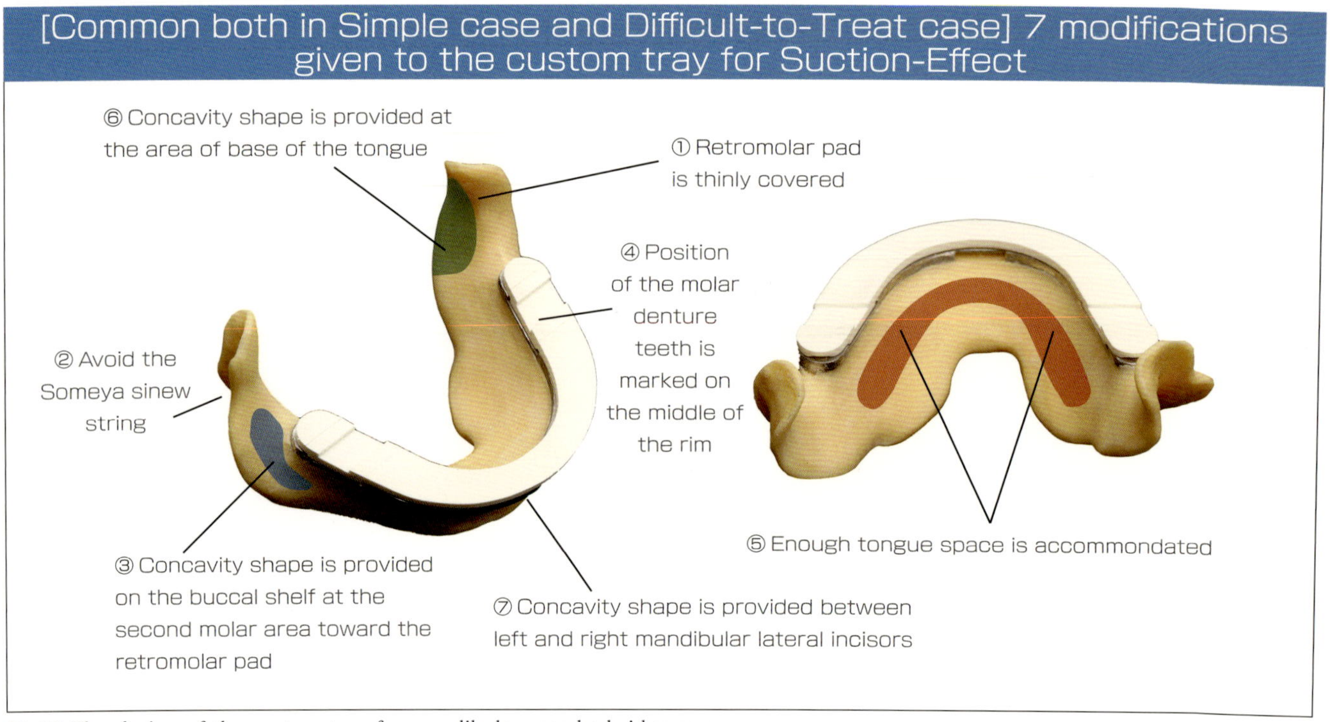

Fig22 The design of the custom tray for mandibular resorbed ridge case.

(5) 7 features on the custom tray, which are essential for successful mandibular suction-effective final impression

These features are same for both simple case or difficult case. They are shown in Fig 22.

(6) Providing thickness to the custom tray to increase suction-effect

Thickness of the custom tray border is adjusted according to each patient's ridge shape (Fig 23).

Thicker border is provided for the unfavorable ridge shape. The tray border of the sublingual fold region is thickened for the patient who lacks spongy tissue in the sublingual fold region or has habit of retracting the tongue strongly while opening the mouth. Buccal border of the tray is rounded and thickened for the purpose of increasing occlusal support of buccal shelf region if resorption of posterior ridge is severe. Stable lip support is achieved by thickening the tray border of anterior region for the case with shallow lavial vestibule, where the mentalis muscle is located on the superior portion of the ridge due to ridge resorption.

(7) Setting Gnathometer M

Gnathometer M is one of BPS products, which allows final impression and Gothic arch tracing on the same day. If Gnathometer M is not available, final impression

Thickness of the tray is changed according to each patient

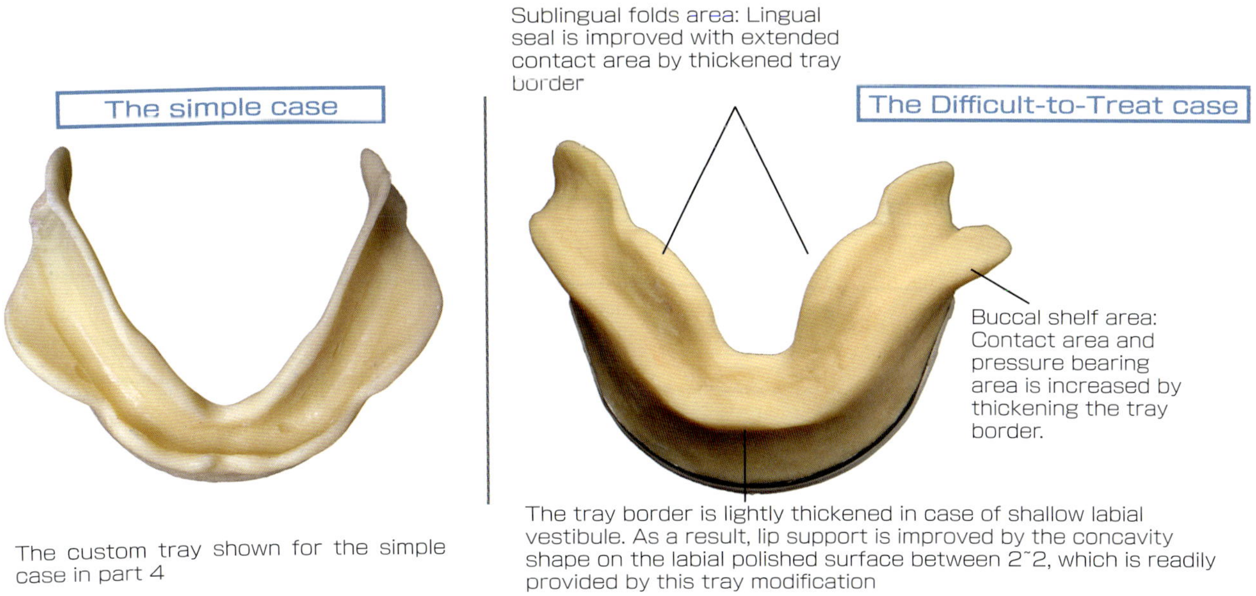

Fig23 Basic tray design is the same regardless of the ridge shape. Modification is provided to the thickness of the tray border according to each patient.

Setting of the Gnathometer M

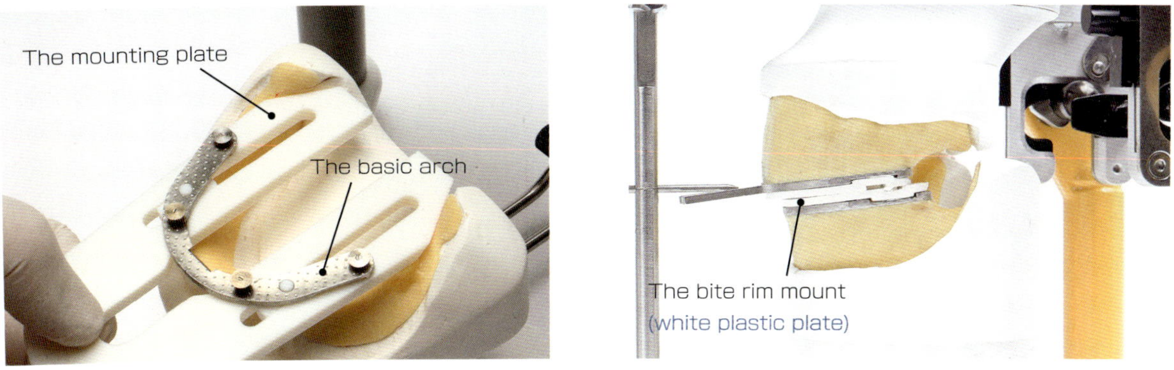

Fig24 Setting of the Gnathometer M.

and bite registration are taken using the custom tray with the wax rim attached (Fig 16 right below) first, and then confirm the horizontal mandibular position later using the Gothic arch tracer fabricated on the master cast. Metal basic arch is attached to the base resin by auto cure resin using the mounting plate. The white plate is called the Bite rim mount, which is part of the Gnathometer M. The Bite rim mount can be replaced by the Gothic arch tracer right after the impression is taken (Fig 24).

The anterior reference point for the basic arch of the maxillary Gnathometer M or for positioning of the wax rim.

The basic arch (white plate) or the arch of the wax rim is set at 7mm for male and 9mm for female in average from the incisive papilla

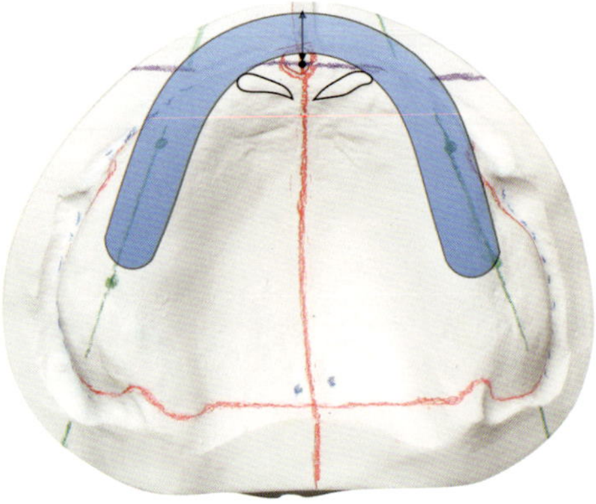

The case with favorable alveolar ridge Introduced in part 4

The arch is set about 10mm anterior to the position, the mal-located incisive papilla supposed to be, in the case with displaced maxillary incisive papillae and unclear palatal rugae in addition to maxillary ridge resorption

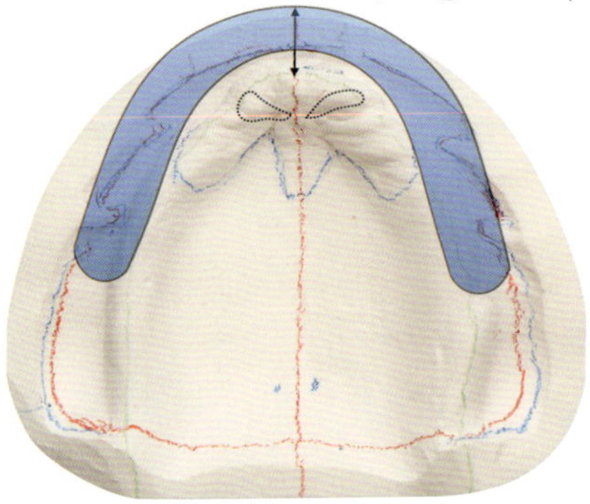

The case with unfavorable alveolar ridge

Fig25 The anterior reference point for the basic arch of the maxillary Gnathometer M or for positioning of the wax rim.

The anterior reference point for the basic arch of the mandibular Gnathometer M or for positioning of the wax rim

The anterior reference point for the wax rim or the basic arch is set at the transverse line of the anterior region of the alveolar ridge in the case with favorable alveolar ridge

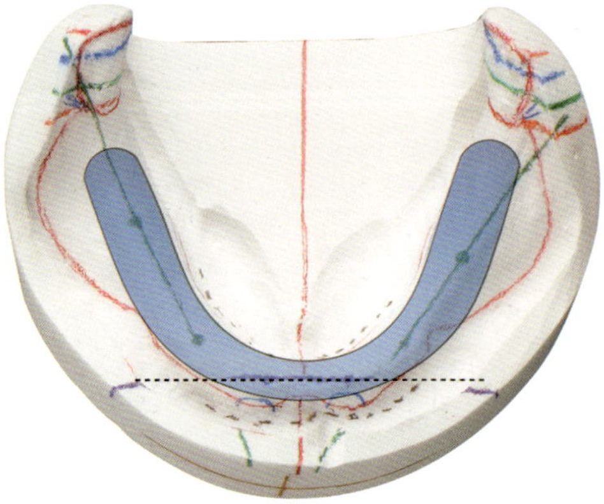

The case with favorable alveolar ridge in part 4

The bisected line of the anterior alveolar ridge in labiolingual direction is set as the anterior reference point for the wax rim or the basic arch in case with unfavorable alveolar ridge and unclear ridge crest

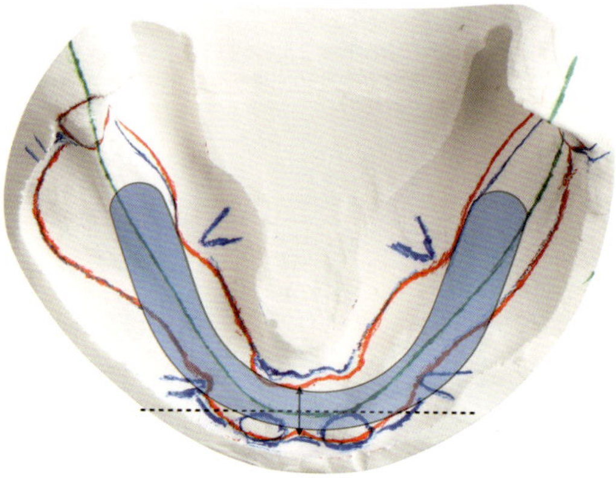

The case with unfavorable alveolar ridge

Fig26 The anterior reference point for the basic arch of the mandibular Gnathometer M and for positioning of the wax rim.

The anterior over-jet and the occlusal plane of the custom tray according to maxillomandibular relationship.

☞The custom tray is fabricated according to each maxillomandibular relationship of Class I, II and III by setting upper and lower basic arches separately.
The occlusal plane: the occlusal plane is set parallel to Camper's line for Class I, toward upper edge of the retromolar pad for Class II and toward 1/2 of the retromolar pad for class III. This is due to the difference in the angle of the maxillary occlusal plane to receive the occlusal force according to the difference in the arch of closure.

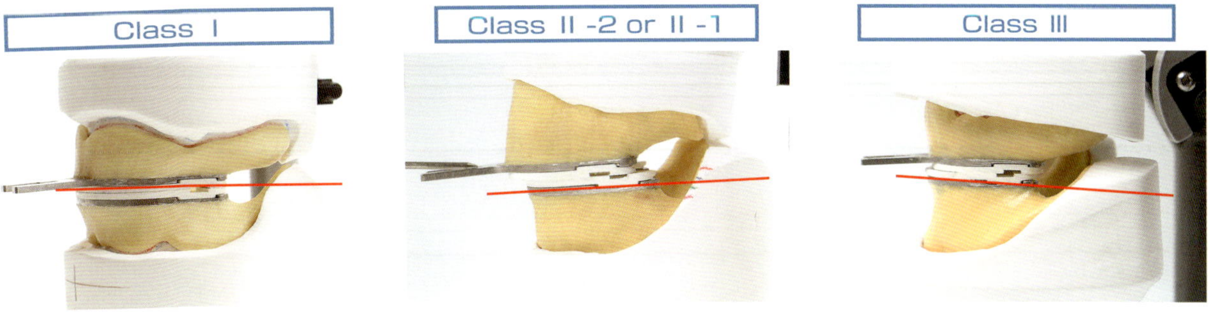

Fig27 The anterior over-jet and the occlusal plane of the custom tray according to maxillomandibular relationship.

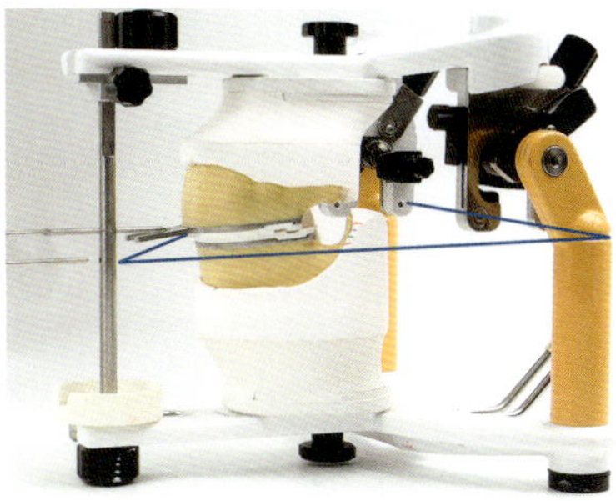

Fig28 The custom tray for Class 2 case with the occlusal plane slightly tilted up posteriorly.

Maxillary and mandibular base resin bases are attached to the Metal basic arch simultaneously in Class I case. They should be attached separately in Class II and III cases, because there is always anterior-posterior gap due to difference in the anatomical landmark for determination of anterior-posterior position of the anterior dental arch between favorable and unfavorable ridges as shown in Fig 25, 26. The gap should not exceed 8mm, which is the width of the Bite Rim Mount (white plate) since the tracing pin could hit the fixing screw on the tracing plate during Gothic arch tracing. Occlusal plane is set acceding to the jaw relationship of Class I, II and III (Fig27, 28).

Three things needs to be checked before the final impression
① To check the proper orientation of the occlusal plane of the custom tray

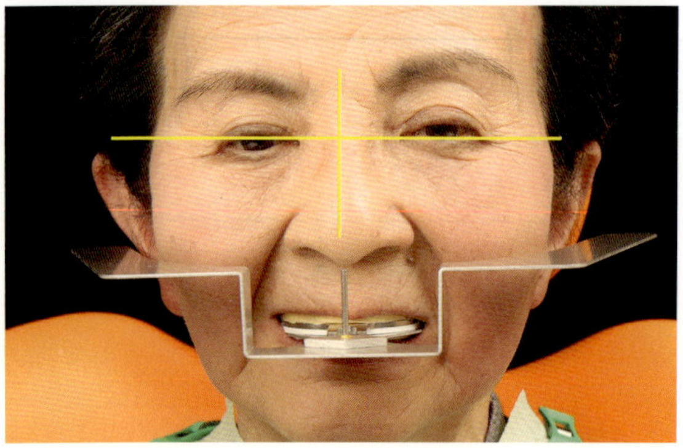

Parallel to the inter pupil line
Consistency of the mid line

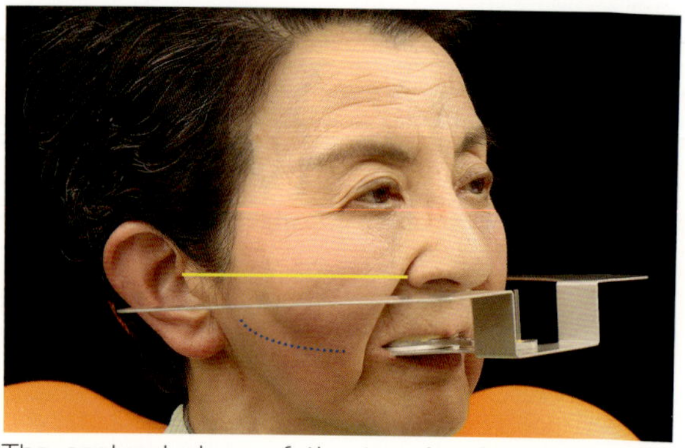

The occlusal plane of the tray is often set to be slightly back downward from Camper's plane, which ends up to be parallel after compensating curve is provided by denture tooth setup

※ Material: Y.N. occlusal plane plate (Senjo, Morita)

Fig29 The patient is asked to bit the occlusal plane plate. Then, the setting of the occlusal plane of the custom tray is checked in relation to the midline, horizontal plane and Camper's plane (nose-ear line).

8 The custom tray try-in

The occlusal plane on the custom tray, accuracy of the initial bite registration record and fit and extension of the border of the custom tray are checked before final impression procedure.

(1) The occlusal plane on the custom tray

The occlusal plane on the custom tray is checked by the Occlusal template, which is bitten on by the patient between maxillary and mandibular trays, in relation to the mid line, horizontal plane and Camper's Plane (Fig 29). The occlusal plane on the tray is often set slightly lower in posterior than Camper's Plane. This discrepancy is compensated when denture teeth are set with the compensating curve.

Once proper plane settings (inter pupil line, mid line and Camper's Plane) are confirmed, next step is initiated. Any discrepancy noticed should be mentioned in the prescription for the dental technician to mount the final impressions and master casts correctly.

Three things needs to be checked before the final impression
② To check errors of preliminary bite registration record by the Centric Tray

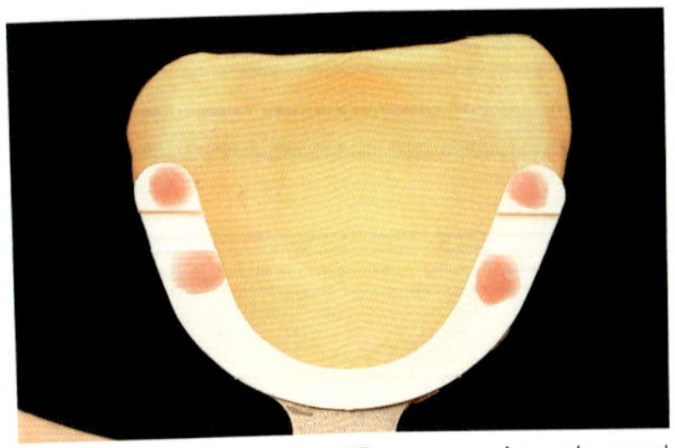

Step1 : The paraffin wax is placed at the position of maxillary first premolars and first molars

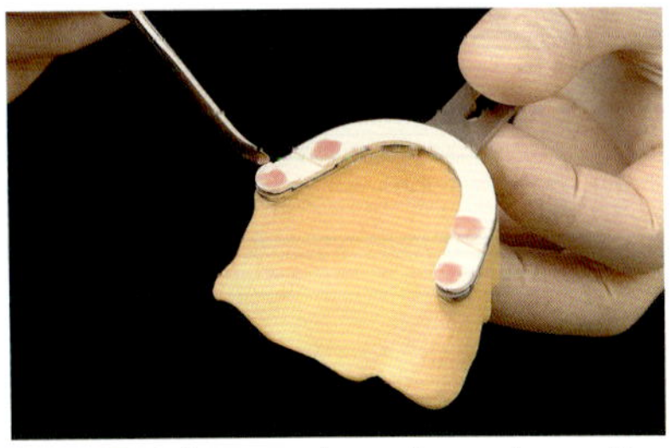

Step2 : The wax is softened and the patient is asked to bite down

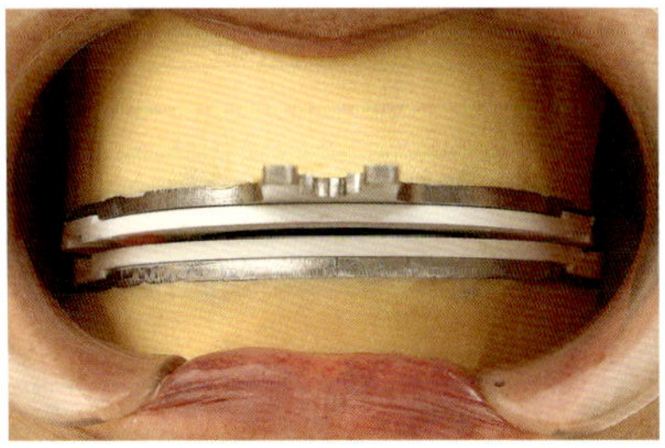

Step3 : Uniform space should be seen between upper and lower plates. If uneven space is found, decision needs to be made if reattachment of Gnathometer M is necessary

Fig30 The patient is asked to bite down on the softened paraffin wax placed at maxillary first premolars and first molars for the purpose of checking the accuracy of the bite registration record.

(2) Errors in the initial occlusal bite registration by the Centric Tray

The bite registration record with the Centric Tray is not so accurate. Even if maxillary and mandibular trays are not in desired position, they often looks like occluding in good position.

The patient is asked to bite on the softened paraffin wax placed on maxillary first premolar and molar areas on both side, in order to check if the initial bite registration record is accurate (Fig 30).

Move on to final impression procedure once the wax is removed from the plate, if the even space between maxillary and mandibular plates is confirmed. Final impression can be taken with the wax kept on the plate even with uneven space, as long as the discrepancy is small. These 4 point wax allows even pressure on maxillary and mandibular ridges during final impression procedure. Slight change in VDO does not influence the quality of the final impression, since final definitive VDO is determined by adjusting the length of the stylus of the pin tracer after the final impression. Small discrepancy between maxillary and mandibular plates in all direction does not influence the accuracy of the final impression either. Only if significant amount of discrepancy between maxillary and mandibular plates or uneven space is observed, new bite registration record is taken using the custom trays and the the Gnathometer M is reattached.

Three things needs to be checked before the final impression ③-1 To check fit of maxillary custom tray

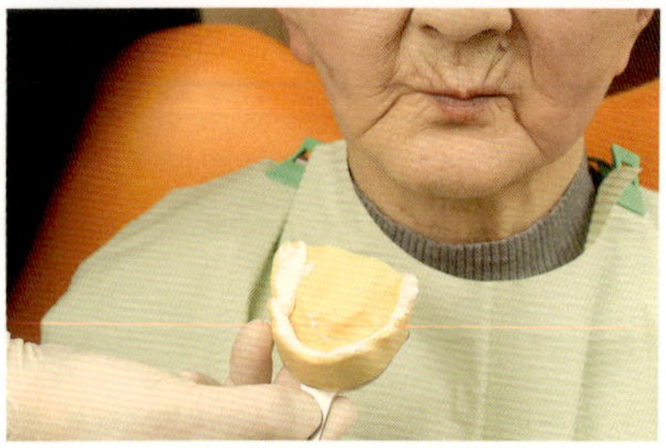

Step1 : Fit of the tray is checked by finger pressure with the Fit-checker(GC) only around the border area, since more extensive area is blocked out on the model with wax in flabby ridge case. Fit of the tray is checked in occlusion if it is indicated

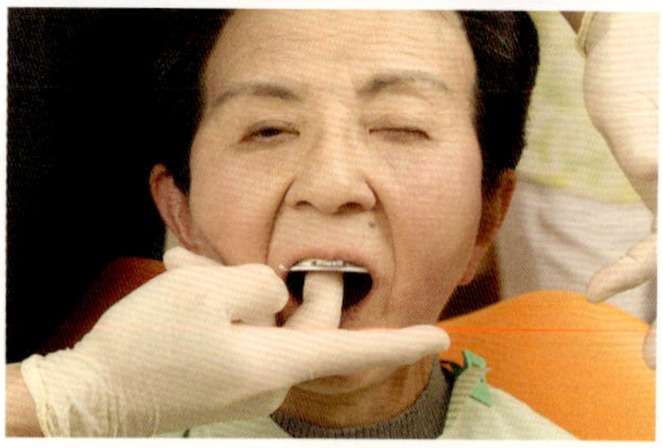

Step2 : Fit check with finger pressure

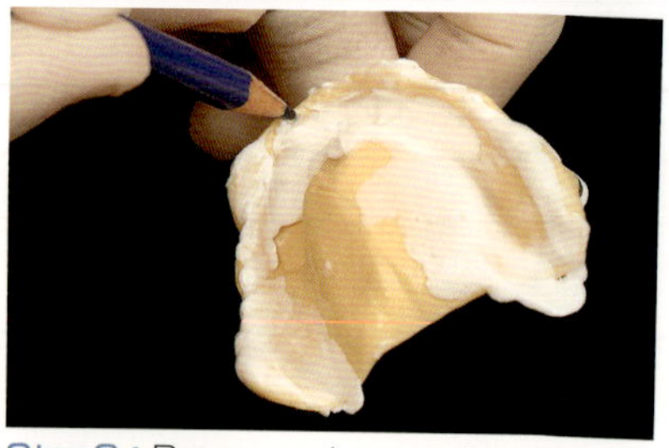

Step3 : Pressured area is marked by the pen and adjusted with the bur

Fig31 Fit check of maxillary custom tray.

Three things needs to be checked before the final impression ③-2 To check fit of mandibular custom tray

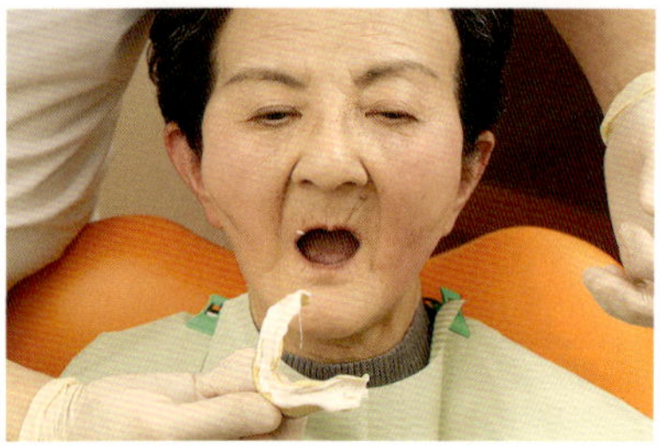

Step1 : Fit-checker is applied on the entire internal surface of the tray

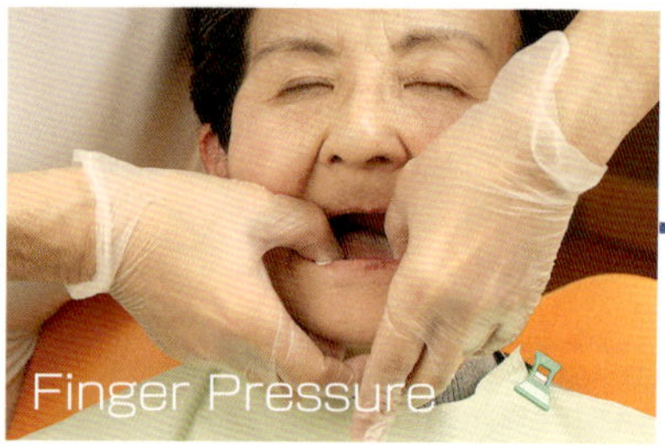

Step2-a : The tray is inserted in the mouth and pressured area where the fitchecker get thinner should be confirmed when applying pressure by operator fingers. The tray position error should be avoided in a case with poor ridge form

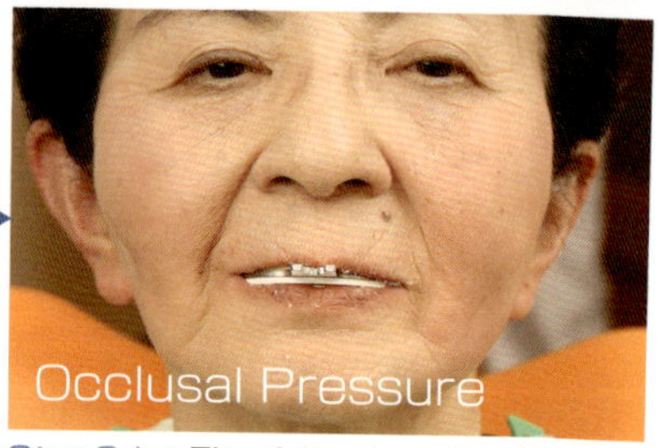

Step2-b : Fit of the tray is checked in occlusion with Fit-checker after grinding pressured area off in the previous manner

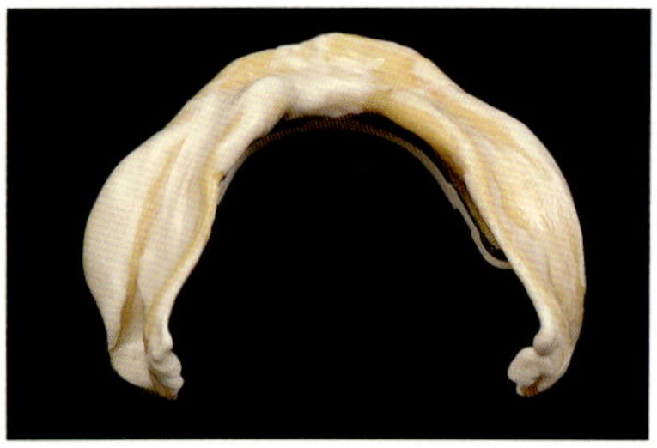

Step3 : Pressured area is observed while considering the blocked-out area with wax on the model

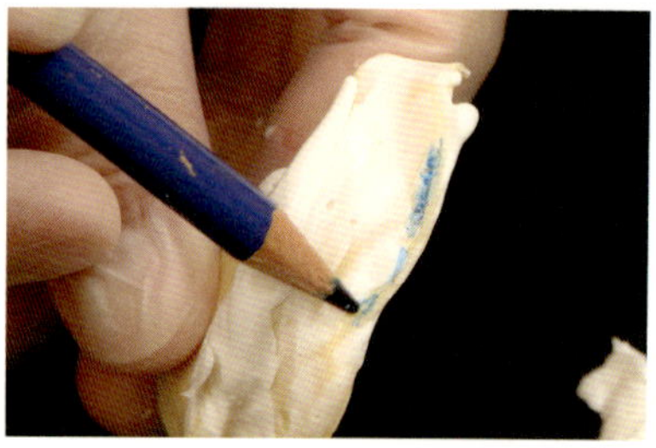

Step4 : Mark with a pen

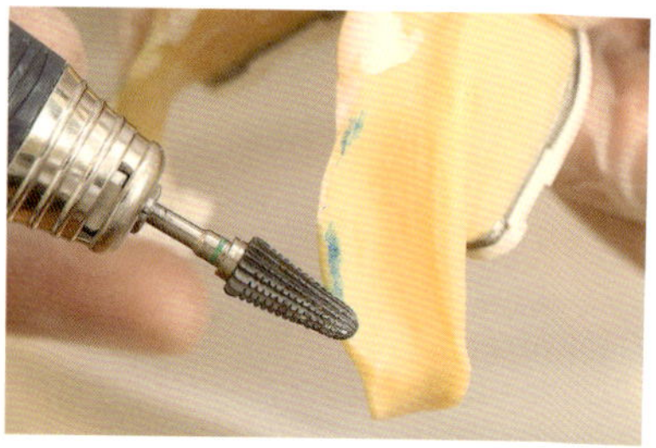

Step5 : Scrape off with a bur

Fig32 Fit check of mandibular custom tray.

Adjustment of the poor-fit part of the tray around the retromolar pad region (Self-curing resin)

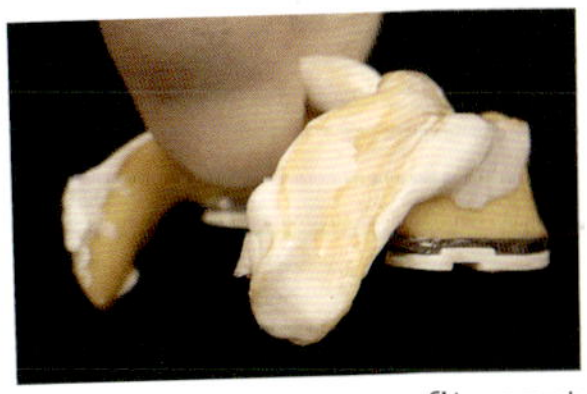

Step1 : The poor-fit part of the tray around the retromolar pad region is observed

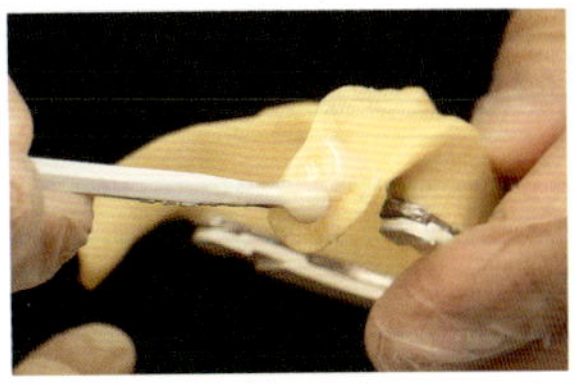

Step2 : Self-curing resin is applied on that part of the tray in order to adjust the shape of the tray proper to the final impression

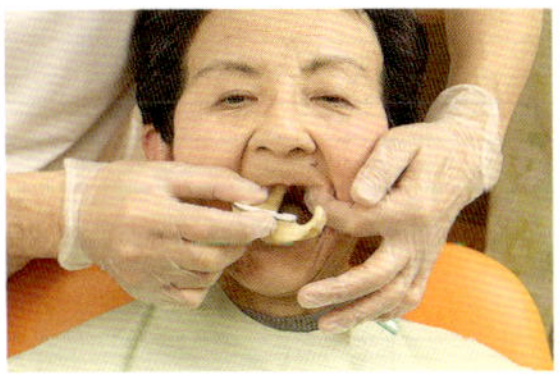

Step3 : The tray applied self-curing resin is inserted into the mouth

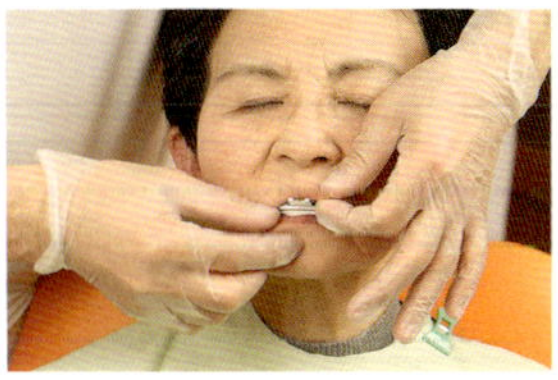

Step4 : The static shape of the retromolar pad is captured with the self-curing resin in the closed mouth. The tray should be removed from the mouth before the self-curing resin starts setting and put in the water until it completely has set

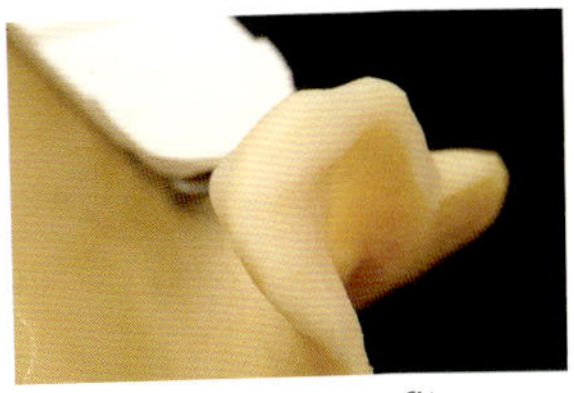

Step5 : The poor-fit part of the tray is clearly observed

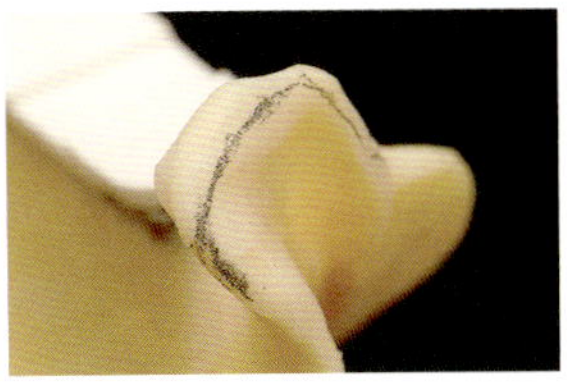

Step6 : Draw the exact outline of the retromolar pad with a pen

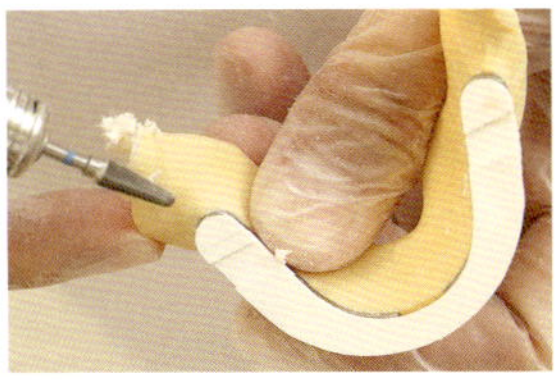

Step7 : The tray should be trimmed off following its exact line

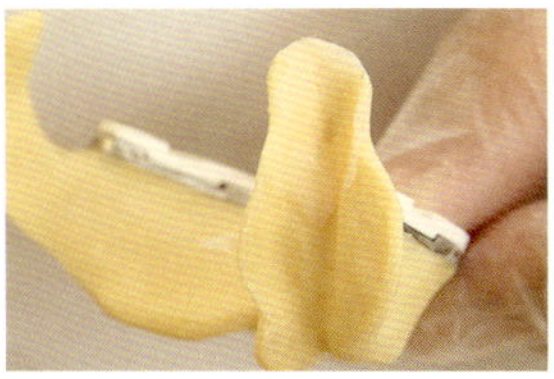

Step8 : Adjustment of the tray is completed

Fig33 Adjustment of the poor-fit part of the tray around the retromolar pad resion.

(3) Fit of the custom tray and extension of the tray border

Fit of the custom tray and extension of the tray border are checked using GC Fit Checker (GC) and adjustment is made accordingly. Finger pressure is used for maxilla for the first check and occlusal pressure is used with the mandibular custom tray in for another check if it is required (Fig 31). First check for the mandible is carried out under the operator's finger pressure and the second check is under the occlusal pressure between maxillary and mandibular tray (Fig 32).

Fit of the custom tray in the retromolar pad, the most difficult area to achieve the seal, is the most important factor in the Difficult-to-Treat case. If the retromolar pad is soft without fibrous immobile tissue in anterior third as shown in this case, it is easily deformed under pressure from the maxillary tuberosity area during the preliminary impression even with a Frame Cut Back tray is used. If the fit of the tray is not ideal, the retromolar pad area of the tray is modified using self-cureing acrylic to improve the fit according to the shape of the retromolar pad in closed mouth condition (Fig 33).

9 Skills for successful final impression of maxillary flabby ridge - For successful suction-effect of the maxillary complete denture

It is evident that flabby ridge would be persistent, even though impression technique with no pressure for flabby ridge or surgical excision of flabby tissue are employed, unless the cause of the flabby ridge is treated properly (Fig 34). On the other hand, flabby ridge should heal up by itself once the cause is removed (Fig 35).

As mentioned in the section of maxillary custom tray, maxillary anterior inflammatory flabby ridge is the result of excessive irritation of the ridge mucosa due to repetitive push up of the maxillary denture by habitual anterior chewing. Enough amount of anterior clearance needs to be provided establishing stable bilateral posterior occlusion and this condition has to be maintained in order to eliminate the habitual anterior chewing. Inflammation of flabby ridge area will be resolved as the irritation on anterior region is decreased (Table 1). Appropriate thickness of the anterior border of the tray needs to be provided to minimize the migration of the maxillary denture during chewing.

(1) The first step of impression taking

Heavy body impression material is applied in the tray, where the flabby ridge will be, and then the tray is inserted and pushed lightly posteriorly. The flabby ridge, which is tucked forward, is pushed back straight with this technique to restore its shape (Fig 36). Inflammation subsides faster with the flabby ridge being straight up without tucking. Impression material of the upper part of the flabby ridge is trimmed away carefully using the sharp instrument leaving the impression material of anterior part of the flabby ridge intact.

(2) The second step of impression taking

The second step is border molding using heavy body impression material (Fig 37). Only one layer of heavy body impression material is applied on anterior region, since enough thickness is already provided to the custom tray.

The condition of the mucosa of this patient is categorized as the soft cheek. Two layers of heavy body impression material is required for the patient with extensive ridge resorption and soft cheek (the mucosa is easily extended buccaly with the finger) in order to establish thick enough denture flange border to restore the lost tissue. The upper lip of many patients with flabby ridge tends to be thin, which is the result of prolonged weakened activity of orbicularis oris muscle. It is the preventive self maneuver for maxillary denture fall. This is the reason why thickening the impression of the anterior border would not be problematic.

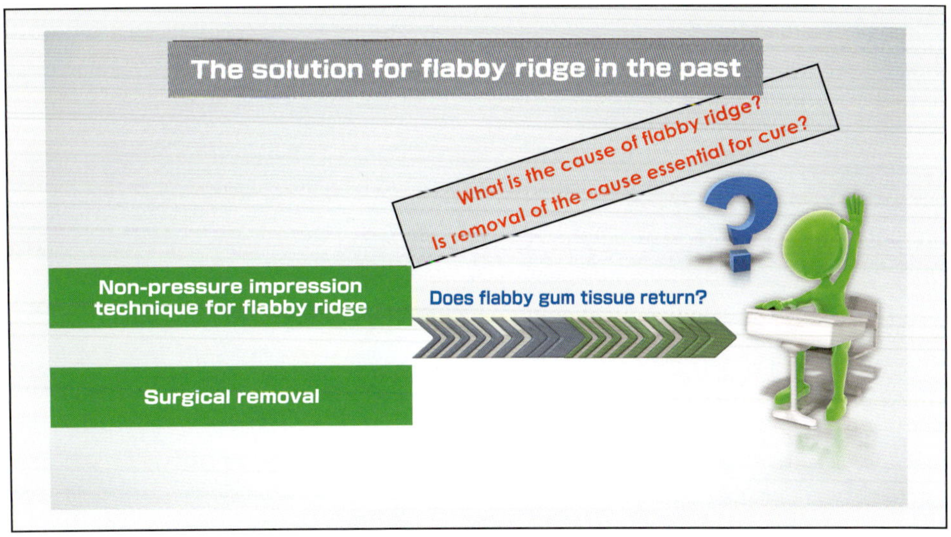

Fig34 Non-pressure impression technique for flabby ridge or surgical resection of flabby ridge has been recommended. However, it is clear that flabby gum tissue would return if the cause of it is not treated properly.

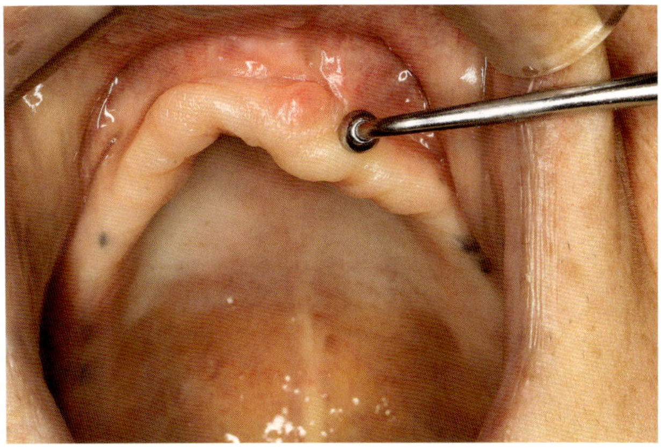

Fig35 The main cause of inflammatory flabby ridge is excessive occlusal pressure due to anterior chewing.

Healing process of maxillary anterior flabby ridge

【The cause】

Excessive pressure to maxillary anterior ridge by habitual anterior chewing

↓

【Elimination of the cause】

Excessive pressure is controlled by eliminating the habitual anterior chewing and providing 1.5～2.0 mm clearance in anterior region

↓

【The technique】

①Upward-forward shift of the denture is decreased by thickening the denture border at anterior region

②Occlusion is adjusted periodically so that maxillary and mandibular denture do not contact each other at anterior region

↓

【The result】

Inflammation subsides and flabby tissue is atrophied and firmed after the pressure on anterior ridge is decrease

Table 1 Healing process of maxillary anterior flabby ridge.

Final impression steps for maxillary Difficult-to-Treat case ① Pushing up the tuck of flabby ridge posteriorly

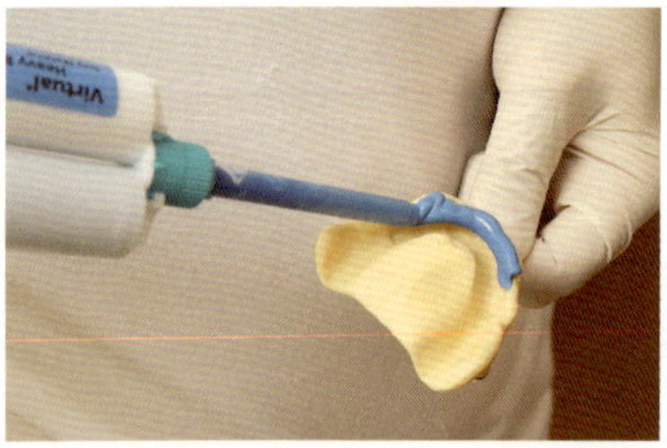

Step1 : Heavy body impression material is applied to the tray in the area equivalent to the flabby ridge

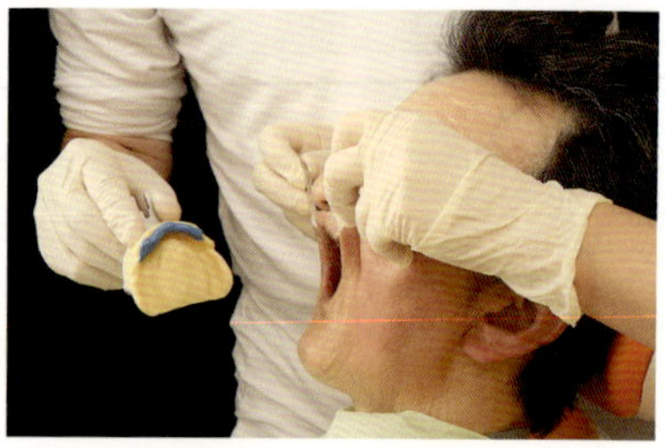

Step2 : The ray is inserted

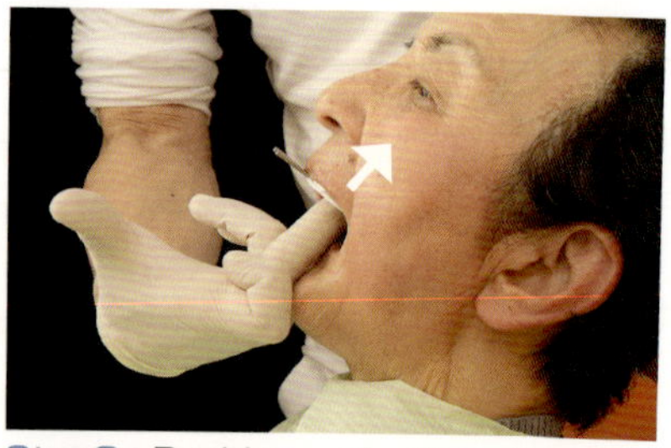

Step3 : Position of the tray is checked and pressure is applied vertically

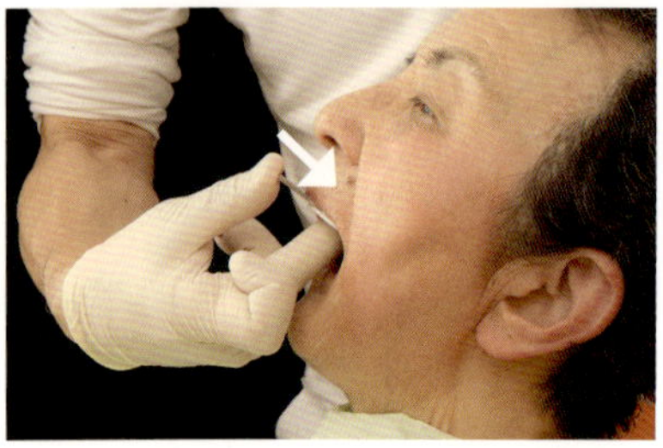

Step4 : Flabby ridge, which is tucked forward, is straightened up posteriorly by pushing the tray gently backward

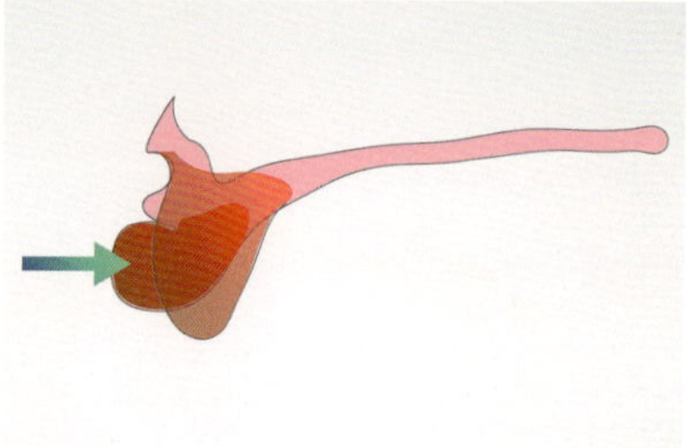

Step5 : Inflammation of the flabby ridge would not regress easily with the tucked condition

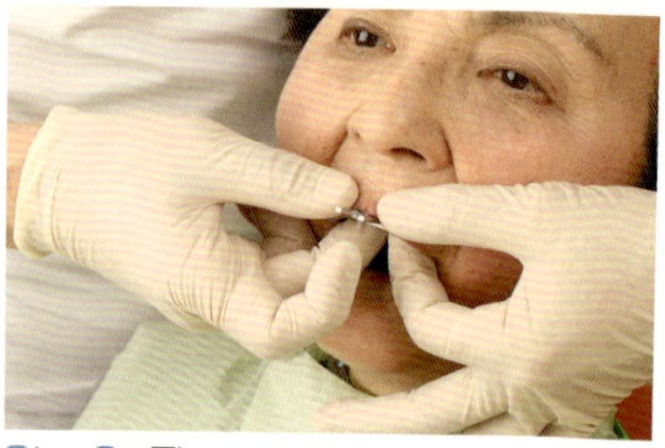

Step6 : The upper lip should not be pulled down vigorously to secure thickness of anterior impression

Fig36 Final impression steps for maxillary Difficult-to-Treat case ① .

Small amount of heavy body impression material is placed as the stopper on the middle of the palate to maintain the space, which was relieved by the wax for flabby ridge. Anterior shift of the tray during impression procedure is prevented as well.

Attention must be paid not to pull the upper lip down too strong or let the patient suck the finger of the operator vigorously in order to form the border region thick enough.

Next, movement of the coronoid process is recorded on the external surface of the impression in the tuberosity area by asking the patient to move the mandible right and left.

Impression of the functional movement of the maxillary buccal and lip area is recorded by having the patient make the move [purse the lips] [retract the corner of the mouth] (Fig 38, 39).

Final impression steps for maxillary Difficult-to-Treat case ② Border molding using heavy body impression material

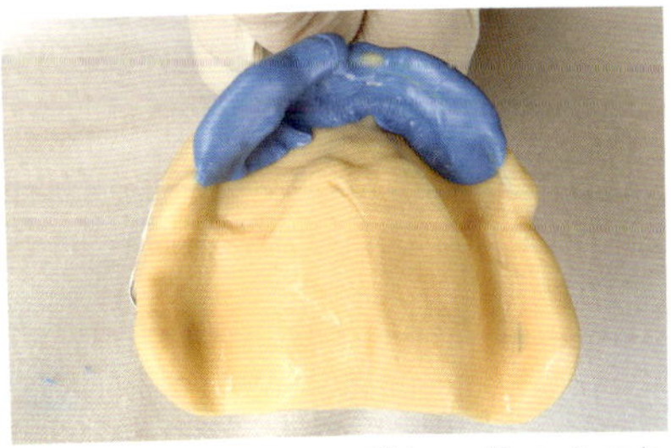

Step1 : The condition the tuck, which is straightened up posteriorly

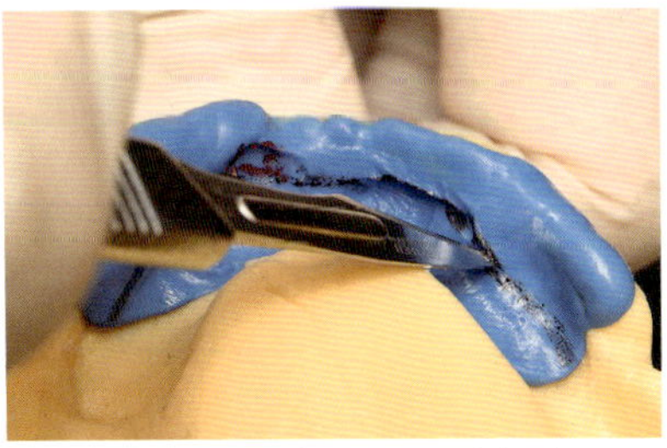

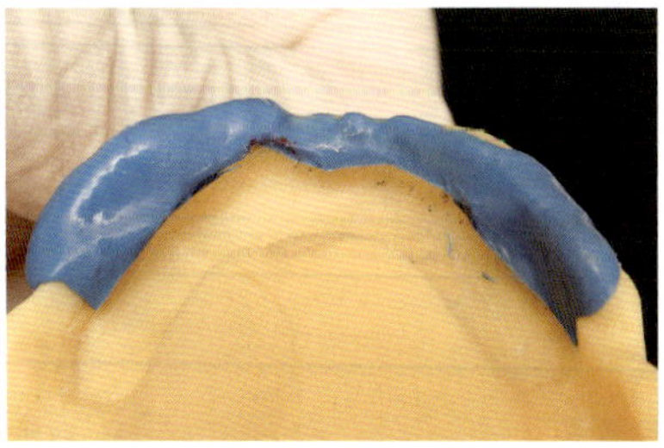

Step2 : Impression material of upper portion of the flabby ridge is carefully trimmed away using scalpel

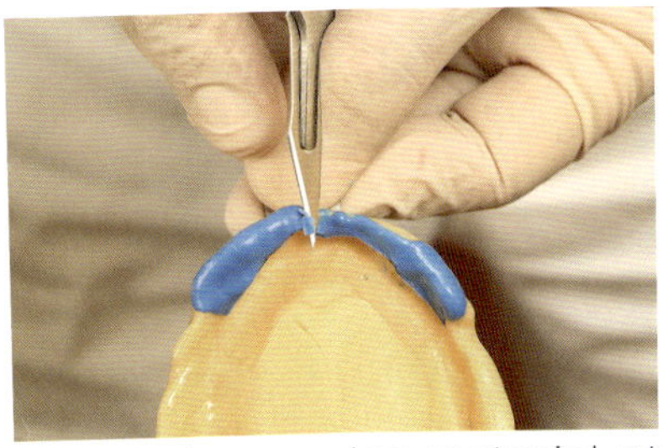

Step3 : Impression material at the superior labial frenum area is trimmed away

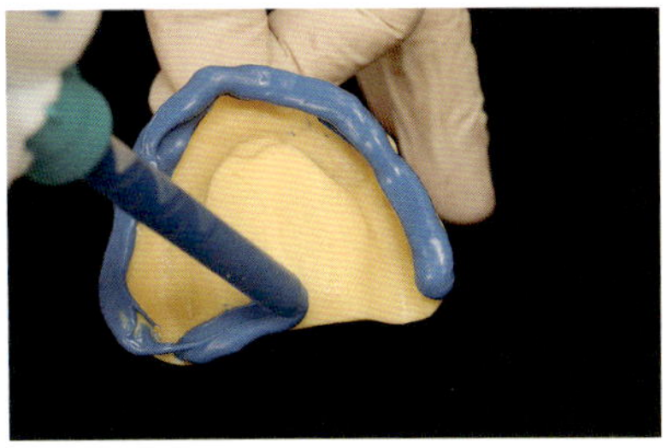

Step4 : One layer of heavy body impression material is applied

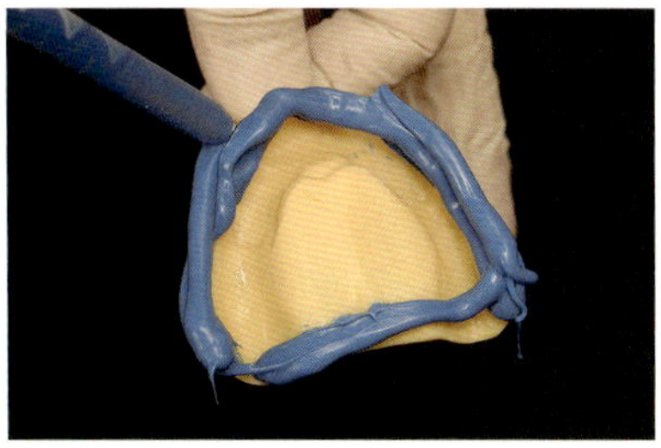

Step5 : Two layers of impression material is applied to molar region if the patient's cheek mucosa is very soft

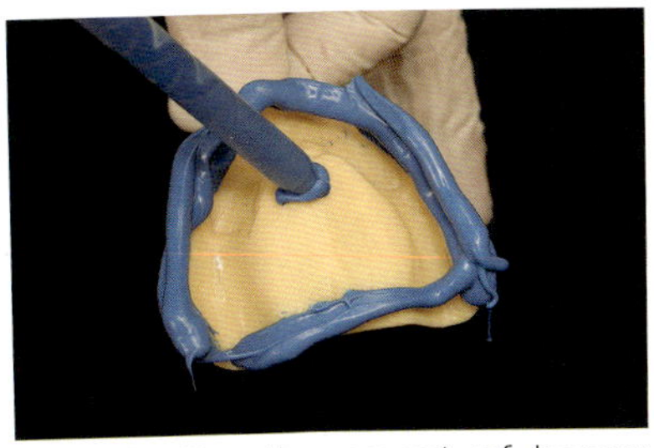

Step6 : Small amount of heavy body impression material is applied on mid palatal area as a stopper

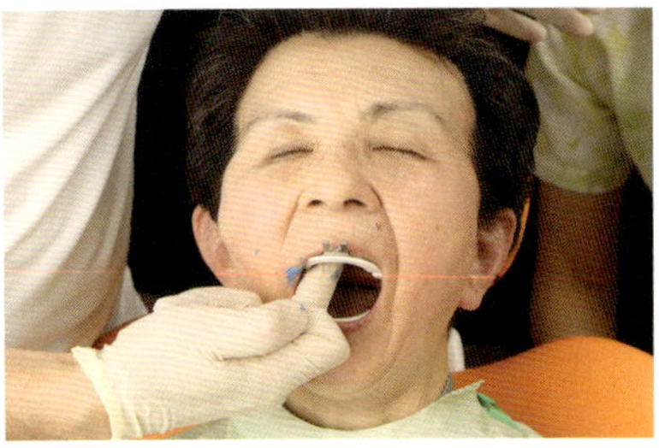

Step7 : The tray is inserted in the proper position and pushed upward

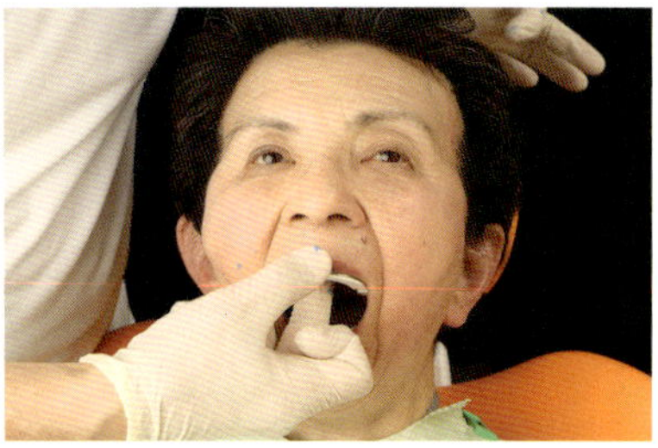

Step8 : Subsequently, tucked flabby tissue is straightened up posteriorly again by pushing the tray posteriorly keep it still with gentle pressure

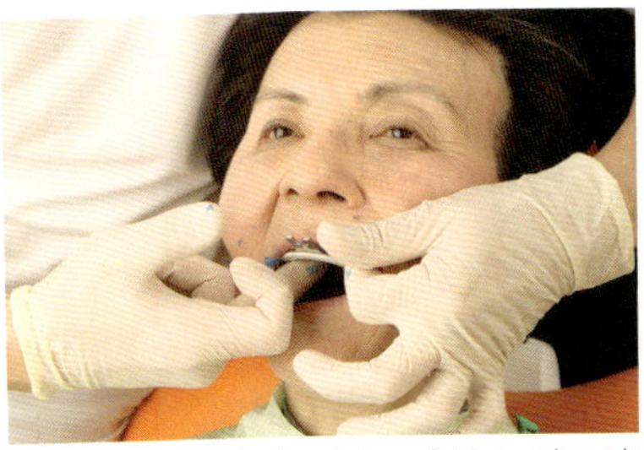

Step9 : Pull left side of the cheek down

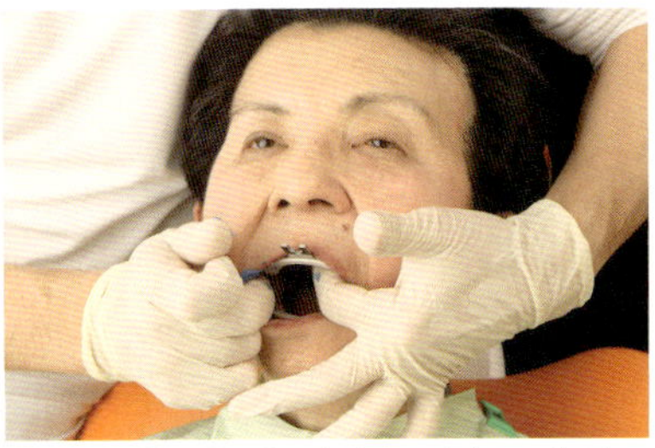

Step10 : Pull right side of the cheek down

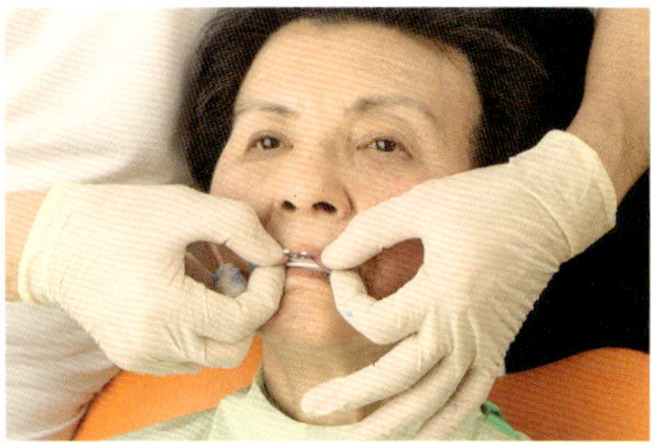

Step11 : The upper lip should not be pulled down vigorously to secure thickness of anterior impression

Fig37a Final impression steps for maxillary Difficult-to-Treat case ② (to be continued to following page).

Final impression steps for maxillary Difficult-to-Treat case ② Border molding using heavy body impression material

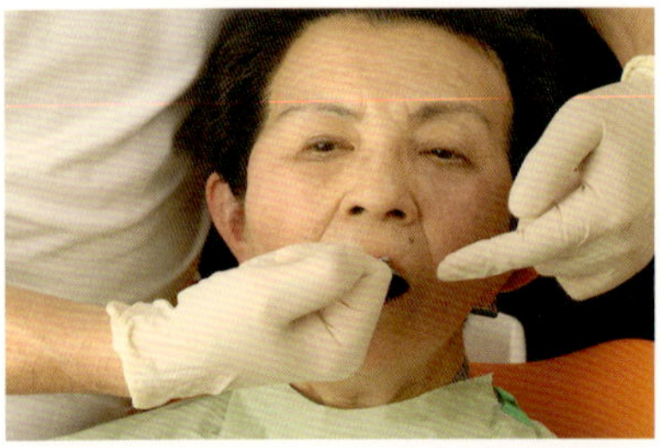

Step1 : Move the mandible right to left direction to avoid the coronoid process from hitting the tray

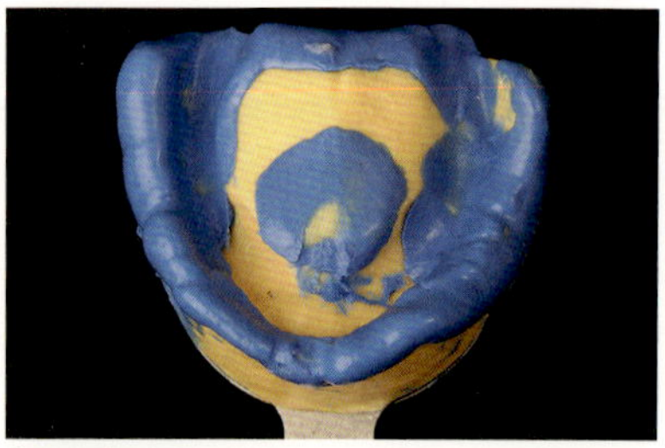

Step2 : The impression with the border, which is thick enough in areas of upper lip and molars

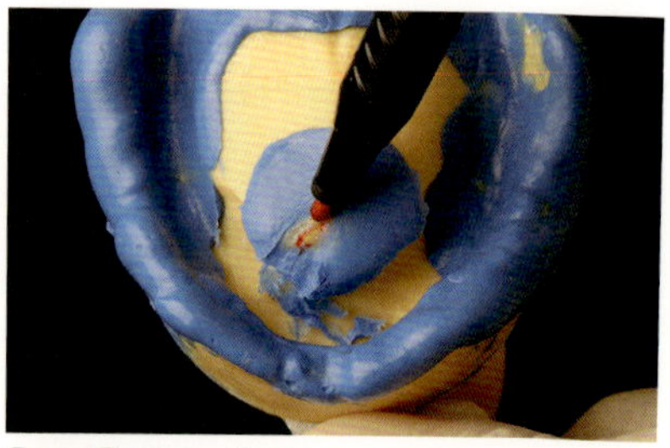

Step3 : Interfering area on the palate is marked with the pen

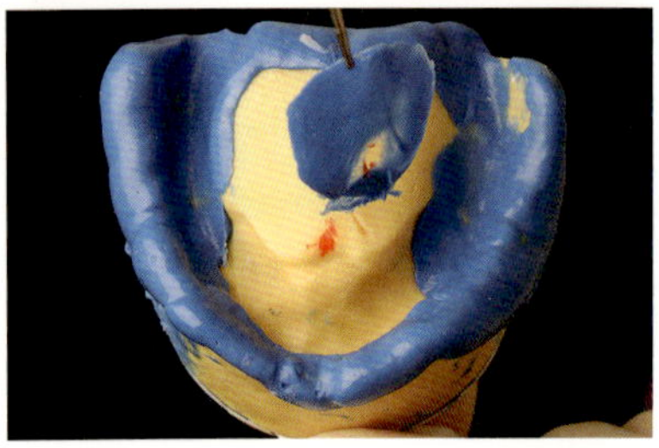

Step4 : The impression material on the palate is removed and interference is relieved

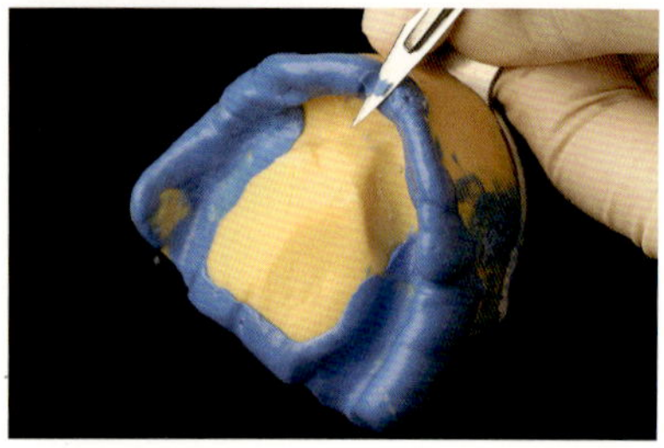

Step5 : The impression material at superior labial frenum region is trimmed away

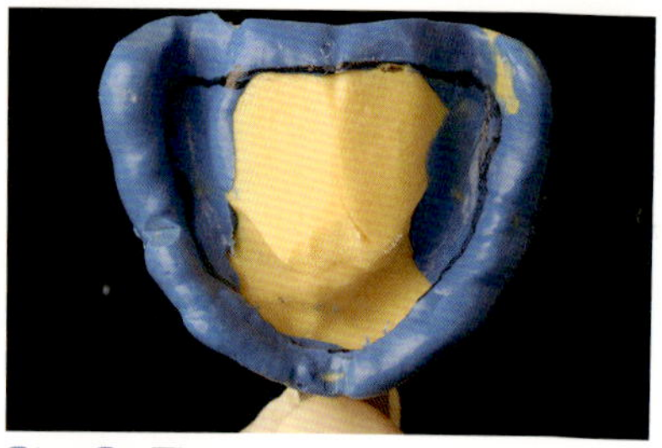

Step6 : The impression material at the ridge crest area is removed considering the difference in compressibility

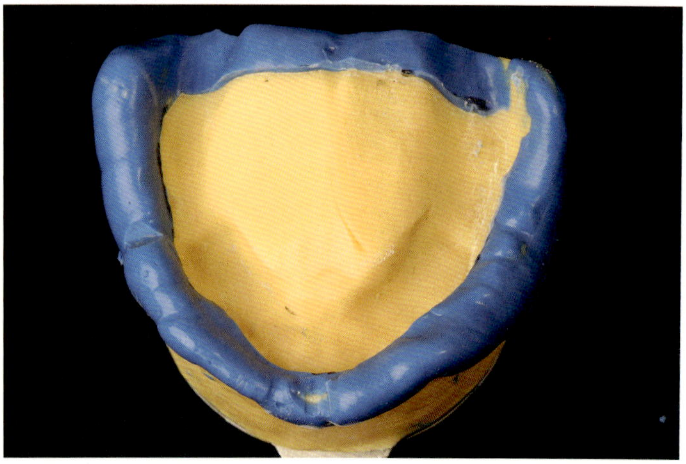

Step7 : Completed border mold

Fig37b Final impression steps for maxillary Difficult-to-Treat case ②. Border molding using heavy body impression material (continued from the previous page).

Final impression steps for maxillary Difficult-to-Treat case ③ The final impression using light body impression material

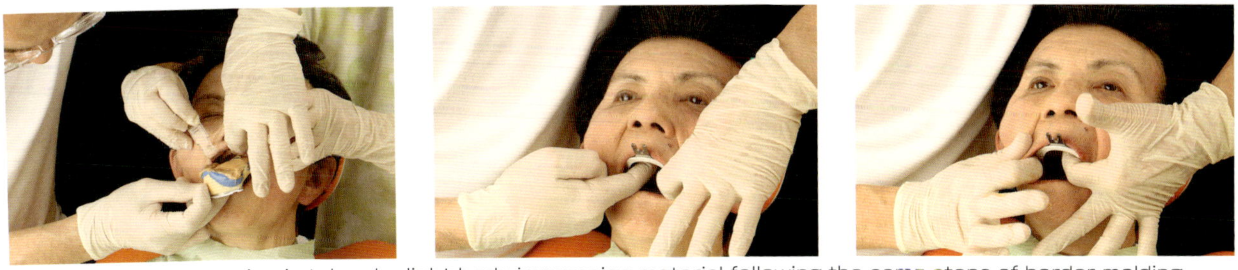

The final impression is taken by light body impression material following the same steps of border molding procedure with heavy body impression material

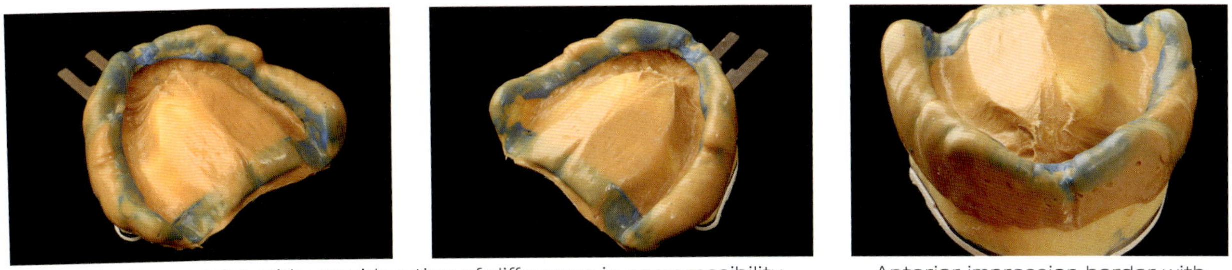

The final impression with consideration of difference in compressibility

Anterior impression border with enough thickness

Fig38 Final impression steps for maxillary Difficult-to-Treat case ③.

Final impression steps for maxillary Difficult-to-Treat case ④ The result

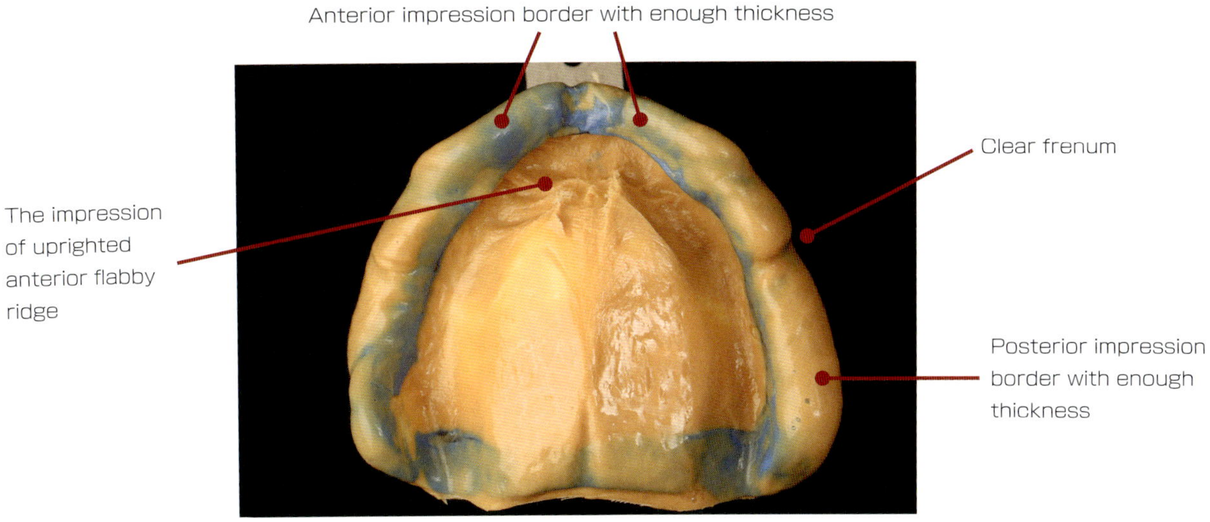

Fig39 Final impression steps for maxillary Difficult-to-Treat case ④. The final impression with consideration of difference in compressibility.

10 Mandibular suction-effect impression for the difficult-to-treat case

(1) Mandibular suction-effect impression for the difficult-to-treat case

This is the difficult case with conditions of severe ridge resorption, extensive tongue retraction when the mouth is opened, the genial tubercle and lack of spongy tissue in the sublingual fold region.

Retromolar pad area and lingual side are two regions difficult to be sealed in mandibular complete denture. As mentioned previously, in order to achieve a close contact closure between the internal surface of the tray and the retromolar pad tissue, it is important to improve the fit of the custom tray with self cure acrylic resin prior to the final impression (P105, Fig 33).

And also lingual border seal is easily broken because of the movement of the tongue when the tongue is retracted significantly upon opening the mouth and when the sealing area of the denture border is too small in the case lacking spongy tissue in the sublingual fold region. Moreover, it is difficult to determine the shape of lingual denture base border around the lingnal frenum since functional movement of the oral mucosa is not clearly defined due to existence of the genial tubercle.

(2) Final impression process of difficult-to-treat case

Choice of optional impression technique is determined depending on the result of intra oral exam (P74, Table 1). It is highly recommended to check it before impression procedure. Possible additional optional impression steps in this case are

1) Optional lingual border formation for lingual seal for Difficult-to-Treat case (silicone putty).

2) Optional mandibular labial border formation (silicone putty).

Subsequently, border molding is performed all around using heavy body material followed by final impression under the 5 movement using light body impression material.

It is recommended to use the impression material, which has silicone putty, heavy body (hard), monophase (medium), light body (soft) and extra light body (extra soft).

(3) Optional lingual seal technique for Difficult-to-Treat case using silicone putty

Border molding technique to seal lingual border using silicone putty is introduced. The purposes are to fill the space created as the result of the tongue retraction upon opening mouth and to record the movement of the mucosa covering the genial tubercle spine using silicone putty (Fig 40).

Mixed silicone putty is elongated and placed on external surface, where the

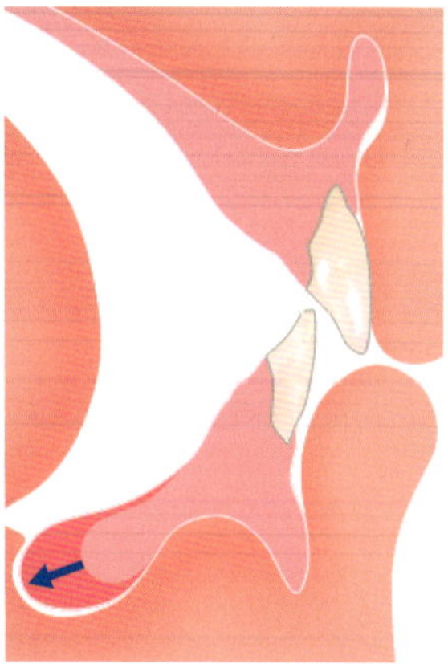

Fig40 The space is created at the lingual border area due to retraction of the tongue upon opening the mouth. Silicone putty is used to fill this space.

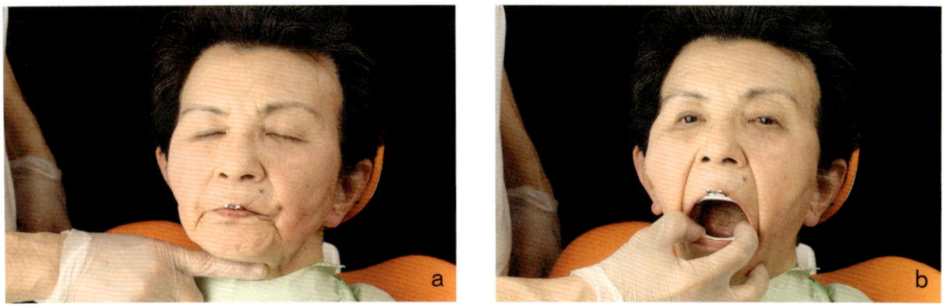

Fig41a, b [Swallowing] (a) and [Opening the mouth slightly larger] (b) are 2 movements, which the patient is instructed to do for sealing technique of lingual side using the silicone putty.

adhesive is applied, of the lingual aspect of the custom tray. The putty should be flattened so that the movement of the tongue is well recorded.

The patient is asked to make 2 movements of [to swallow] and [to open the mouth rather widely] repeatedly (Fig 41).

The patient is asked to keep the mouth closed once the putty starts to harden. Water is provided with the dropper, since swallowing is difficult without saliva. Steps of this technique is shown in Fig 42.

(4) Optional mandibular labial border molding optional technique

As resorption of the mandible progresses, location of the attachment of mentalis muscle changes toward the crest of the anterior alveolar ridge, which limits the thickness of the denture base causing instability of the mandibular denture even with subtle movement of lower lip. The impression of border area should be made rather thick intentionally aiming for expansion of sealing area at the labial border and increase of lip support.

The technique using the silicone putty, same as border molding technique for the optional lingual border seal, is presented. Mixed silicone putty, formed in long narrow shape, is placed external surface of labial aspect of the custom tray, where the adhesive is applied. The silicone putty is formed in flat, which allows more precise adaptation to functional movement (Fig 43).

The patient is asked to do two movements of swallowing and opening the mouth rather widely after adapting the impression material more intimately by lifting the

Border molding of lingual side for lingual seal of Difficult-to-Treat by 2 movements (with silicone putty)

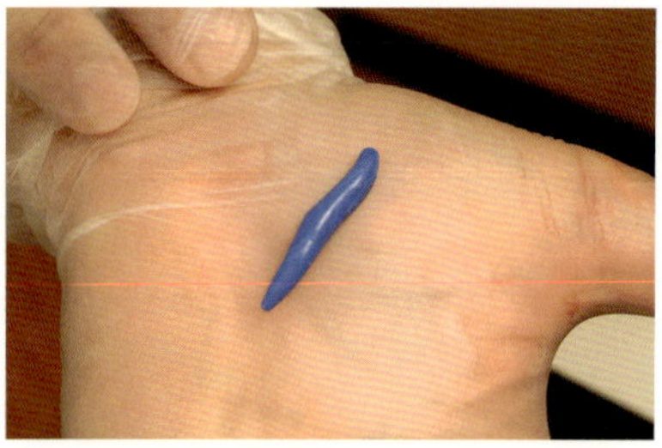

Step1 : Mixed silicone putty is molded to sausage shape

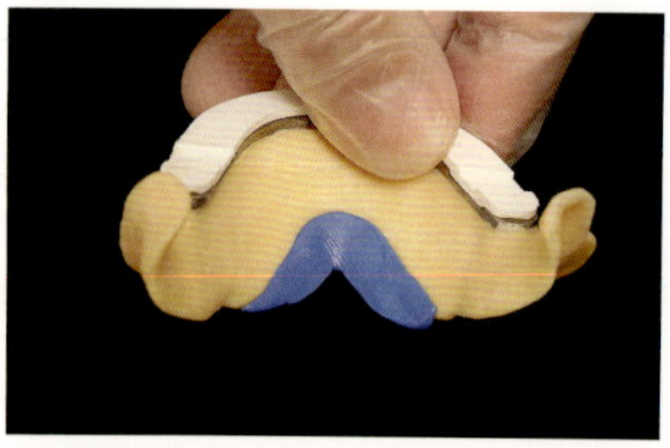

Step2 : The putty is placed between deflection points of S shape curve after application of adhesive on anterior lingual region of the tray

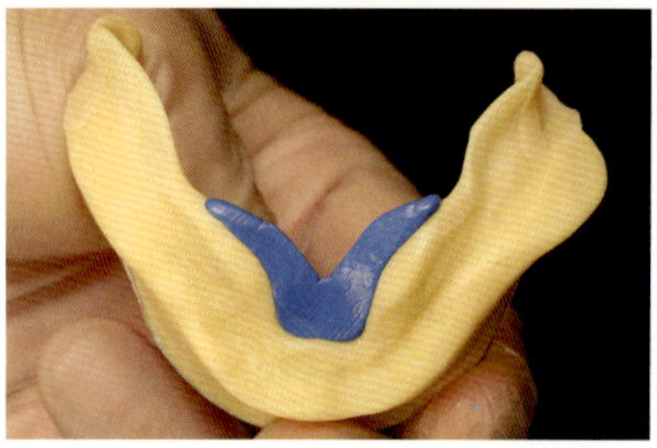

Step3 : The trick is to mold the putty flat

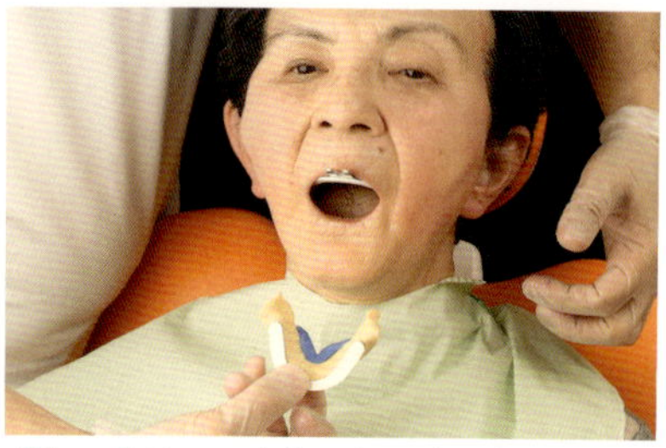

Step4 : Insert the tray in the mout

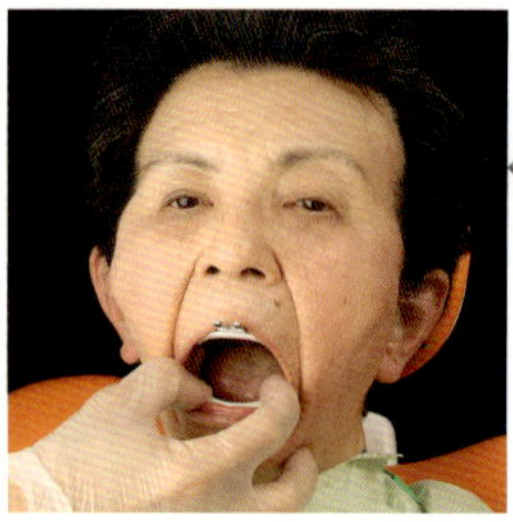

Step5

Repeat 2~3 times

Patient is asked to swallow, then open slightly larger and wait for 10 seconds to swallow again. This movements are repeated 2~3 times

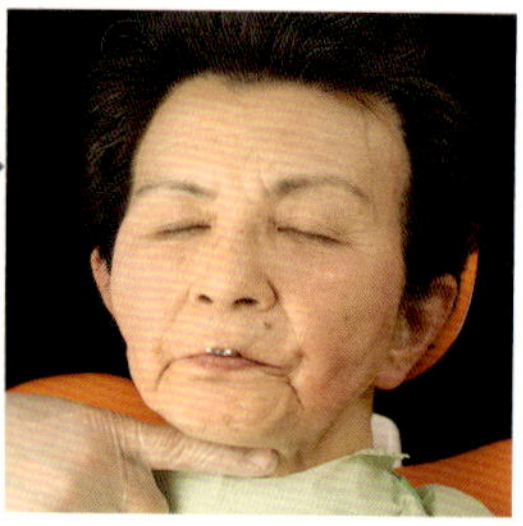

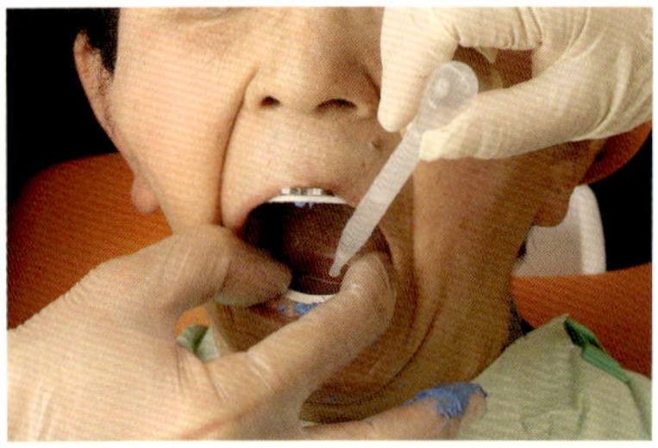

Step6 : Water is applied with the syringe

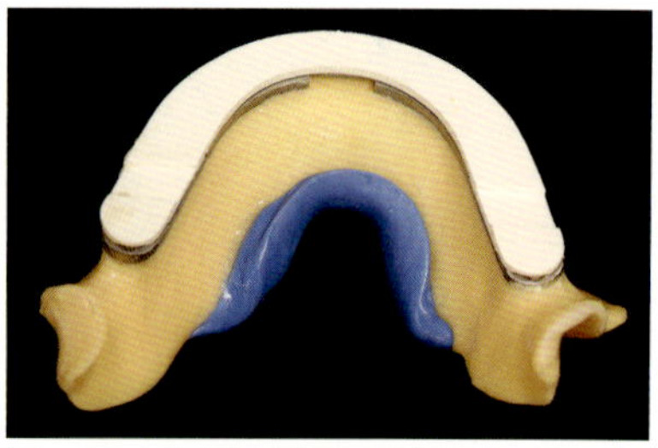

Step7 : Molded lingual border by 2 movements (occlusal view)

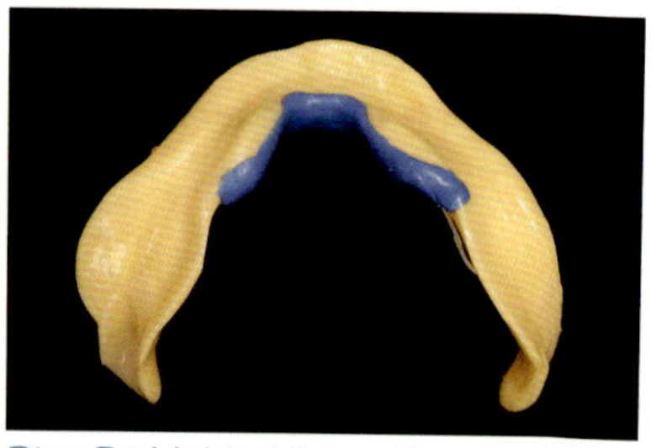

Step8 : Molded lingual border by 2 movement (lingual view)

Fig42 Border molding of lingual side for lingual seal of Difficult-to-Treat by 2 movements using the silicone putty.

Mandibular labial border molding by 2 movements (with silicone putty)

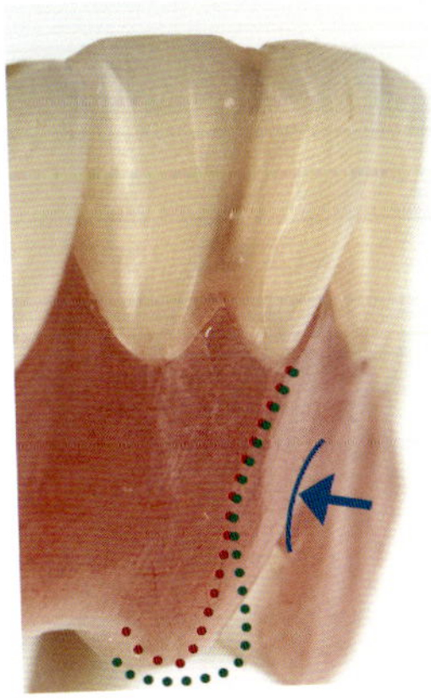

Contact area to mucosa In border area is increased by thickening the border of mandibular anterior region. The concavity on the polished surface, which is necessary for lip support, is readily provided with thick border molding

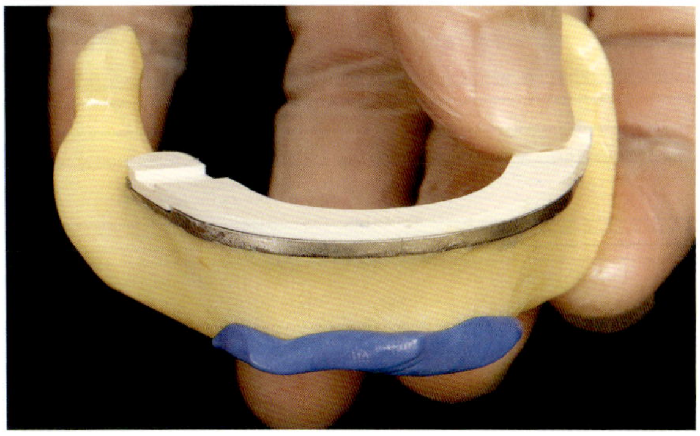

Step1 : Mixed silicone putty is molded to small sausage shape and placed on the external surface of labial side of the tray after the adhesive is applied

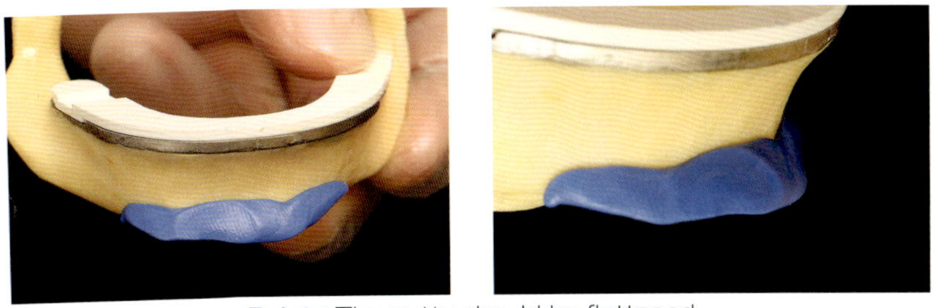

Point : The putty should be flattened

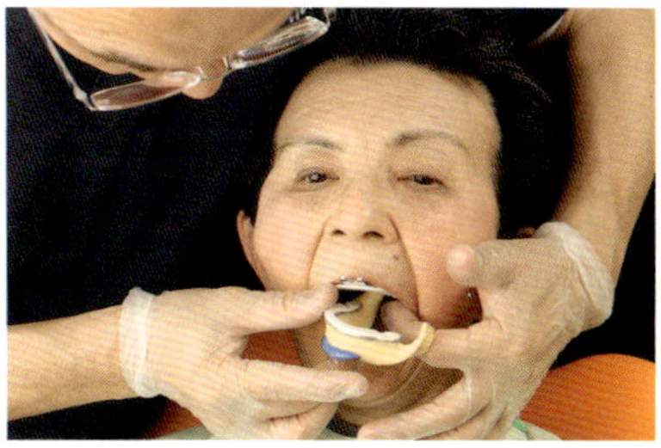

Step2 : The tray is inserted

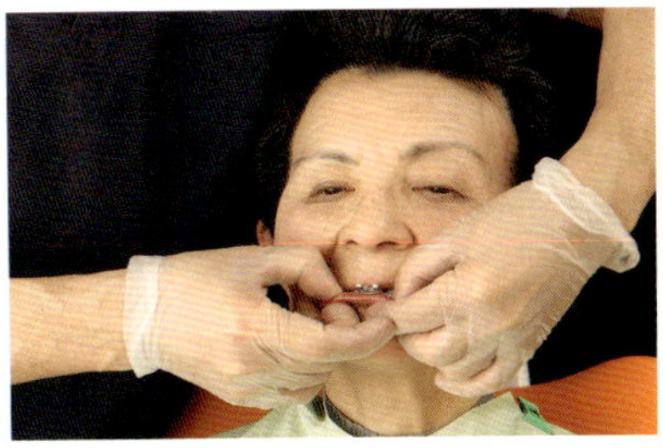

Step3 : Border molding by the operator

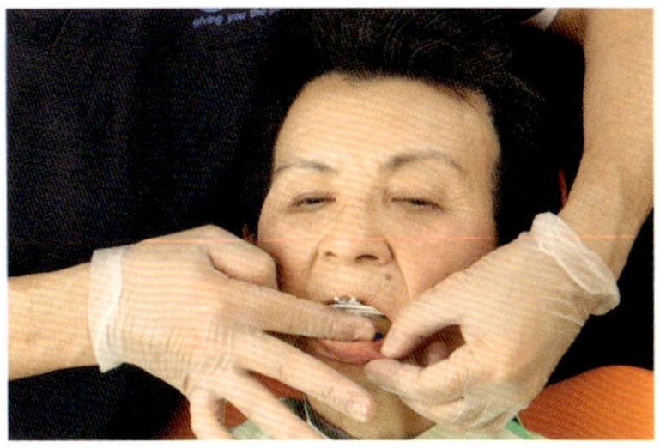

Step4 : The shape of the impression material is modified with fingers

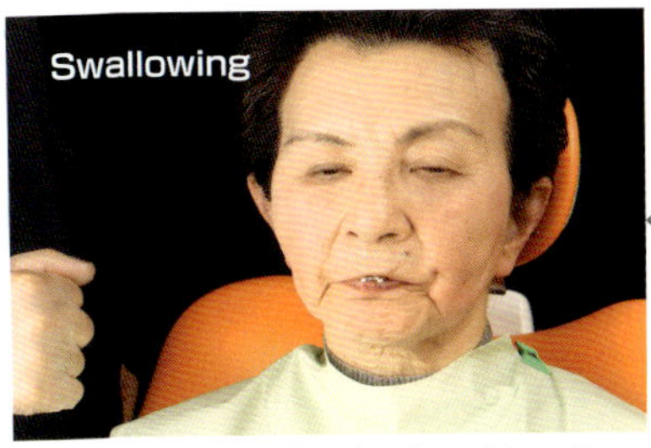

Border molding by functional movement of the patient (swallowing)

Step5 : Repeated

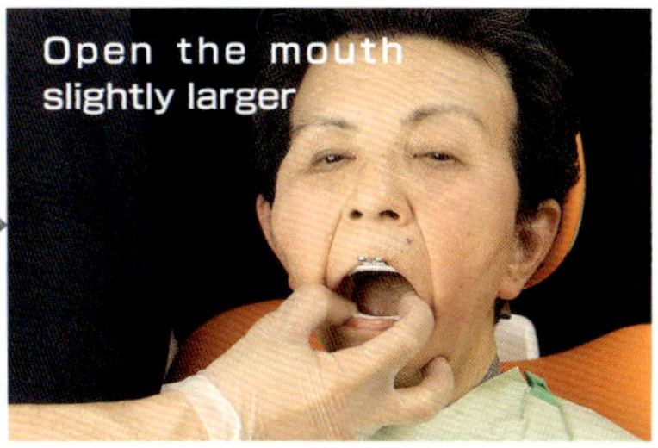

Border molding by functional movement of the patient (opening the mouth)

Fig43 Mandibular labial border molding by 2 movements.

Finishing of the tray after border molding

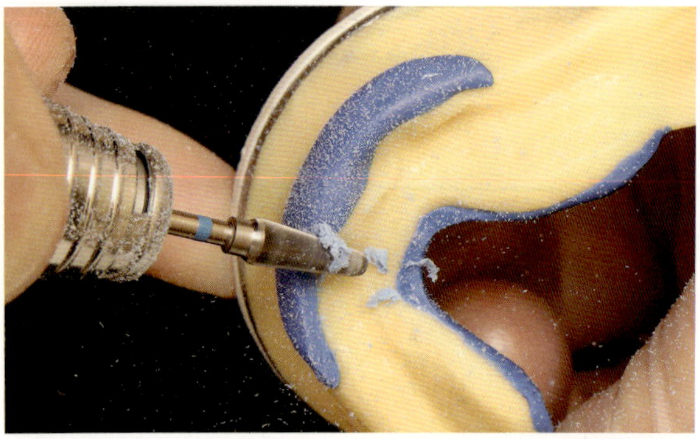

Step1 : It is important to remove impression material inside the tray thoroughly after border molding

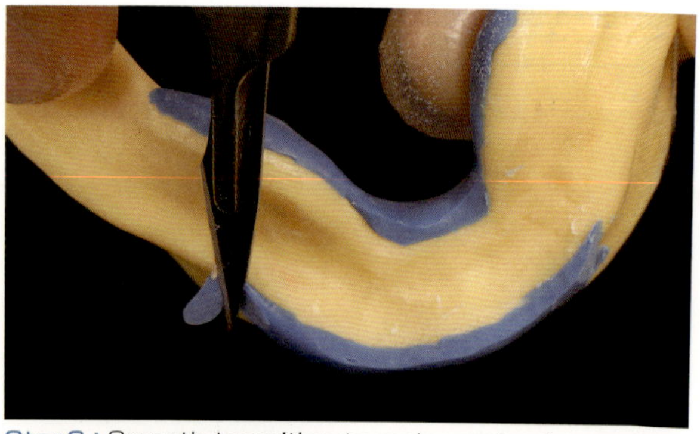

Step2 : Smooth transition to molar region is created

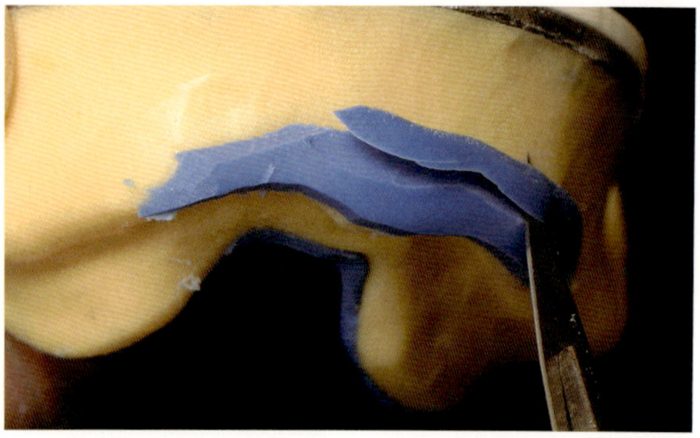

Step3 : Proper concave shape is formed on labial polished surface

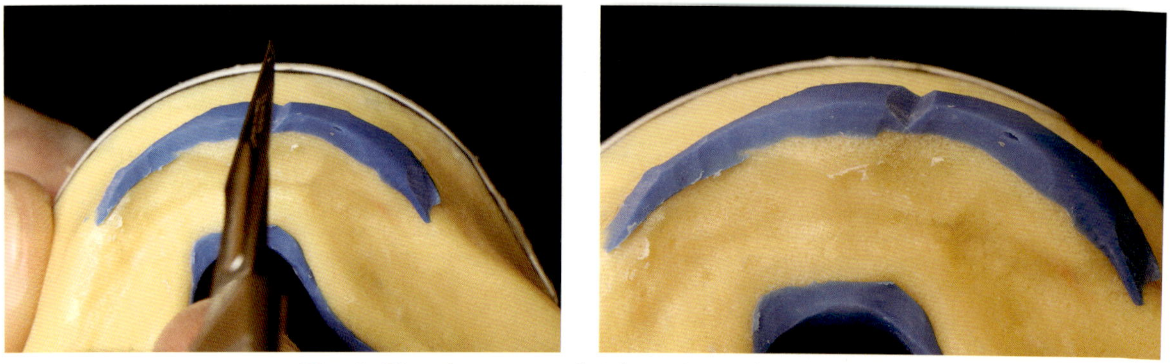

Step4 : Clear frenum area is trimmed away in V shape

Fig44 Finishing of the tray after border molding.

Fig45 Vaseline is applied on posterior portion of the maxillary tray as part of the preparation for mandibular final impression.

Preparation for mandibular final impression

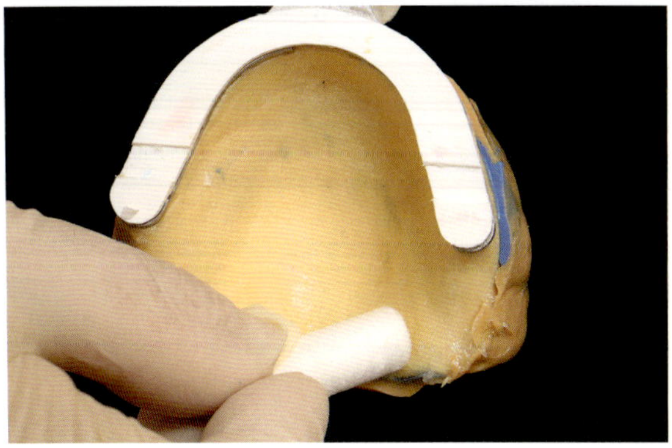

Posterior portion of the maxillary tray to prevent adhesion of excess impression material of mandibular impression

lip up or molding it by the operator's finger since activity of the mentalist muscle is rather subtle only being activated during swallowing. The mandibular denture is pushed strongly posteriorly by tension of the lower lip upon opening the mouth. This activity needs to be recorded in the impression. The patient is asked to keep the mouth closed once setting of the impression material is initiated.

Following procedures are important to remove impression material on internal surface of the custom tray, to make V-shaped cut where the impression of lingual frenum is clearly recorded and to make smooth transition toward molar region once the modification of the custom tray is completed (Fig 44).

11 Border molding and final impression of the mandibular complete denture

Vaseline is applied to the posterior surface of maxillary custom tray (Fig 45). All mandibular denture border is molded and final impression is taken under 5 basic movements, which is consistent with those movements for the simple case.

Monophase impression material is used for border molding of the retromolar pad area in order to minimize distortion of the area and heavy body material is used for rest of the border (Fig 46) during the first stage of the functional impression (Fig 47). The order of these movements does not affect the quality of the final impression.

Excess impression material is trimmed away (Fig 48), then the second stage of functional impression is taken with the same 5 movements using the light body impression material (Fig 49, 50).

Final impression and whole circumference border molding with 5 basic movements (Monophase & Heavybody impression material)

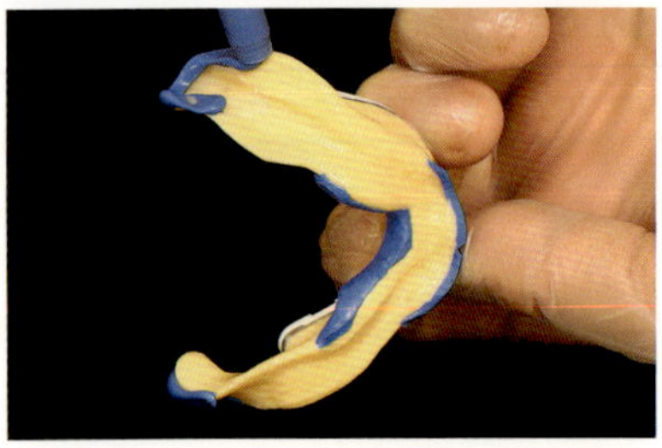

Step1: Monophase impression material is used in the retromolar pad area for the purpose of minimizing compressive deformation due to hardness of the impression material

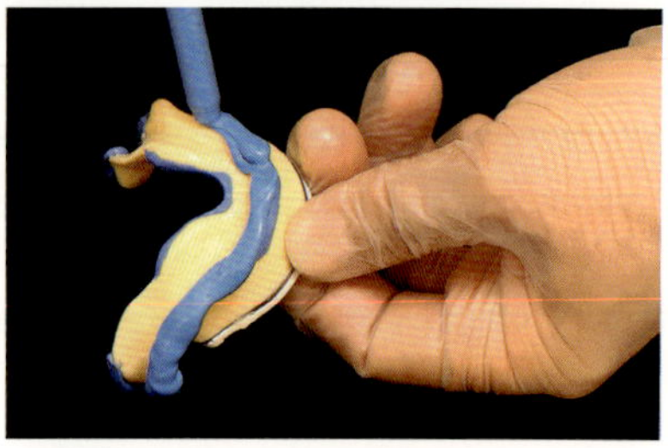

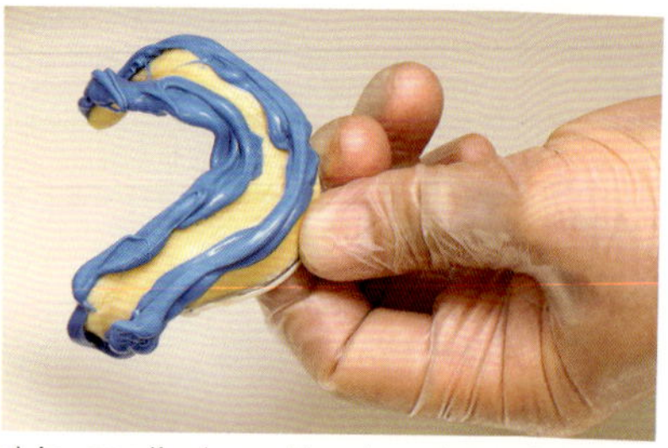

Step2: Heavy body impression material is applied on the border of other areas. layers of heavy body impression material is applied in molar buccal shelf region for the purpose of obtaining enough stress bearing area if the patient has soft buccal mucosa, which can be stretched out

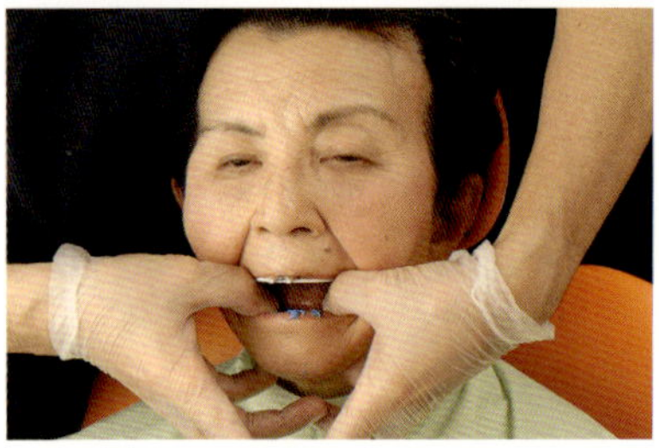

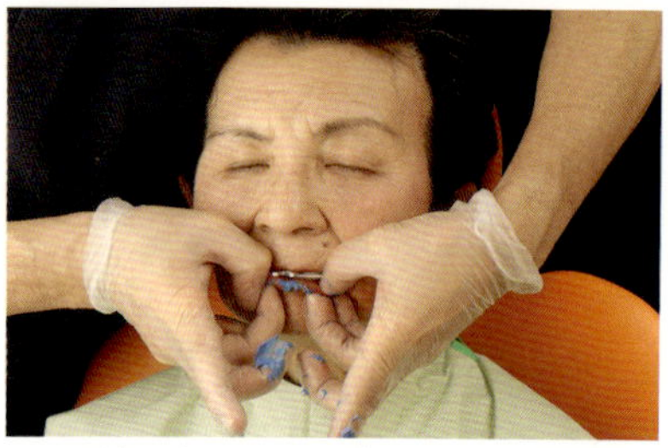

Step3: The tray, filled with impression material, is inserted in the patient' s mouth. Correct positioning of the tray is difficult in severely ridge resorption case. Once the position is confirmed to be correct, the tray is pressed for 7 seconds. The patient is asked to do 5 movements at this point

Fig46 Preparation of the mandibular custom tray for border molding.

5 movements for the basic impression

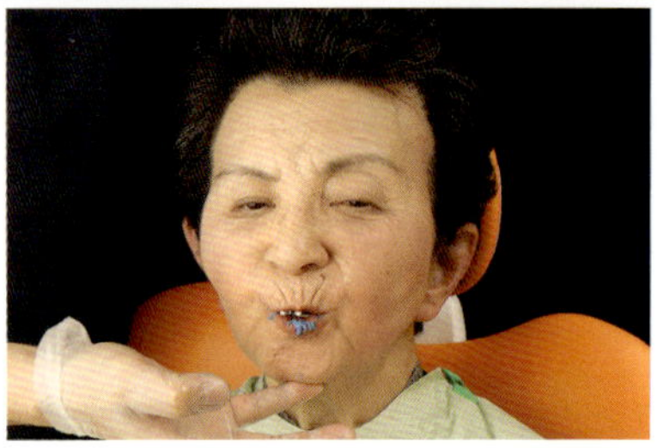

Step1: Let the patient purse the lips: "Woo" (movement of cheeks and lips)

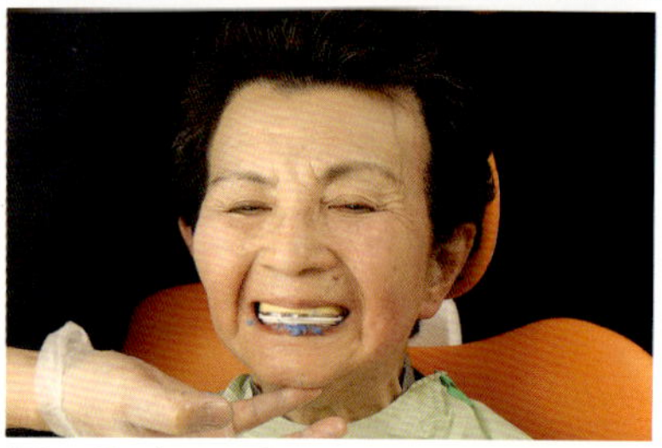

Step2: Let the patient pull the corners of the mouth: "Eee" (movement of cheeks and lips)

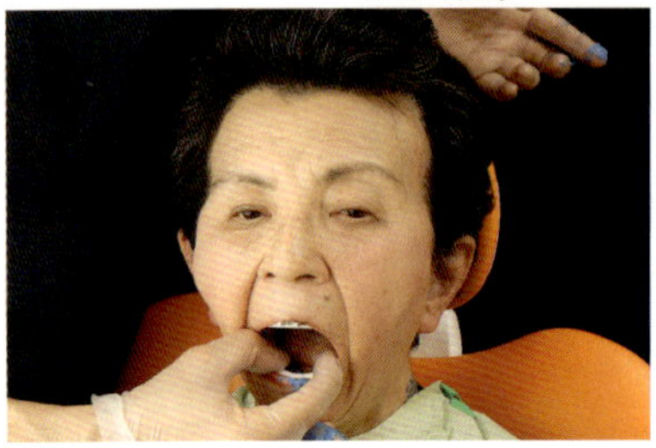

Step3: Let the patient open the mouth and move the tongue lightly from right to left (movement of base of the tongue and lower lip)

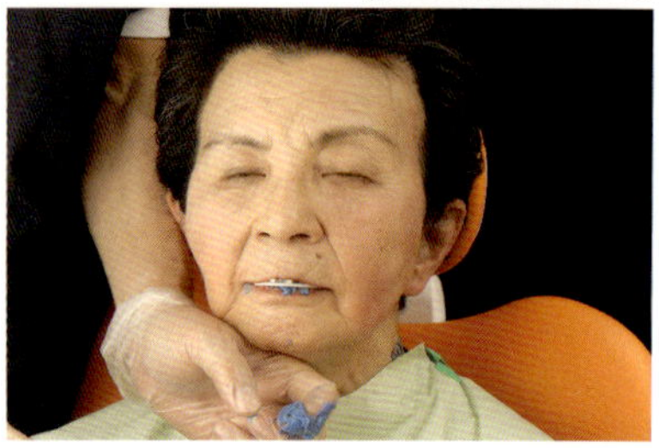

Step4: Let the patient close the mouth and push back of anterior region of the tray with the tongue (the floor of the mouth in tension)

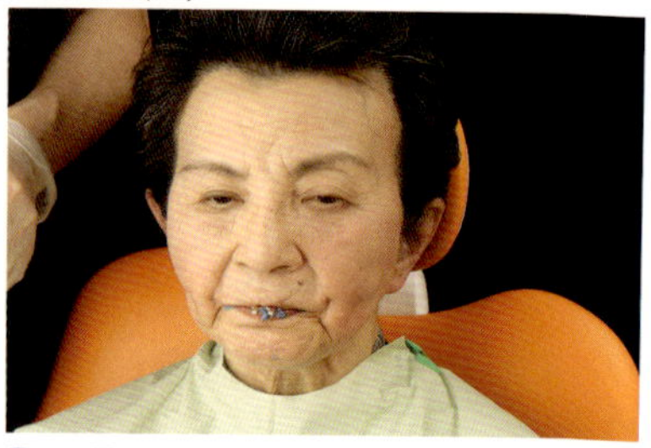

Step5: Let the patient swallow (overall movement of the oral cavity)

Fig47 5 movements for the basic impression.

Finishing after border molding

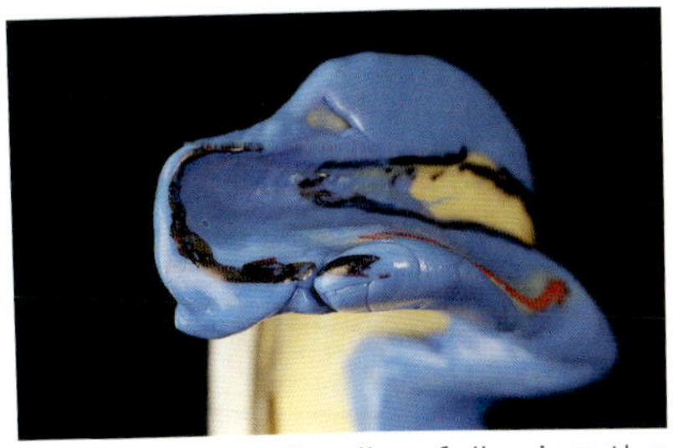

Step1 : Draw the line following the outline of the retromolar pad

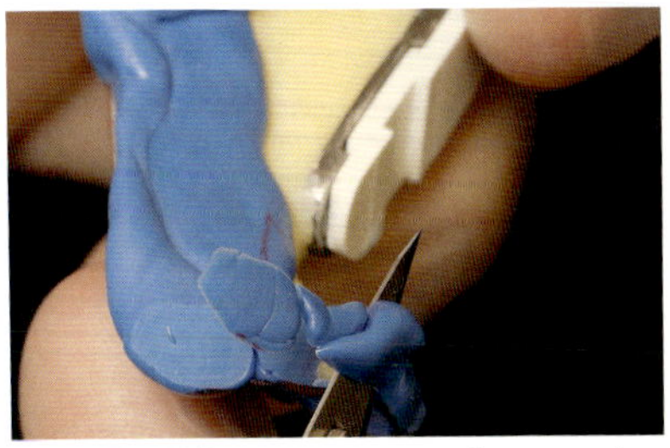

Step2 : Trim excess impression material away following the line

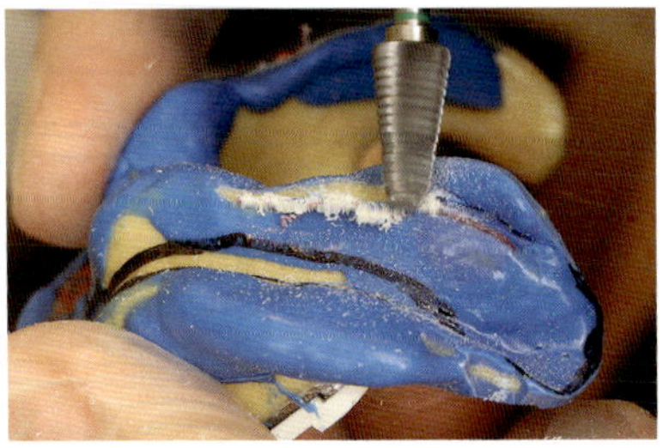

Step3 : Trim the impression material away in the area with compressed area

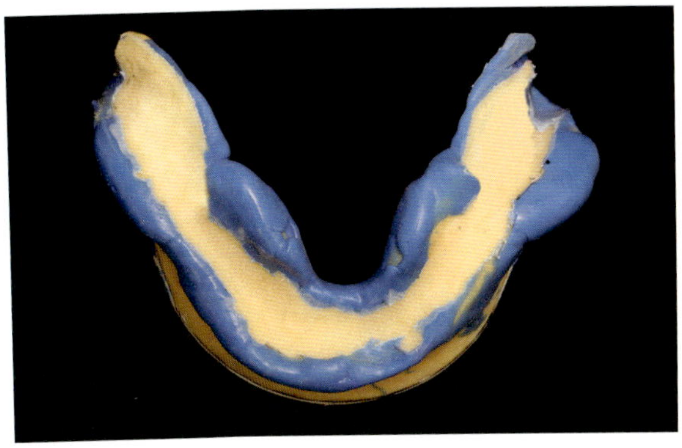

Step4 : Then, impression material of compressed area and ridge crest region with poor displaceability is trimmed away. It is not necessary to relieve anterior 1/2 of retromolar pad with no fibrous tissue as shown in this case

Fig48 Finishing after border molding.

Final impression procedure with basic 5 movements (light body impression material)

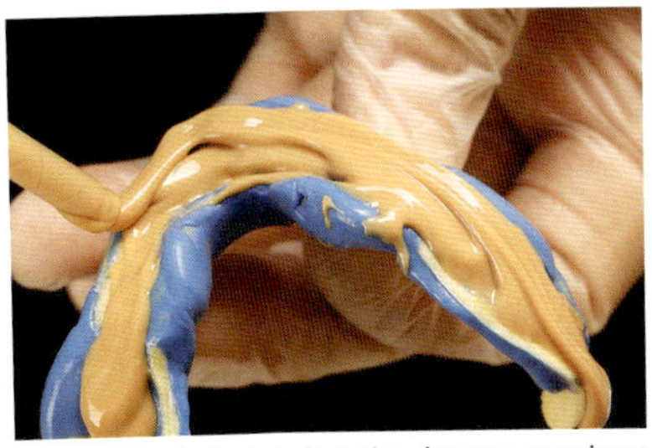

Step1 : Light body impression material is loaded on the tray

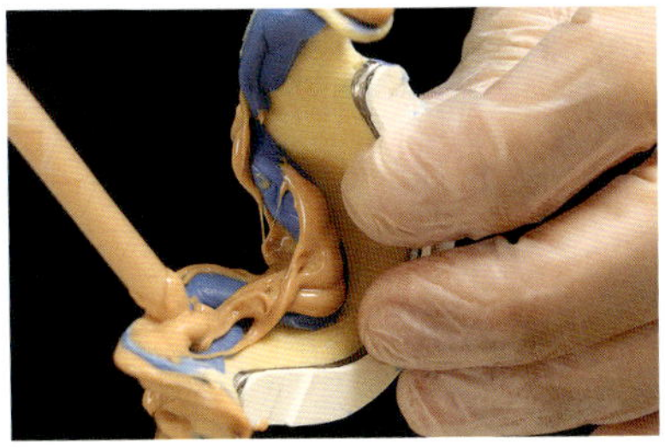

Step2 : Impression material is applied on the extended border molded area of lingual anterior region

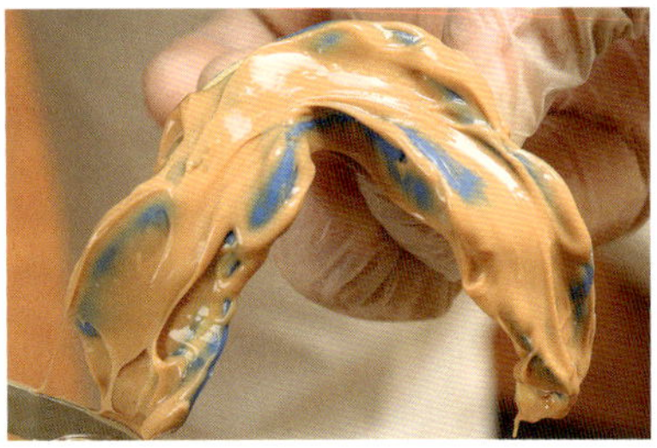

Step3 : Impression material is spread out to buccal and lingual side using the spatula

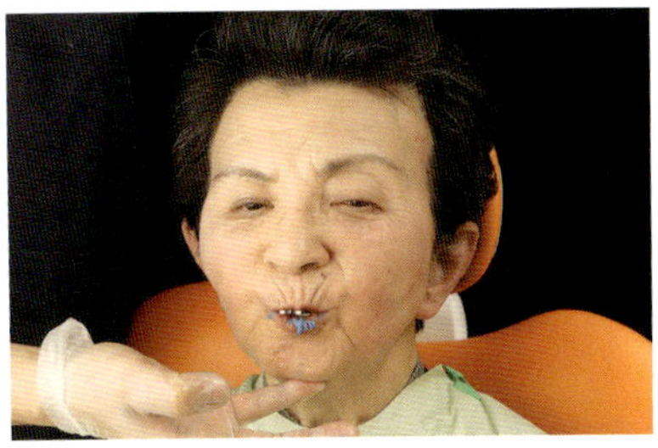

Step4 :

Basic 5 movements, shown in Fig 47, is repeated 2 to 3 times (repeat count depends on the temperature of the operating room or the type of the impression material)

Fig49 Final impression procedure with basic 5 movements (light body impression material).

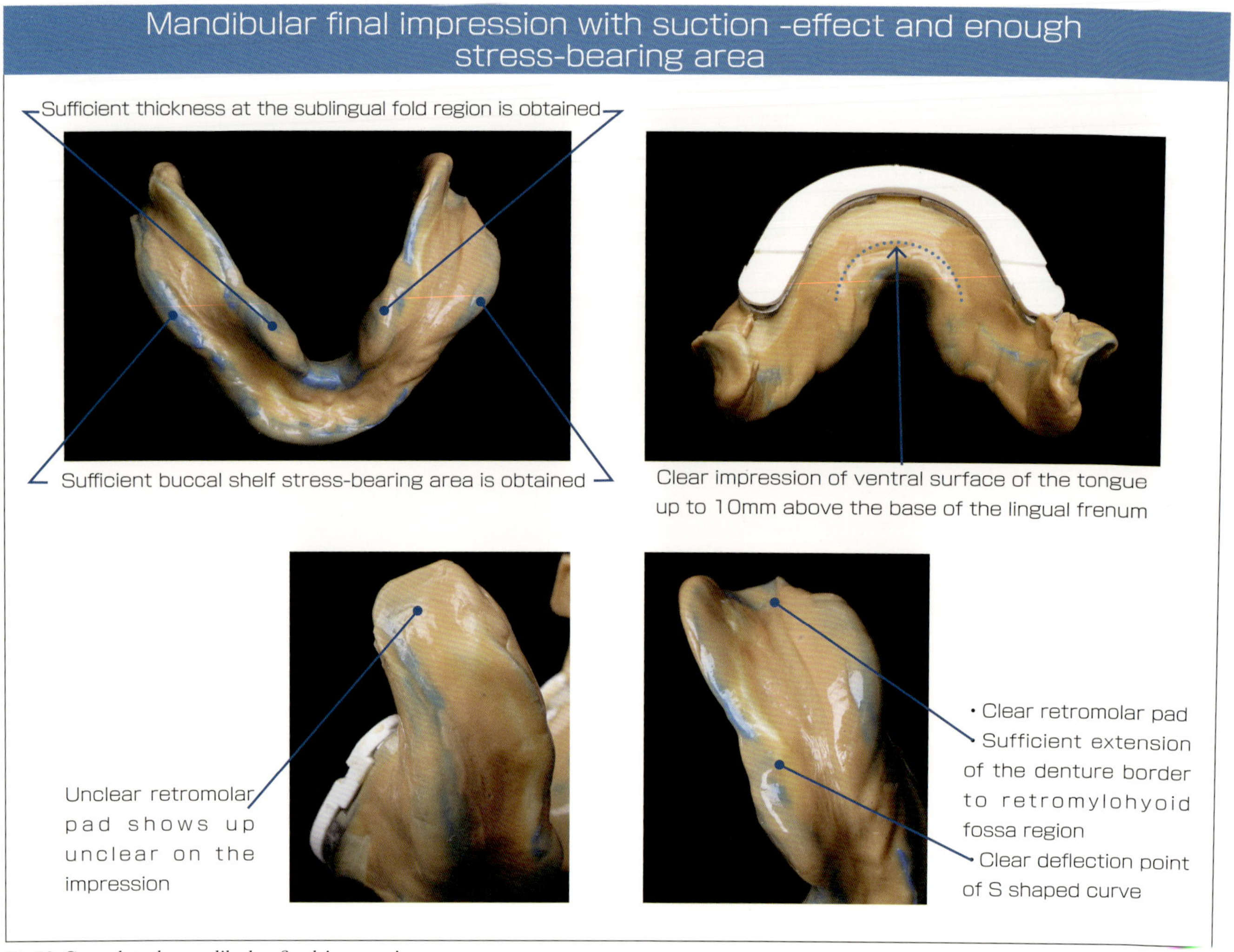

Fig50 Completed mandibular final impression.

12 Boxing

Lingual seal can be easily broken under the combination of conditions of excessive tongue retraction when the mouth is opened and lack of spongy tissue with the existence of the genial tubercle. In order to achieve adequate seal at the lingual frenum area in such as this case, it is required to increase the contact area to ventral surface of the tongue utilizing polished surface of the lingual border area for the seal. Boxing line is set 1cm above the border and this area is reproduced into the final denture resin to facilitate the seal. Lingual denture border of this area is rather thick, but patients seldom complain about pain or discomfort (Fig 51, 52).

Fig51 Boxing position for the case of tongue retraction. Most important information is contained in the area between the impression border to 5mm above to it. Suction-effect of the final denture is usually achieved by replacing this area of 5mm accurately by the resin.

Contact seal between ventral surface of the tongue and polished surface of the denture is necessary to prevent air leak from lingual denture border area in Difficult-to-Treat case. Boxing line is higher than usual since about 10mm from the border needs to be replaced by the resin.

Boxing for the case, with which lingual suction-effect would be difficult to achieve ①

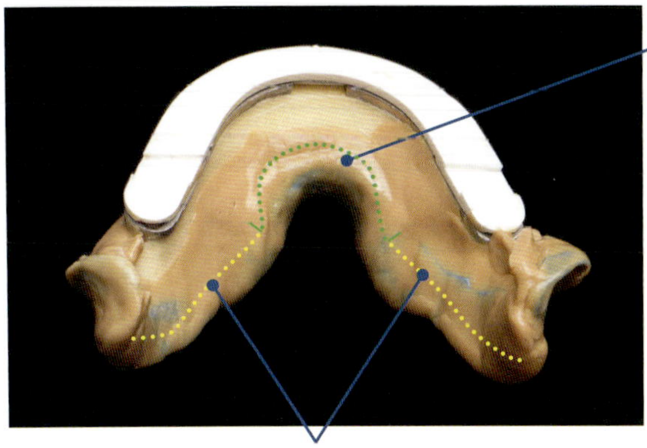

Boxing for the case, with which lingual suction-effect would be difficult to achieve ② : using the model block

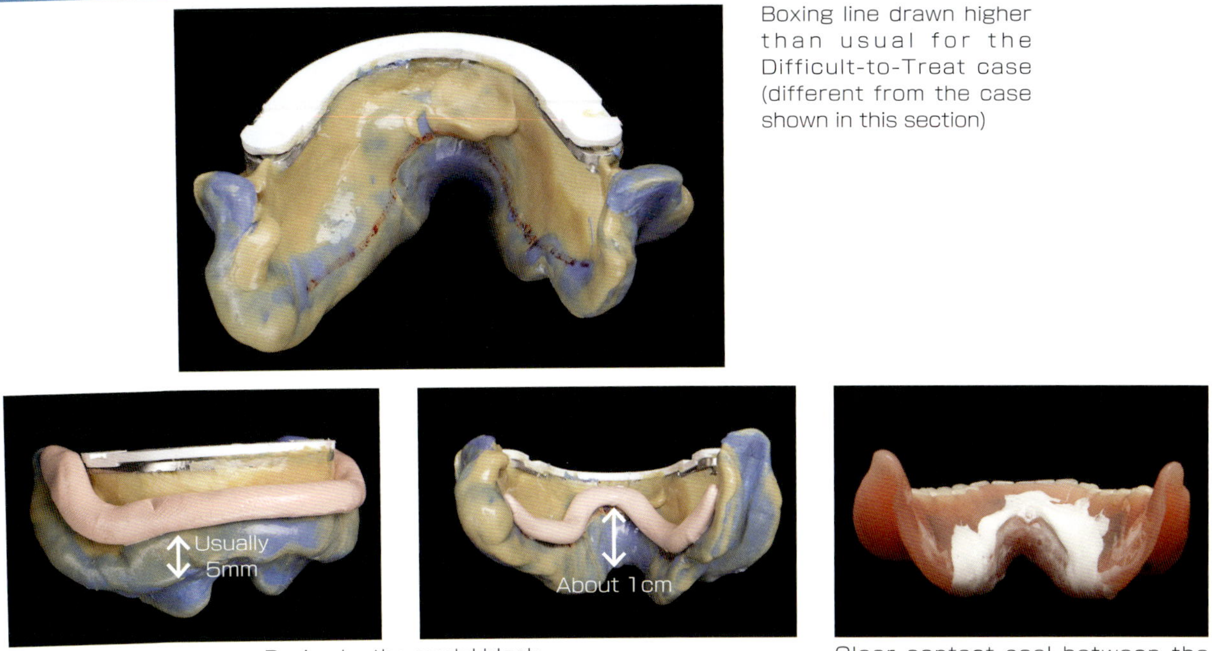

Fig52 Example of boxing for the case of retruded tongue with another case.

13 Functional post dam for the difficult-to-treat case (maximizing the posterior seal of maxillary complete denture)

(1) The role of functional post dam in the difficult-to-treat case

There are two techniques for providing post dam. One is conventional technique by curving in the soft palate part of the master cast, which has higher displaceability than hard palate so that the denture base of the area sinks into the soft palate, which is considered to be the conventional method. The other technique, functional post dam technique, is rendered directly in the patient's mouth (Fig 53). While waiting for the final impression of the mandible to be completed, it is often found that suction-effect of maxillary impression becomes weaker. This is because the completed maxillary impression is pushed in anterior-upward direction.

Close contact closure of maxillary posterior border tends to be broken due to upward-anterior rotation of maxillary and mandibular impression unit in occlusion in cases with maxillary flabby ridge or anterior open bite. Providing the post dam arbitrarily on the cast would not be sufficient for difficult-to-treat cases, since it is difficult to anticipate the degree of rotational displacement of the impression unit and related seal break for each case. Functional post dam technique, which is achieved by asking the patient to swallow with the monophase impression material applied on posterior region of the final impression, is utilized for these cases to improve seal-effect (Fig 54).

Posterior border seal according the degree of inclination of the denture in occlusion can be achieved with this technique. The author employs functional post dam technique for most of cases except for severe open bite case with severe flabby ridge, in which both functional and conventional post dams are provided.

2 Types of post dam

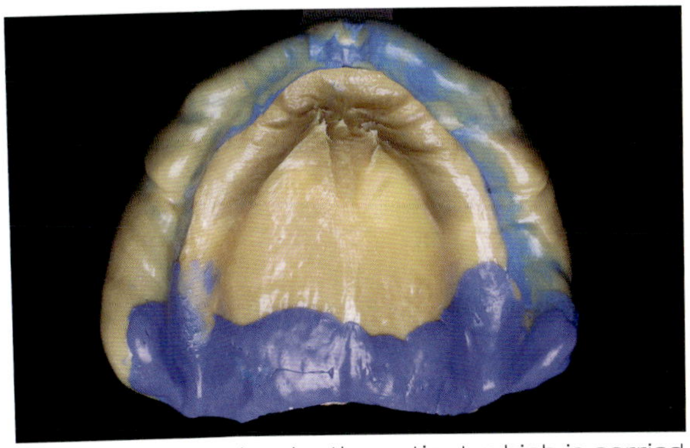

Functional post dam by the patient, which is carried out after the final impression

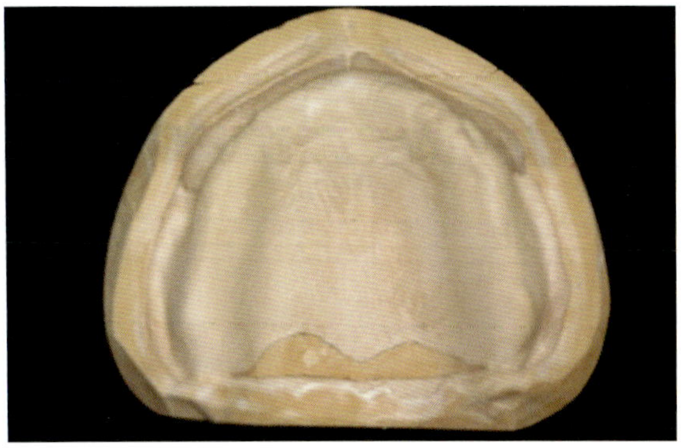

The post dam curved on the model by the technician

Fig53 2 Types of post dam.

Clinical steps of functional post dam

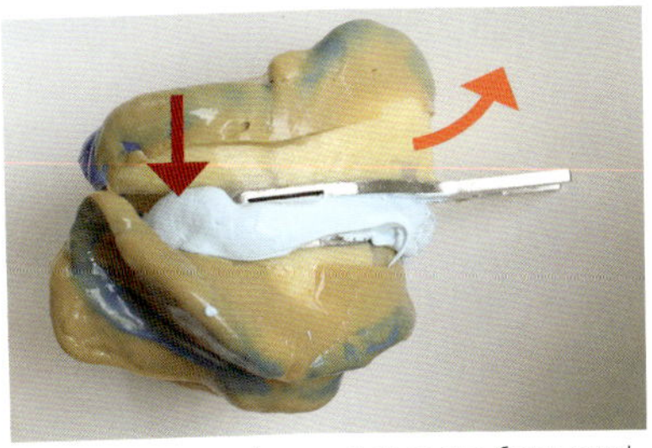

Border is weakened due to forward-upward rotational movement of the maxillary/mandibular impression in cases with maxirally flabby ridge

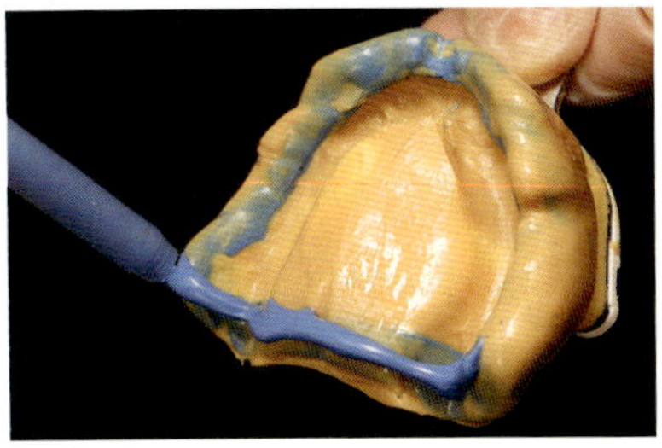

Step1 : One layer of monophase silicone impression material is applied on posterior border area of the maxillary impression

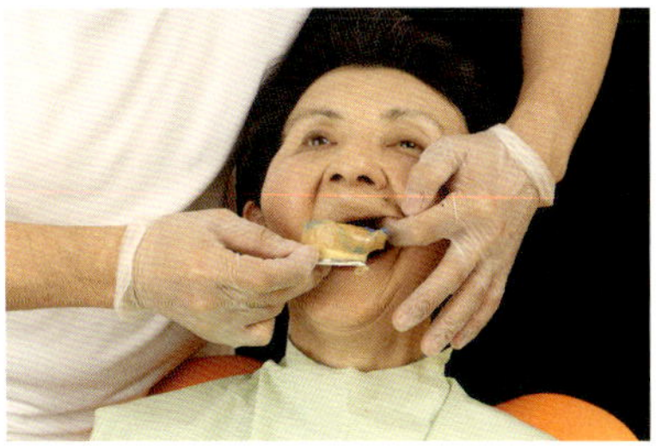

Step2 : It is inserted in the mouth

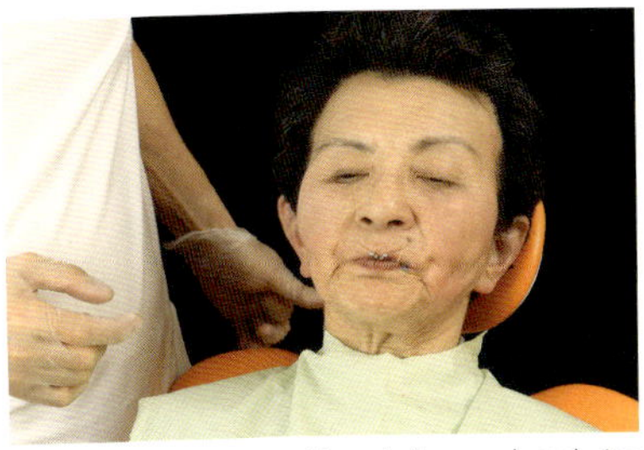

Step3 : The patient is asked to swallow and wait until the impression material is set with the mouth closed and lightly in occlusion

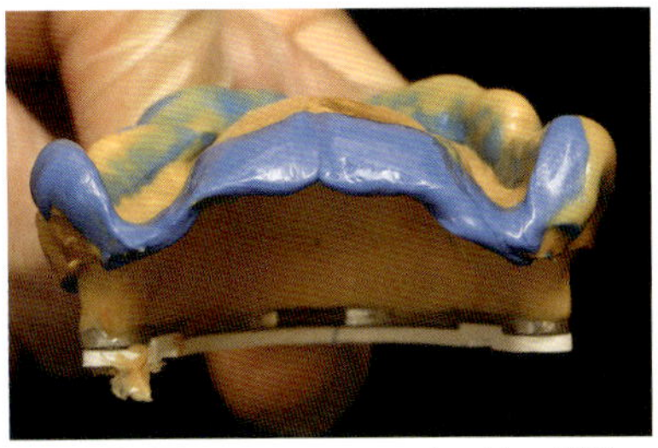

Step4 : The space created by tilting of the impression is filled with the impression material

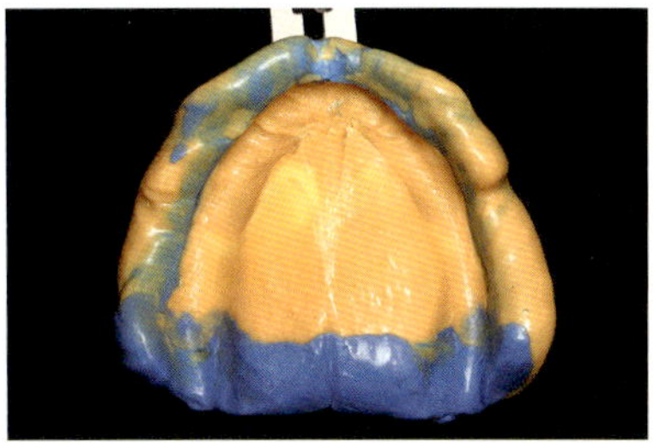

Step5 : Completion of functional post dam

Fig54 Clinical steps of functional post dam.

14 Confirmation of occlusal vertical dimension (VDO) and Gothic arch Pin-Tracing

Maxillary and mandibular impression unit is removed out of the mouth and excess impression material is trimmed away before Gothic arch tracing is carried out. VDO is confirmed then by utilizing vertical dimension at rest, air-blow technique or phonation technique.

(1) Gothic arch

Three dimensional movement of the condyle is recorded on the horizontal plane by Gothic arch tracing. There are 2 purposes of Gothic arch tracing for edentulous case. The first purpose is to find the correct position for the cast to be mounted on the articulator so that denture teeth can be set properly. The second purpose is to grasp the functional condition of the patient's temporomandibular joint from the Gothic arch tracing and reflect it to occlusal adjustment during mandibular movement[71-72].

(2) Disadvantages of bite registration with record base and wax rim

Bite registration procedure without Gothic arch tracing just with occlusal wax rim and record base has some disadvantages.

1) The procedure is performed without eliminating the memory of the patient's habitual mandibular position.
2) Fit of the record base is not as good, since it is made on the master cast relieved with the wax.
3) It is difficult to soften the wax rim evenly.
4) Information of temporomandibular joint cannot be obtained.

(3) Gothic arch tracing using the Gnathometer M

Sensory Deprogramming[73-75] and taking bite registration record with impression unit, which should have superior fit, are the significant advantage of using Gnathometer M, which is a part of BPS system (Fig 55-57). The memory of the patient's habitual mandibular position from the existing denture is almost completely eliminated during the one hour of the final impression procedure. Gothic arch tracing is carried out right after the final impression is taken in BPS denture fabricating system using Gnathometer M.

First, VDO is taken arbitrarily with Centric Tray. Next, VDO is taken more accurately right after final impression is taken. Finally, horizontal mandibular position is taken with Gothic arch tracing. It is the unique characteristics of BPS system that the accuracy of the record improves as the procedure progresses.

Final measurement of VDO after the final impression

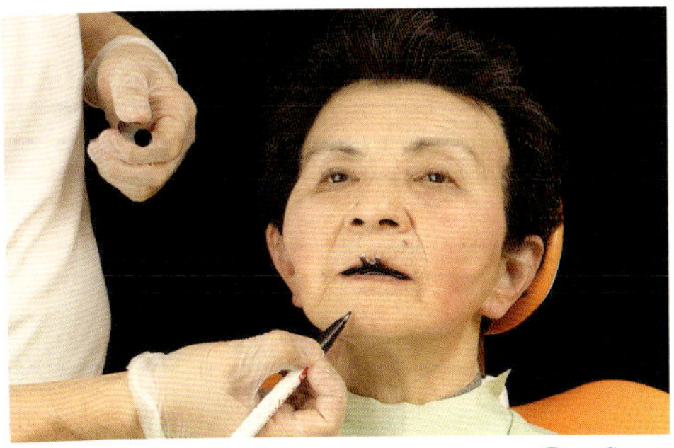
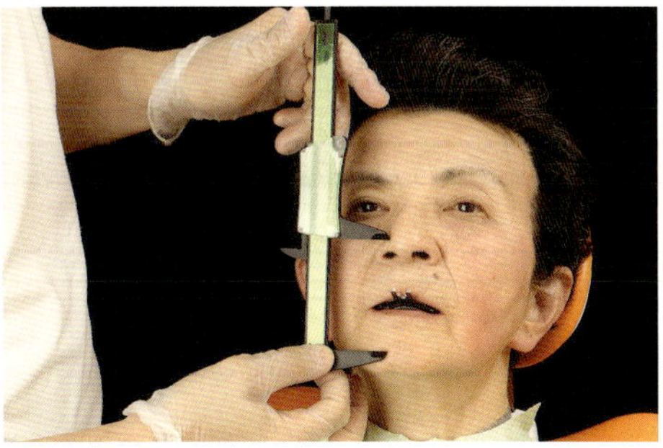

Confirmation of VDO

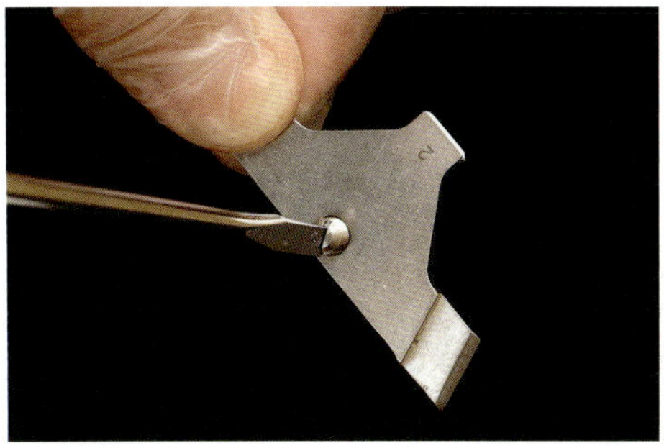

Adjustment of VDO (the tracing pin moves 1mm by full turn, adjustable between -2mm ~ +6mm)

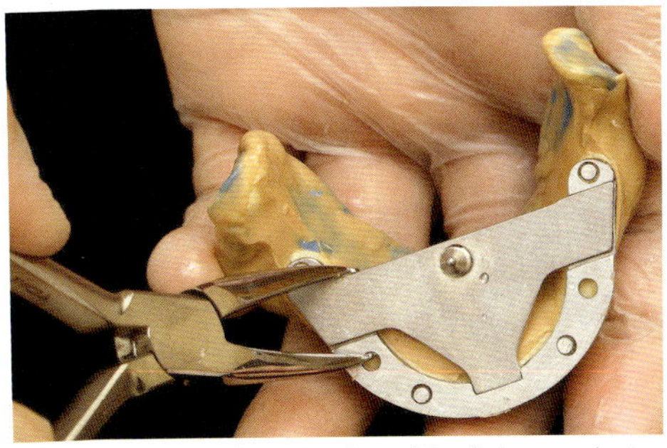
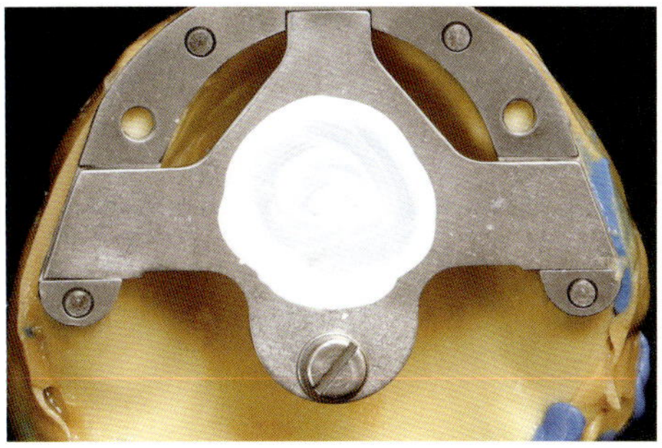

The registration stylus (Gothic arch tracing pin) of Gnathometer M is set on the mandibular tray and the registration plate, which is painted, is set on the maxillary tray

Fig55 Final measurement of VDO after the final impression.

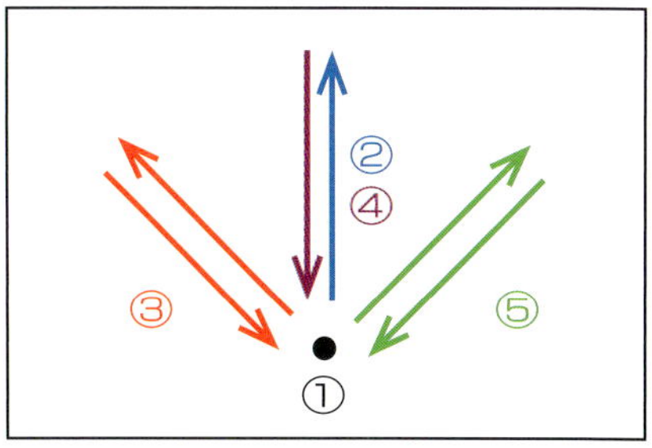

Fig56 Gothic arch tracing order by Baba[88].

(4) Apex point and tapping point

The tapping point and the apex point, which is the tip of the Gothic arch, coincide in only 12% of edentulous people. The tapping point is located at 0.5 ~ 1.0 mm anterior to the apex point in majority of edentulous people[76, 77].

The tapping point is adopted as the treatment position which is optimized by the occulusal adjustment, if it is stably positioned anteriorly within 2 mm of the apex point.

Many edentulous patients carry various types of structural problems of the temporomandibular joint and functional problems of condyle due to deformation of the condyle or the glenoid fossa, such as rounded apex area of the Gothic arch, more than 5 mm of discrepancy between the apex and the tapping points, discrepancy in outward and inward path or asymmetric lateral border movement. The treatment denture utilizing flat tables is useful to find the stable mandibular position before transition to the definitive denture[78, 79]. The obtained information of the condyle path is reflected on adjustment of occlusal surface, such as a choice of denture teeth, occlusal scheme or establishment of wide centric or long centric. Number of patient's visit for denture adjustment decreases as a result[71].

(5) Clinical technique for efficient Gothic arch tracing

Active method, in which the Gothic arch is drawn by patient's unforced movement, is adopted at present time rather than the passive technique, in which the patient's mandible is guided by the operator forcefully[80]. The position, obtained by forced guidance, is not necessarily the comfortable and functional position for the edentulous patient, whose glenoid fossa is loose and mandibular condyle is deformed.

It is effective to indicate the direction of the movement just by touching the chin of the patient.

Baba's method is the most effective tracing order to learn[81] (Fig 56), which is described below. The most retruded position after tapping → anterior position → the most retruded position → right lateral movement → posterior position → anterior position → left lateral movement. It is important to adopt anterior - posterior movement prior to to each lateral movement for resetting of the memory of the other lateral movement in order to have the patient draw shape properly in a short period of time.

Gothic arch tracing (upright position)

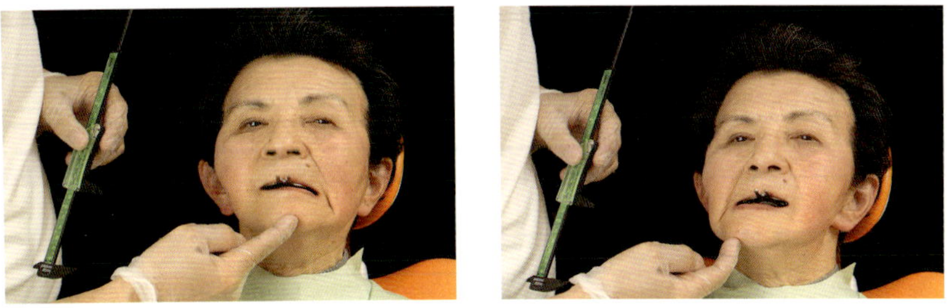

Step1 : Training: It is checked if the tracing pin does not collide to the screw, which stabilizes the tracing plate on the maxillary tray. Interference during movement between maxillary tuberosity and retromolar pad is checked as well

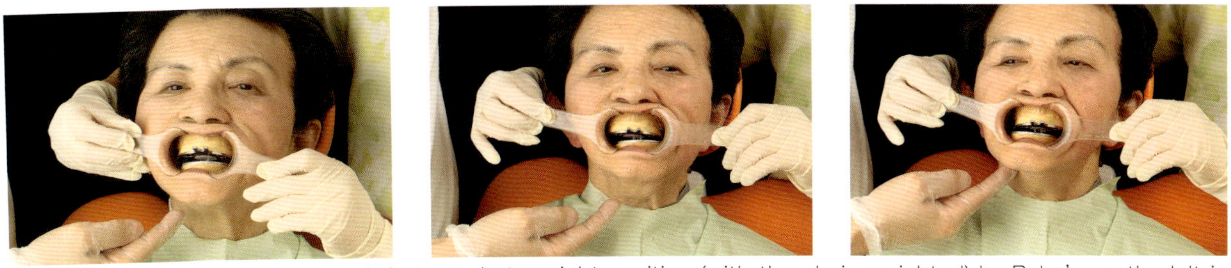

Step2 : Clinical steps: Gothic arch is traced at upright position (with the chair uprighted) by Baba' s method. It is important not to guide the patient' s mandible forcefully. The tapping point is marked with the occlusal paper after gothic arch tracing is confirmed

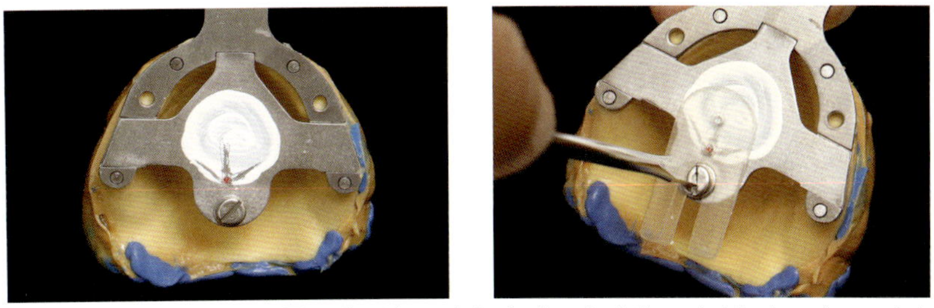

Step3 : Clinical steps: The fixation plate is fixed at the stable tapping point, after Gothic arch tracing by Baba' s method

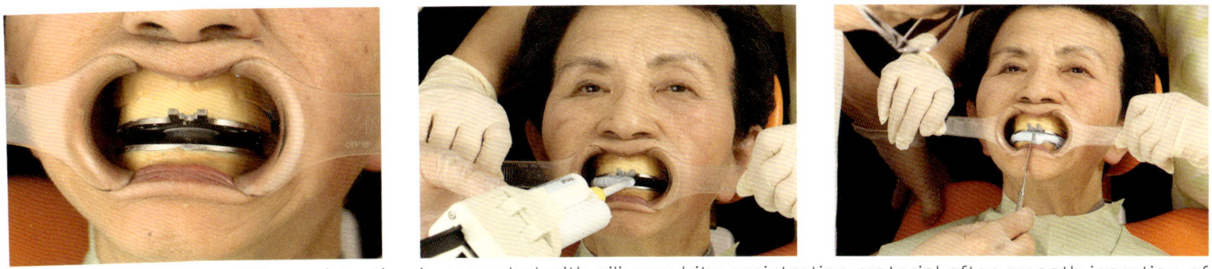

Step4 : Clinical steps: Bite registration is recorded with silicone bite registration material after smooth insertion of the stylus pin into the hole of the fixation plate without interference is confirmed when the patient is asked to close the mouth

Fig57 Steps of Gothic arch tracing.

Face bow transfer

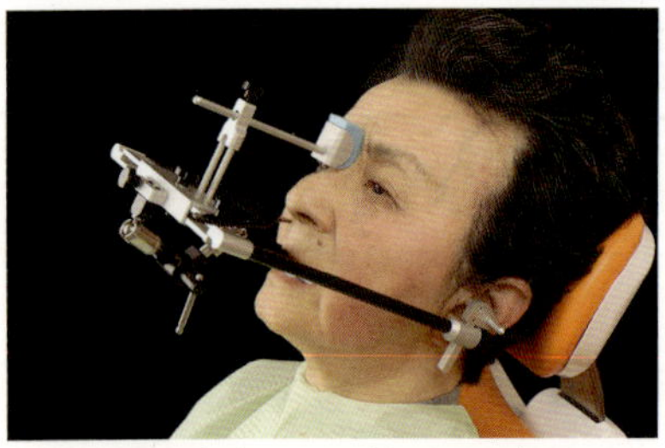

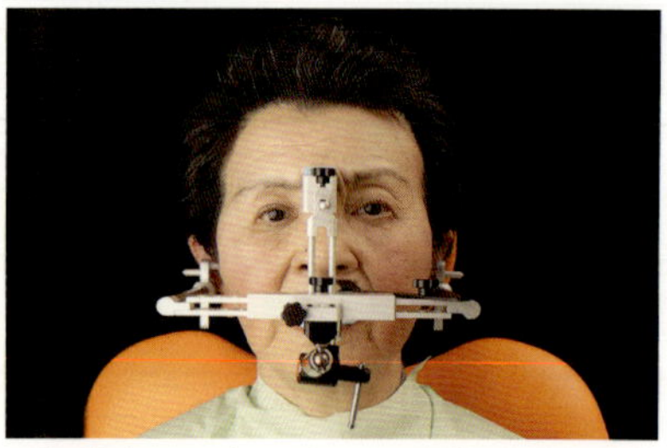

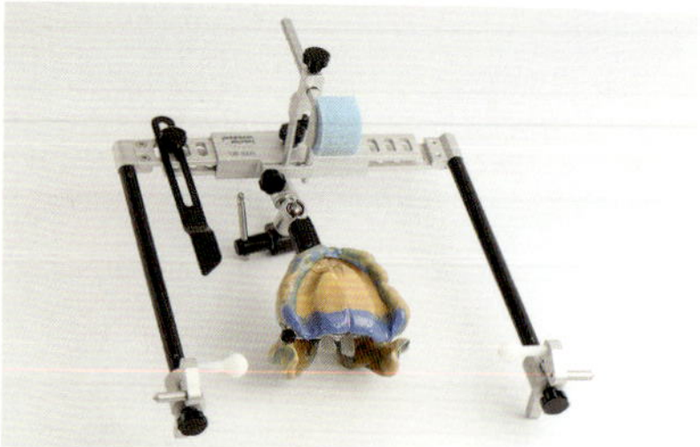

Position of the maxilla in relation to the facial cranium is transferred to the articulator. Registration joint (Ivoclar Vivadent) of UTS (Universal Transfer bow) is sent to the laboratory

Fig58 Face bow transfer.

15 Facebow-transfer (UTS)

The position of the maxilla in relation to the skull can be transferred to the articulator by using facebow-transfer (Fig 58).

The model is not mounted in the center in many cases when the facebow is used, since our face is rarely symmetrical. This asymmetric positioning sometimes makes it more difficult to set up denture teeth symmetrically.

More accurate articulator (such as Stratos 300, Ivoclar Vivadent) and three dimensionally mobile 3D Template (Icoclar Vivadent) are required to overcome this problem.

16 Model analysis in the Difficult-to-Treat case

Model analysis and denture tooth set up by the master technician will be expounded in this section. The midline marked on the silicone putty of the bite registration is the most reliable reference to set up anterior mid reference point for the difficult-to-treat cases without reliable landmark, such as extensive resorbed ridge or flabby ridge. Posterior reference point is determined by mid palatine raphe, mid point of the fovea palatinae and mid point between the right and left maxillary tuberosity (Fig 59).

Mandibular model analysis of difficult-to-treat case places emphasis on identifying the ridge crest line, a line bisecting the buccolingual width of the ridge, sagittal

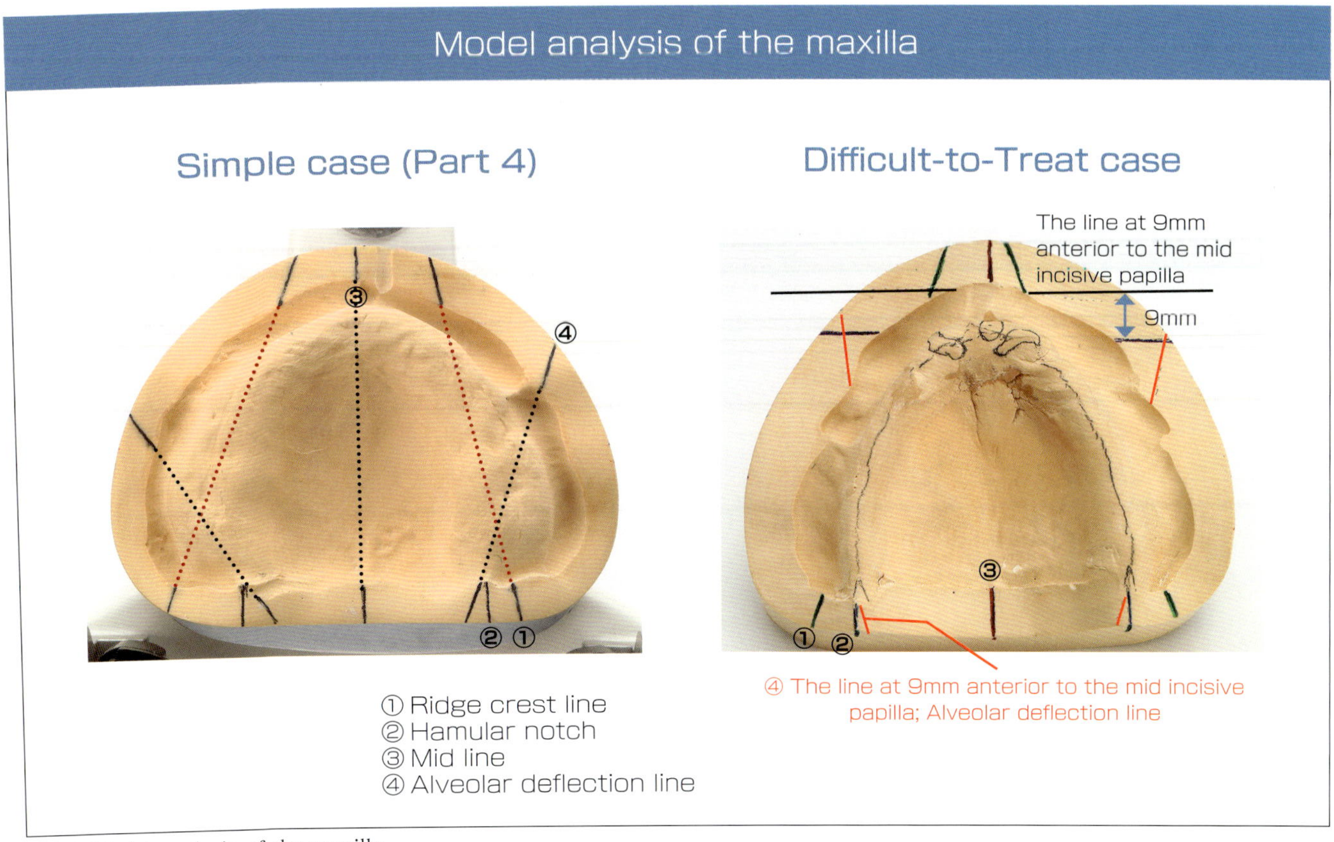

Fig59 Model analysis of the maxilla.

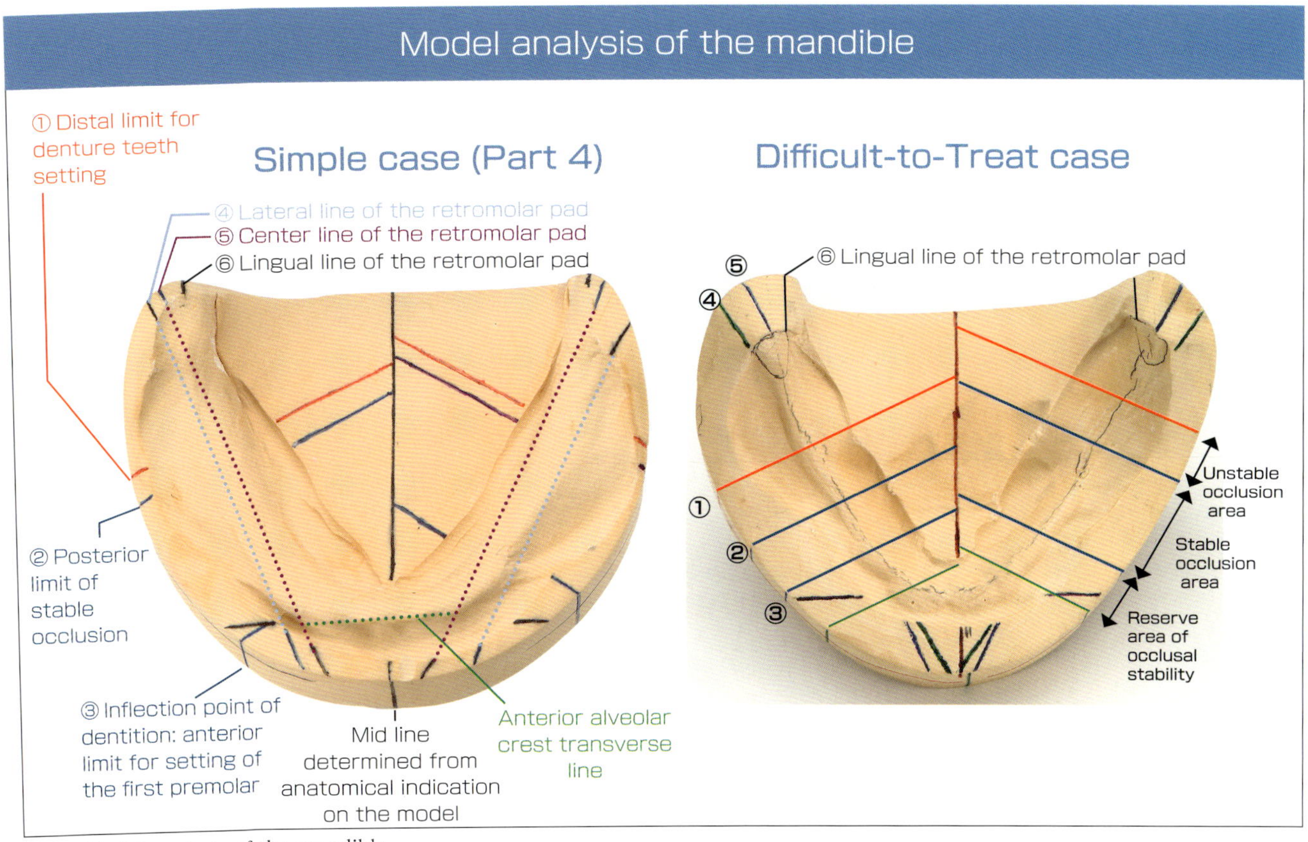

Fig60 Model analysis of the mandible.

Anterior denture tooth setting for Difficult-to-Treat case

Provide intentional winging rotation to central incisors

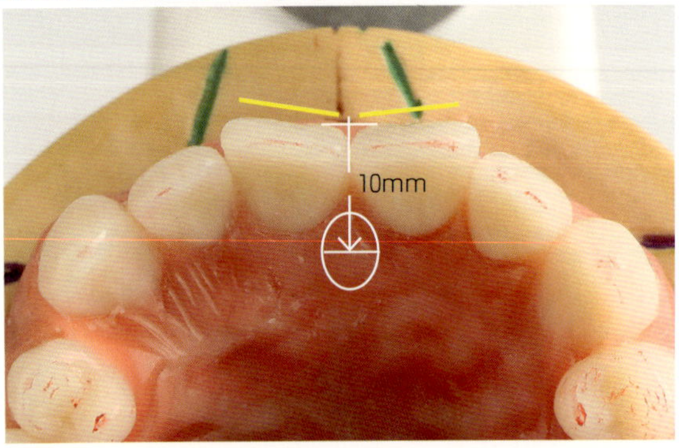

Central incisors are set so that the labial surface is 10mm forward from the middle of incisive papilla (butterfly like alignment)

Incisal edge of central incisors are positioned 2mm lower than usual

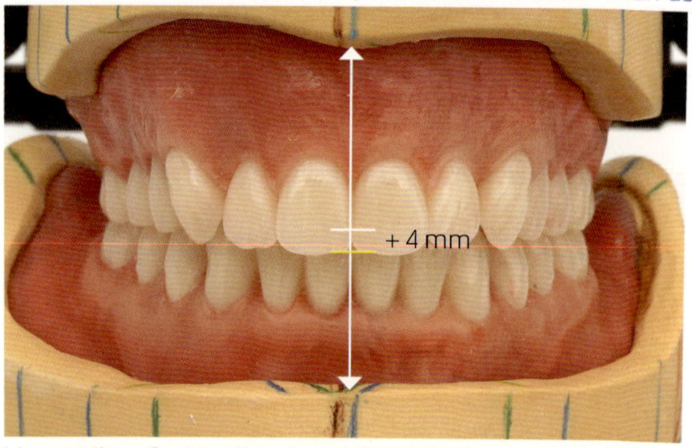

Upper lip of elderlies tend to sag down and don' t show while smiling. In such cases, incisal edge of central incisors are positioned lower than usual so that the patient shows teeth while smiling

Esthetic teeth setting for ClassII division2

Esthetics improves when central incisors are set so that the labial contour of the central incisor is directed toward the mandibular flange.
Maxillary molars were set first and mandibular anterior teeth were set lastly in the simple Class I case(Part 4). Mandibular anterior teeth were set before maxillary posterior teeth to facilitate three dimensional balance of teeth setting in this particular case, which is Class II - 2

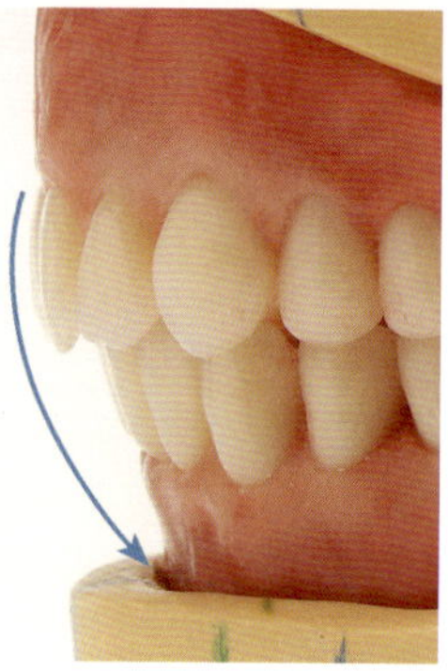

Fig61 Tips for setting anterior denture teeth for Difficult -to-Treat case.

mandibular inclining line and stable occlusal stress bearing area for setting of posterior denture teeth, which are described in figures (Fig 60).

17 Denture teeth setting for The Difficult-to-Treat case

(1) Denture teeth setting for the Difficult-to-Treat case (maxillary anterior)

Anterior-posterior space for denture tooth setup is larger in the case with resorbed ridge than in the case with less extensive ridge resorption. It is important to picture the condition before the ridge resorption and set anterior denture teeth esthetically (Fig 61). Average distance between the labial surface of the maxillary central incisor and center of the incisal papillae in the simple case is 7mm in male and 9mm in female. Central incisors in Difficut-to-Treat case are set

Posterior denture teeth setting for Difficult-to-Treat case

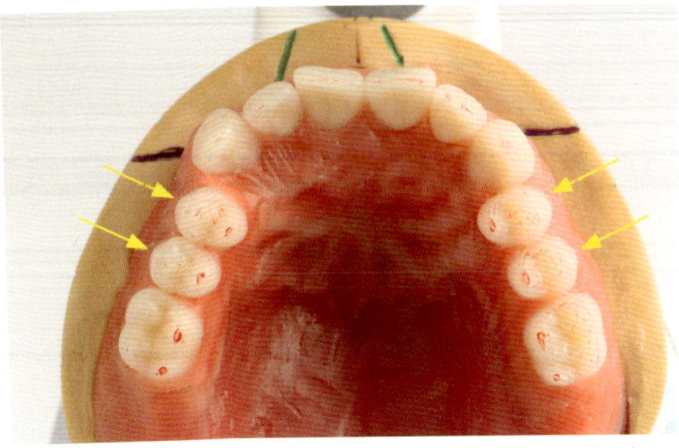

Maxillary first and second premolars are set close alveolar ridge crest in the cast with flabby ridge

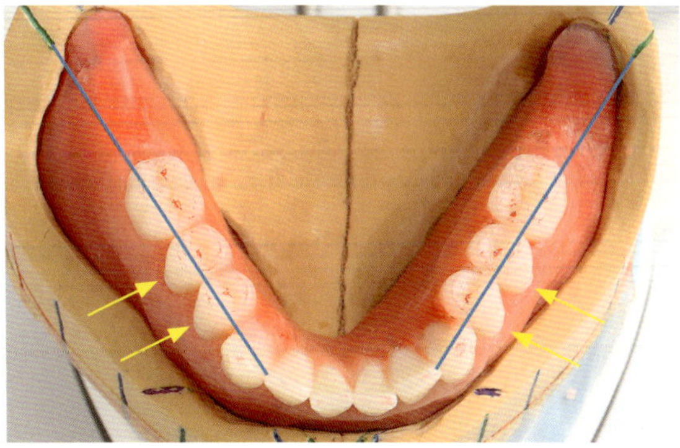

Mandibular teeth are set according to the maxillary first and second premolar teeth, which are set to alveolar ridge crest (blue line : center line directing buccal-lingual width of the alveolar ridge)

Fig62 Posterior denture teeth setting for Difficult-to-Treat case.

further forward, but not to exceed the anterior border of the flange on the model. Not only the denture esthetics would be compromised, but also the chance of dislodgement is increased by doing so. Decent esthetics would be achieved by setting central incisors in a way that extension of labial contour is directed to the mandibular flange especially in Class II - 2 case.

(2) The technique to prevent for the anterior teeth to be [buckteeth]

Maxillary 6 anterior teeth, which are aligned flat, tend to look protruded buckteeth. Maxillary central incisors are set in rotation so that anterior teeth don't look as protruded.

Average vertical position of maxillary central incisor is 2mm below the mid point of the intervestibular distance considering over bite. The upper lip of majority of elders tends to be sagged preventing maxillary anterior teeth to be shown resulting unfavorable esthetics. Therefore, maxillary central incisors are set 3 ~ 4mm below the midpoint to restore more favorable esthetics. This technique is applicable to the case shown in this section.

Papillameter (Candulor, Rinkai) could be used to mark lower border of the upper lip on the model. However, it often is not applicable to the Difficult-to-Treat case because the upper border of Papillameter does not fit to the model in many cases.

Base lines for teeth setting for the Difficult-to-Treat case with alveolar ridge resorption - in search for the area of occlusal stability-

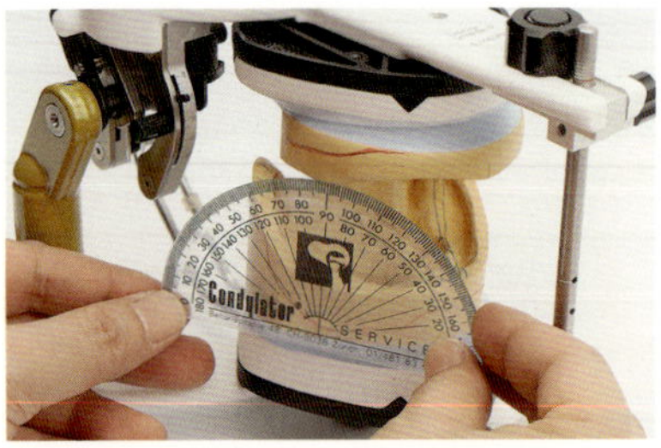

Step1 : Inclination angle of the alveolar ridge is measured using the protractor (The area, measured more than 22.5°: denture teeth are not set in the 'Ski zone')

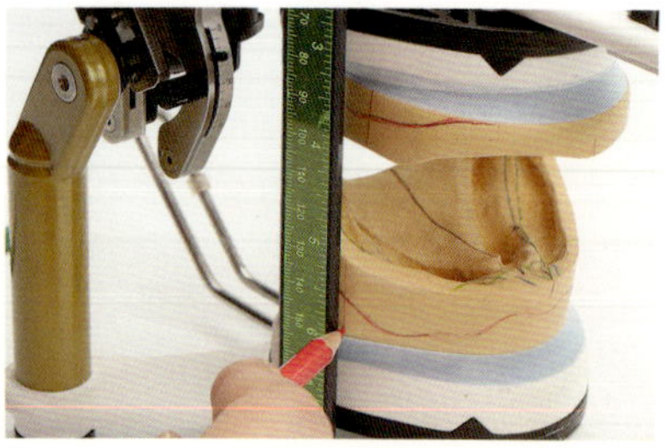

Step2 : Posterior setting limitation line is drawn

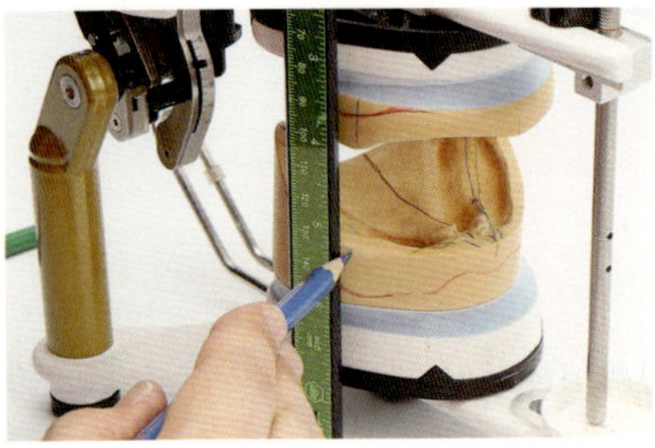

Step3 : The line for areas of occlusal instability is drawn (steep residual ridge slope)

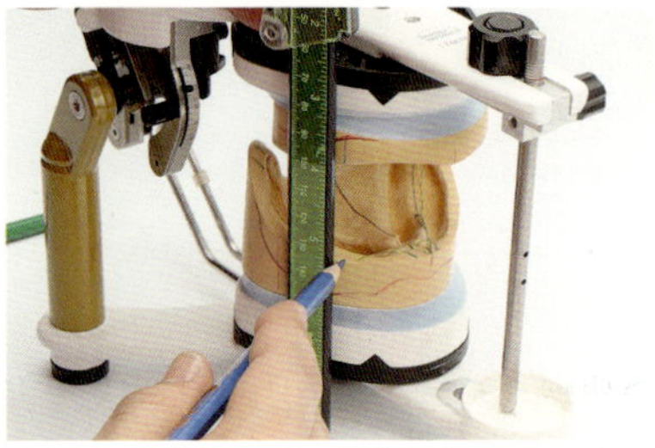

Step4 : The line for posterior area of occlusal stability is drawn (relatively flat area)

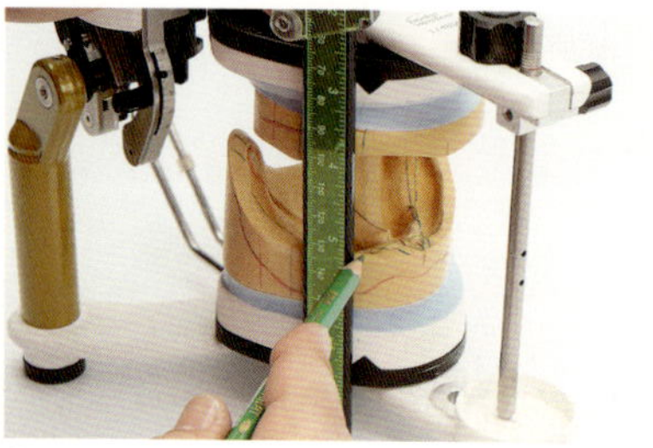

Step5 : The line for anterior area of occlusal stability is drawn (front line of first premolar)

Fig63 Base lines for teeth setting for the Difficult-to-Treat case with alveolar ridge resorption.

(3) Setting maxillary and mandibular premolar denture teeth (setting teeth closer to the ridge crest)

1) The first priority is to prevent maxillary denture dislodgment

Preventing maxillary denture dislodgment is the first priority. Maxillary premolar teeth in flabby ridge Difficult-to-Treat case (including maxillary anterior flabby ridge) are set closer to the ridge crest comparing to the case with favorable ridge (Fig 62). Lateral force, which causes flip of the denture, can be decreased by setting denture teeth closer to the ridge crest.

2) The second priority is to stabilize the mandibular denture by suction-effect

The second priority is to stabilize the mandibular denture by suction-effect. Stable area on the resorbed ridge for premolars are identified and proper three dimensional position is determined. Stability is obtained by setting the fossa of mandibular premolars inside the baseline between mesial corner of the canine and external edge of the retromolar pad intentionally. Final setting is completed considering the relationship with the mandibular premolar teeth to balance the force. Thus, extra consideration is required for setting denture teeth for Difficult-

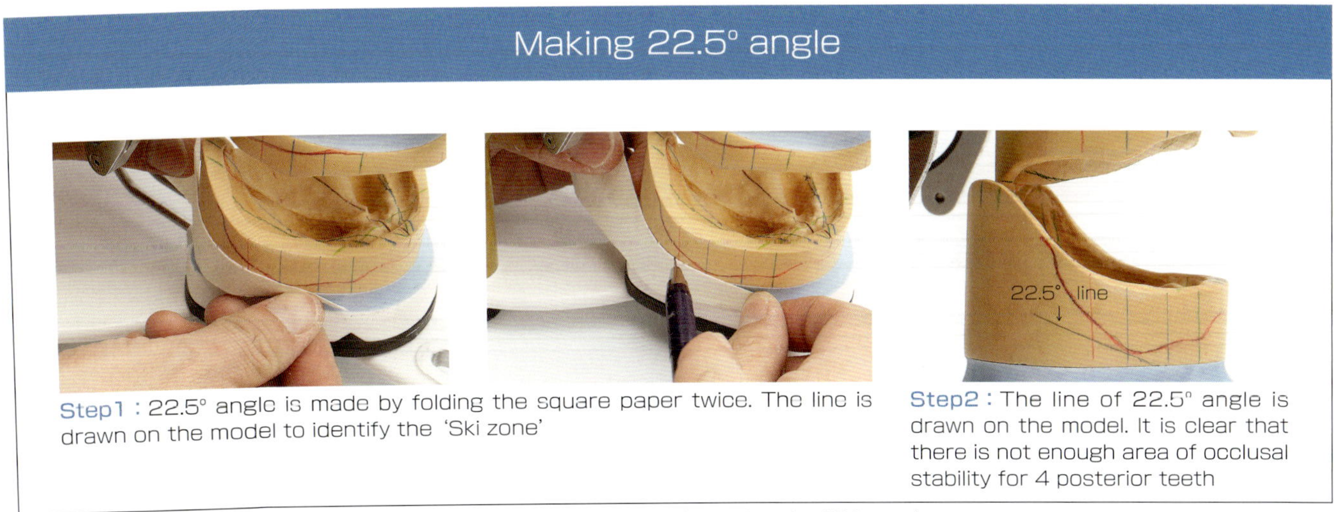

Fig64 Simplified technique to mark 22.5° angle on the model to determine the 'Ski zone'.

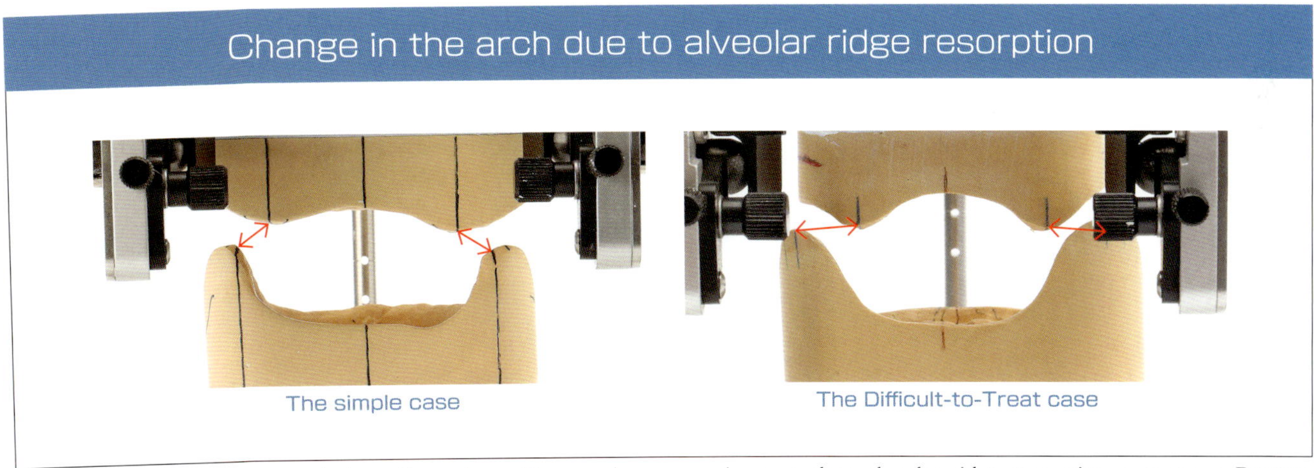

Fig65 Mandibular arch expands laterally and maxillary arch narrows in general as alveolar ridge resorption progresses. Denture teeth are set in cross bite relationship if the angle between maxillary and mandibular molars exceeds 80° in order to avoid constriction of tongue space. it was border line between normal occlusion and cross bite occlusion in this case.

to-Treat case.

(4) Setting mandibular molar denture teeth for the Difficult-to-Treat case (to establish occlusal stability)

1) Importance of Mandibular molar tooth setup based on the area of occlusal stability to be found by the model analysis

Model analysis is critical for the Difficult-to-Treat case with extensive ridge resorption for both arches such as this case, since anatomical landmark is limited for denture teeth set up. More favorable tooth set up area is determined by drawing lines of posterior tooth setup limit zone, occlusal stable and unstable area, front line of the premolar teeth(Fig 63).

Denture teeth should not be set too far inside over the Pound line

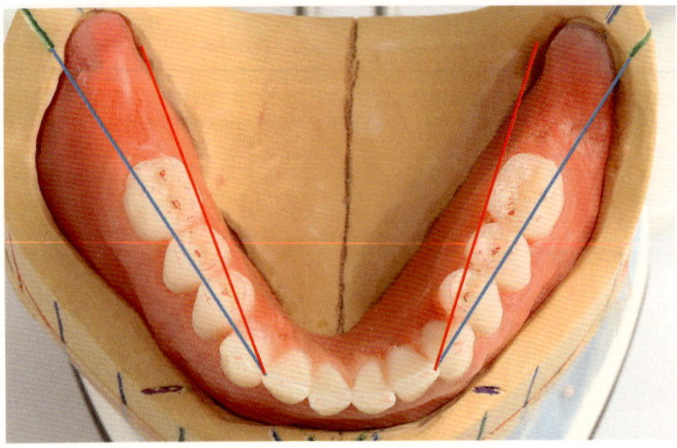

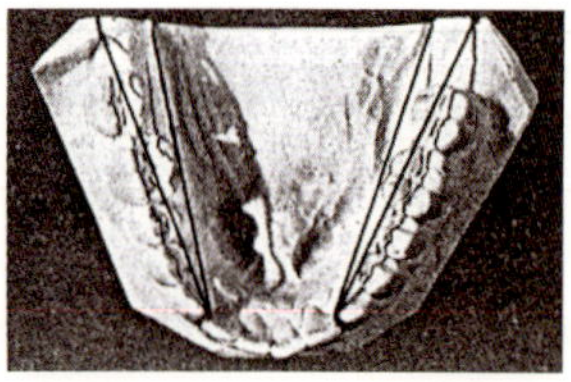

Quote from Pound E. Conditioning of denture patents. J Am Dent Assoc 1962; 64: 461-468.

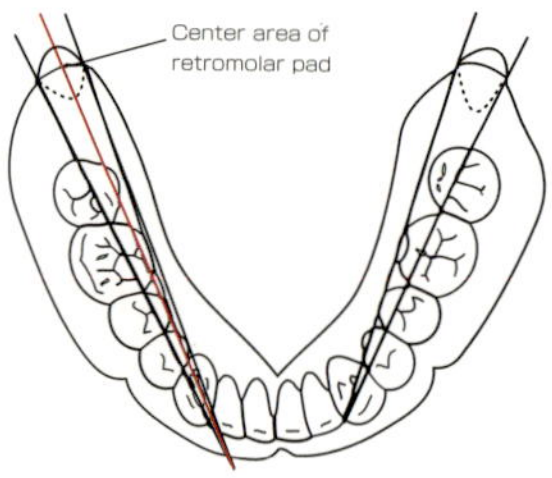

Fig66 Denture teeth should not be set too far inside over the Pound line even it leaves large gap between maxillary and mandibular arches. If denture teeth, which are set too far lingual, hinder the movement of base of the tongue, it is retruded breaking seal at anterior lingual region resulting in denture dislodgment.

The area of the ridge, where slopes more than 22.5°, is considered as occlusal unstable area, since the denture tends to slip forward if the food is bit on in this area. The guide of 22.5° is made by folding the square paper twice. The guide is used to identify the area of the ridge sloping more than 22.5° by drawing the line on the side of mandibular and maxillary model using the base of the model as the base line. Vertical line is drawn at the most anterior point where the slope starts, extending to the each other model (Fig 64). Second molars are not set up in this case because of this limited space.

2) Molars are set in cross bite if the maxillary and mandibular molars are in opposing relationship of more than 80° in frontal view

In general, mandibular ridge arch is widened and maxillary ridge arch is narrowed once ridge resorption progresses (Fig 65). Restriction of tongue space is prevented by providing cross bite denture tooth set up, if maxillary and mandibular first molar opposing relationship exceeds 80° in frontal view. This case was right at the border line.

3) Denture teeth should not be set lingual to the Pound line, even large gap exists between maxillary and mandibular arch.

Difference is clear once it is compared to the simple case. Denture teeth should not be set too far lingual to the Pound line (Fig 66). The tongue is retruded if denture teeth are set up too far lingually preventing free movement of base of the tongue, resulting in broken border seal at area of anterior part of the tongue and dislodgment of the denture.

Lingualized occlusion, which is favorable for the Difficult-to-Treat case

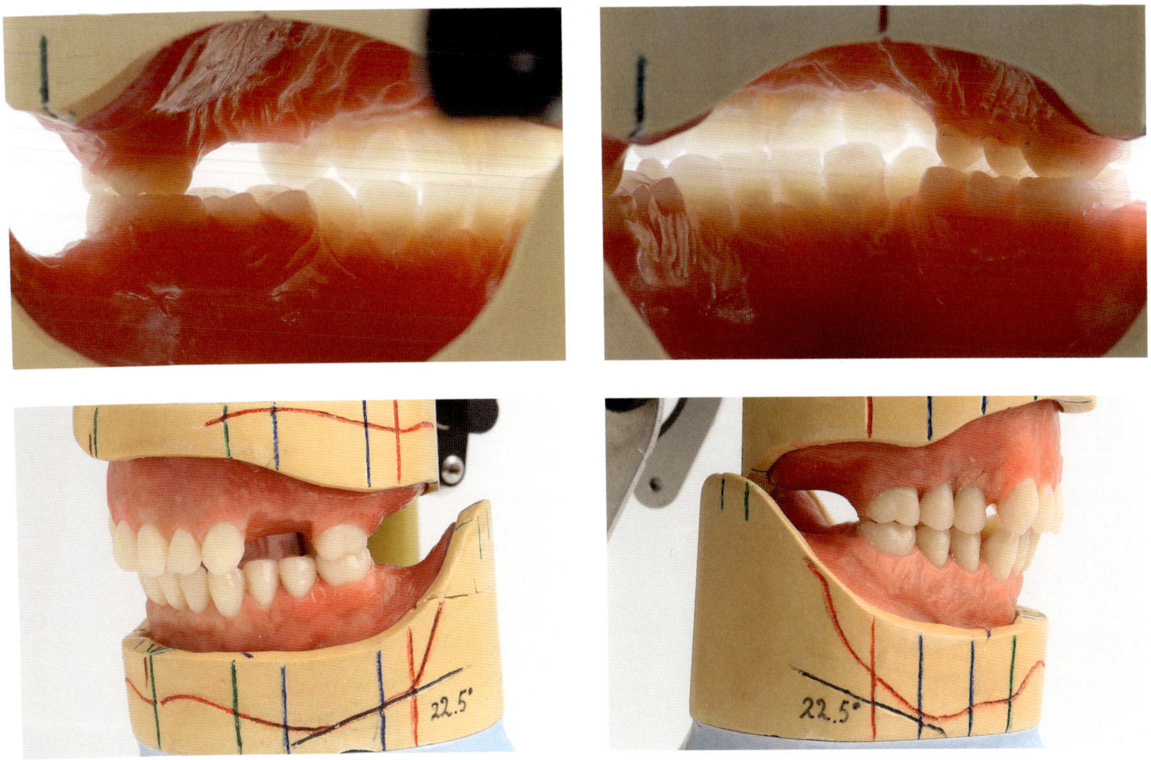

Fig67 Tooth to tooth occlusion of lingualized occlusion. Setting order of maxillary molars are right and left maxillary first molars → right and left maxillary first premolars → right and left maxillary second premolars.

Instructions for 3D template

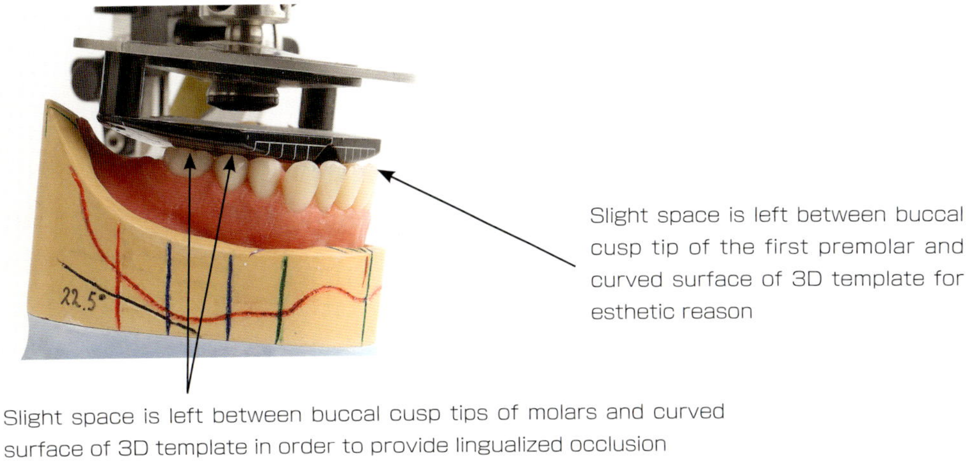

Fig68 Only lingual cusp tips of molars are set to contact curved surface of 3D template. Posterior denture teeth are set according to the marked area of occlusal stability.

Anterior clearance and overbite

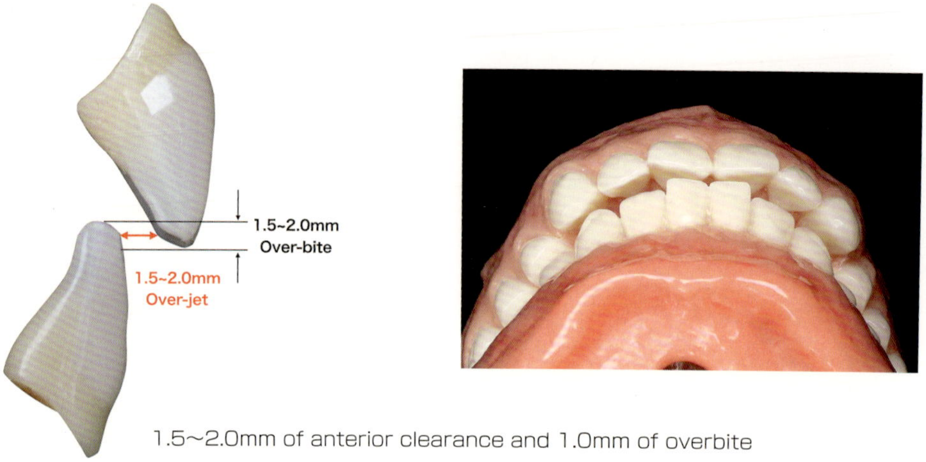

1.5~2.0mm of anterior clearance and 1.0mm of overbite

Fig69 1.5~2.0mm of anterior clearance needs to be kept to prevent contact between maxillary and mandibular teeth in the case with flabby ridge.

(5) Occlusal scheme for the Difficult-to-Treat case

1) Lingualized occlusion

Lingualized occlusion is considered to increase patient's denture satisfaction in cases with extensive bone resorption[82]. Flipping of maxillary denture is prevented by employing lingualized tooth to tooth occlusion because occlusal force can be directed toward the ridge crest even after maxillary denture teeth are set up more buccal than usual. Longitudinal axis of molar denture tooth is tilted buccally establishing contact only on maxillary lingual cusps in lingualized occlusion (Fig 67, 68). Esthetics is improved by making the buccal cusp of the first premolar touch the template closing the space between buccal cusps of maxillary and mandibular first premolars, but not in this particular case.

2) Anterior clearance and over bite

The cause of maxillary flabby ridge is excessive stimulation on the maxillary anterior ridge, which presents low bone density. Inflammation of the flabby ridge will persist and rather deteriorates unless this cause is removed. Hence, 1.5~2.0mm of anterior clearance is maintained despite of tendency of the human being trying to obtain anterior contact (Fig 69). Premature contact of anterior teeth during protrusive movement is avoided by providing shallow over bite and rather prominent compensating curve for Class II division 2 case.

Completed wax denture is shown in Fig 70.

It is important to be conscious about the vector of force on denture base and roots.

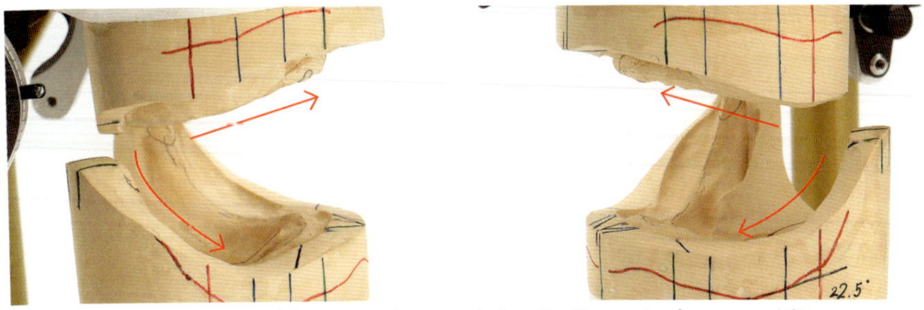

Dentures tend to move forward due to the anterior open bite

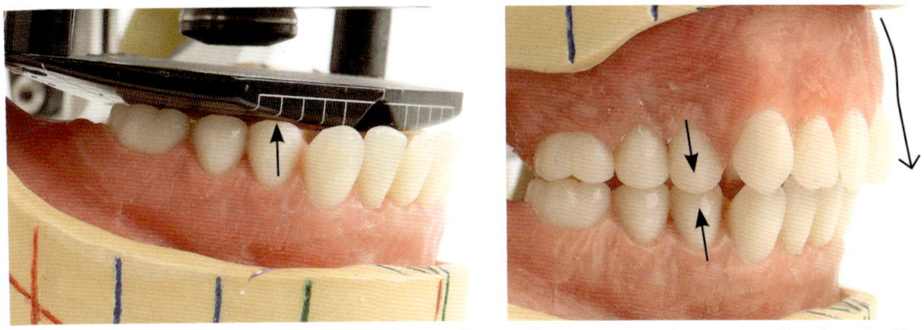

The denture tooth to gingival contour is formed rather straight for female with slight gull wing

Denture teeth are set so that occlusal force is conveyed perpendicular to the maxilla

Completion of denture teeth setup and wax-up

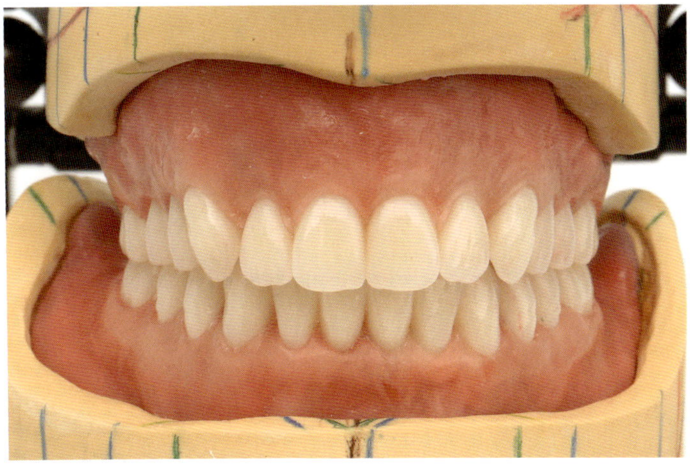

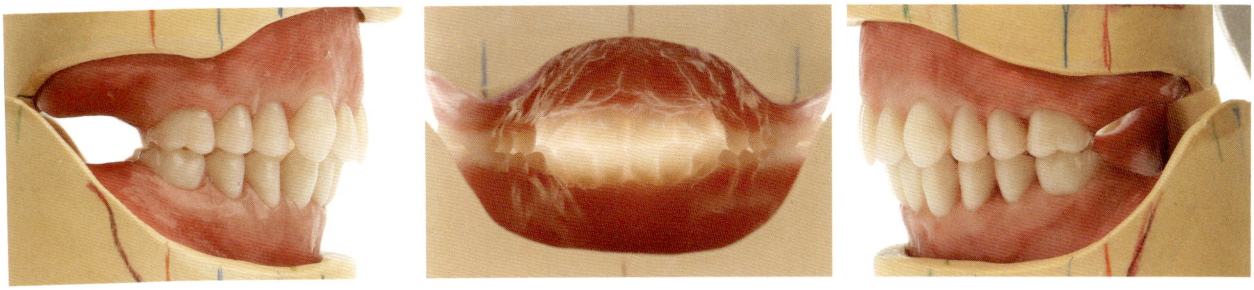

Fig70a, b Completion of denture teeth setup and wax-up.

Class 2 Division II (esthetics) - to provide attractive smile -

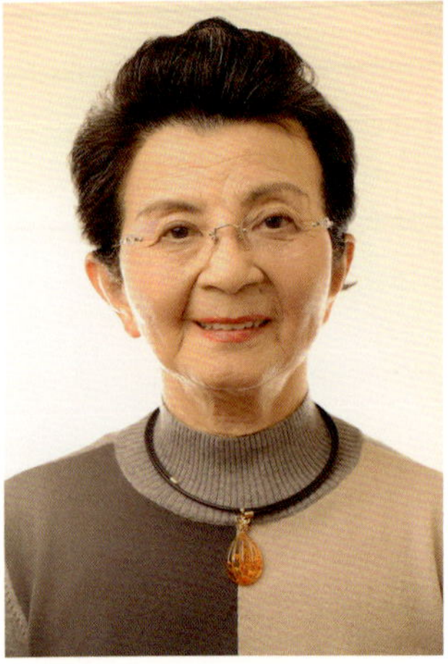

Frontal view at relaxed state.
appropriate Vertical Dimension of Occlusion (VDO)

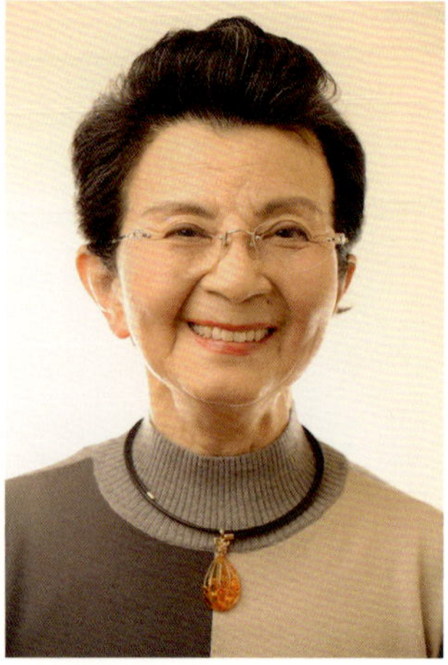

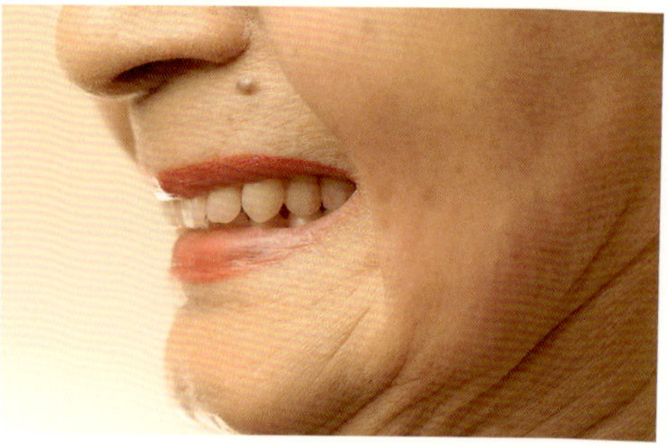

At smile
Upper lip line, well balanced lower lip line and incisal edge line.
Smile looks more attractive when gingiva does not appear while smiling.
There should be appropriate amount of space between the corner of the mouth and denture teeth (Buccal Corridor)

Fig71 Esthetic check points at wax denture try-in.

18 Wax denture try-in

(1) Items to check during wax denture try-in

Wax denture try-in is the only time the patient could participate and give any input.

Denture teeth are set in the average position from the anatomical index for the simple case in BPS system. However, it is difficult to determine the final position of denture teeth only from the model analysis for the Difficult-to-Treat case such as this case shown in this section, which lacks most of anatomical index. Check points during wax-try in are presented below.

1)Check bite registration error (VDO and horizontal mandibular position)

Maxillary and mandibular relationship and VDO are re-confirmed. There could be some discrepancy due to interference of movement of the tongue by the tracing plate. It is essential to check the patient with denture tooth set up.

Stabilization test - to exert full function -

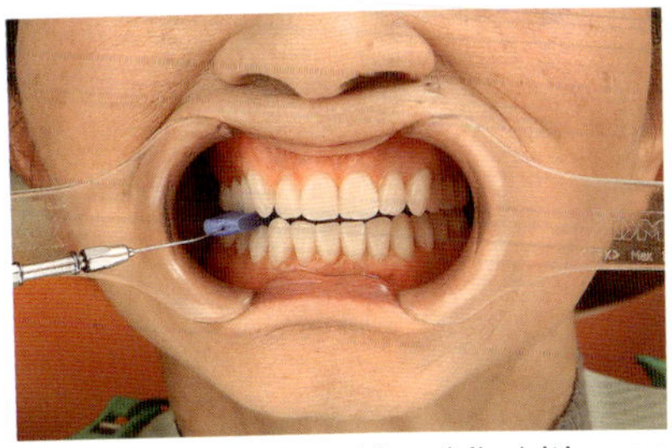

The denture is stable while biting on the silicone on right posterior teeth. Denture teeth set up is considered to be appropriate

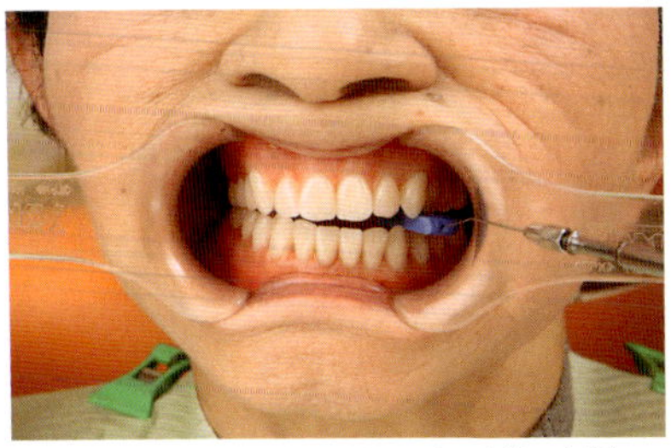

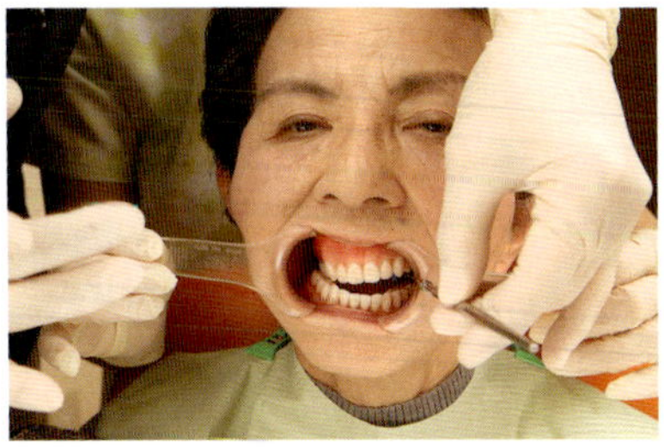

The denture dislodged while biting on the silicone of left posterior teeth. Denture tooth setup was adjusted (further toward alveolar ridge crest) at the chair side

Fig72 It is very important to check denture tooth setup intraorally. The conditions are different between on the stone model and on the elastic alveolar mucosa. It is necessary to prevent dislodgment due to jaw relationship before completion of the denture.

2) Esthetics

Denture tooth setup is checked and confirmed with the patient checking factors such as color and shape of the denture teeth, mid line and horizontal line, harmonized alignment to the face in relaxed state, balance between denture teeth and upper and lower lips in smile and buccal corridor (Fig 71).

3) Stabilization test

Stabilization test is more essential as the case is more difficult. Functional aspect is checked closely (Fig72). Anterior clearance and overbite are adjusted according to the treatment goal of each case (Fig73). Followings are three treatment goals of this case.

a. To control inflammation of maxillary flabby ridge (no contact between maxillary and mandibular anterior entire teeth during function).

b.To set up denture teeth in occlusal stable area for extensively resorbed mandibular ridge (premolars are set up toward ridge crest and do not set up denture teeth in posterior occlusal unstable area).

c.To set up maxillary and mandibular denture teeth so that both maxillary and mandibular dentures are stabilized considering the size gap between maxillary and mandibular dental arch.

Stability of the dentures is checked by having the patient bite down 3mm thick

Anterior clearance and overbite to improve flabby ridge and stabilize maxillary denture

It is important not to create contact between maxillary and mandibular anterior teeth in order to eliminate inflammation of maxillary anterior flabby tissue. Inflammation subsides gradually due to decreased stimulation to flabby area by maintaining the space between maxillary and mandibular anterior teeth. The amount of space should altered intentionally according to the purpose of the treatment.

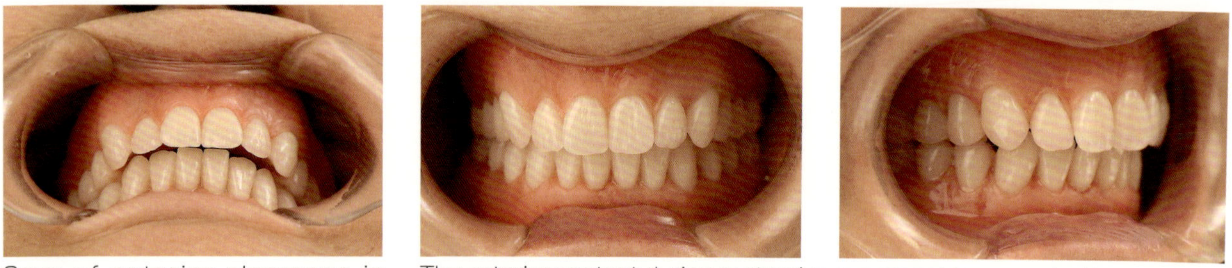

2mm of anterior clearance is provided

The anterior contact during protrusive movement is prevented by providing rather small overbite (1.0mm)

Fig73 The amount of anterior clearance and overbite in order to improve flabby ridge and stabilize maxillary denture.

hardened silicone putty in posterior region. Setup of denture teeth is adjusted to prevent dislodgment by moving teeth toward ridge crest or tilting is tendency of dislodgment is found.

Tongue space and speech are taken into consideration when denture teeth setup is changed.

19 Polymerizing resin

(1) Choice of resin and curing machine

Dental stone is chosen according to the amount of shrinkage of the resin.

IvoBase System (Ivoclar Vivadent) is the auto curing system, which does not require a large scale equipment. Ideal resin polymerization is carried out under programmed temperature (Fig 74, 75).

(2) Necessity of split cast

Split cast needs to be provided to the base of the model for remounting procedure.

Since slight position change of denture teeth due to shrinkage of resin after polymerization is inevitable, remounting procedure is required for occlusal

Investment

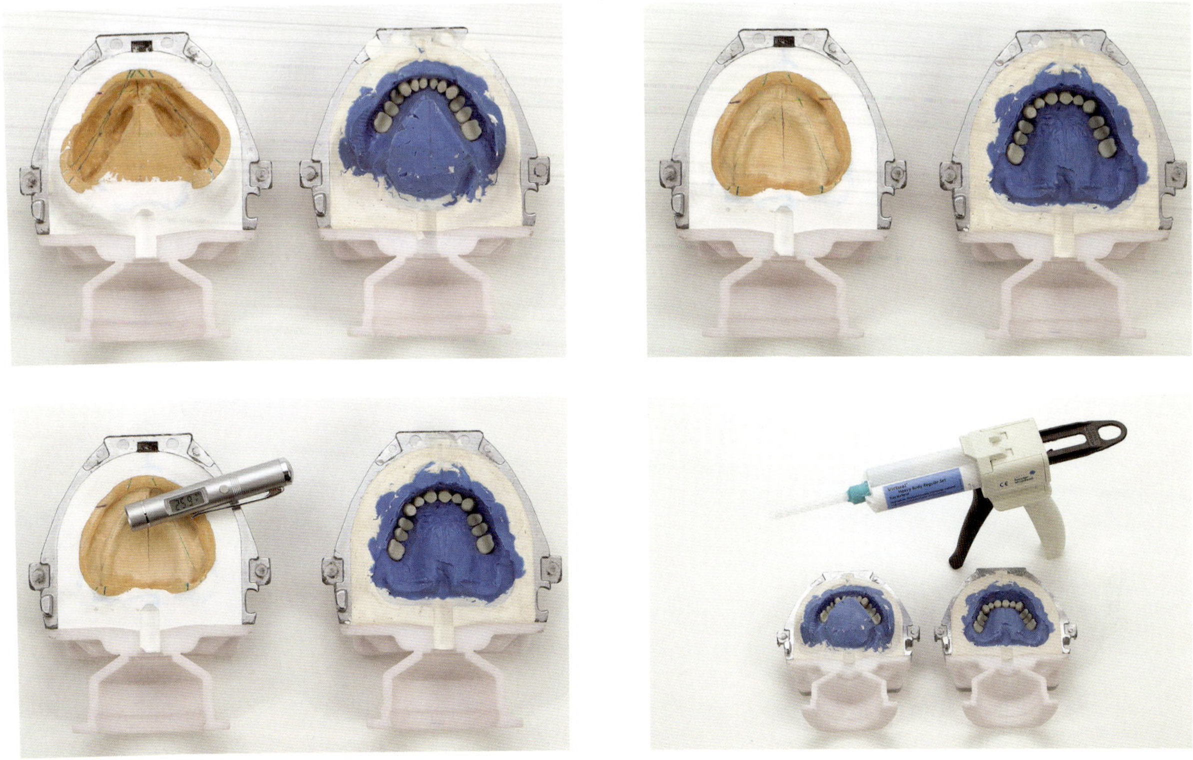

Fig74 Heavy body type (regular) of Virtual is used for the secondary investment. The stone does not adhere to cervical area at the time of deflasking. Mixed stone of Type IV stone and type II stone (2(IV):8(II)) is used for the third investment. Bonding strength is improved by applying resin primer 30 seconds before injection.

adjustment. Time for chair side occlusal adjustment is minimized allowing more time for more detailed adjustment for each patient.

(3) Occlusal adjustment after remounting

Three adjustment in

1) maximum intercuspation

2) lateral movement (bilateral balanced occlusion)

3) protrusive movement

are carried out if clear Gothic arch, which indicates no temporomandibular joint problem, is drawn (Fig 76).

Wide centric or long centric occlusion is recommended, considering immediate side shift, if the apex of Gothic arch is not sharp or tapping point is not stable. It is important to perform occlusal adjustment on the articulator beforehand, since intra-oral occlusal adjustment is not as accurate.

Polymerization using IvoBase System

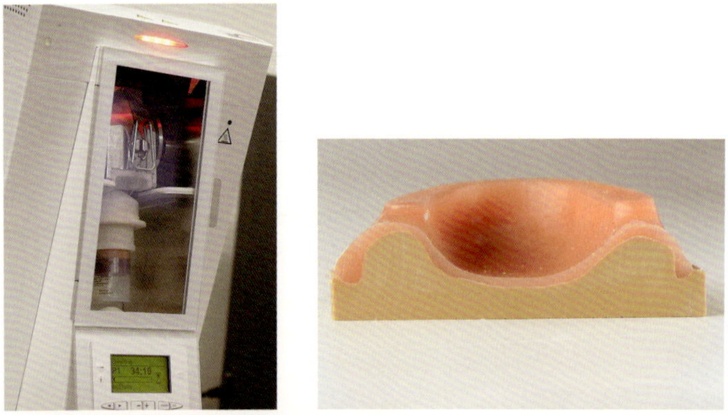

The author does not use the optional Residual Monomer Reduction [RMR] function, when the IvoBase Hybrid Pink is used (all products from Ivoclar Vivadent). Instead, the polymerization unit is pressurized with Polymax 5 (Dreve, Rinkai) under 6 atmospheric pressure at 55°C for 30minutes and then the denture is deflasked after gradual cooling for 12 hours.

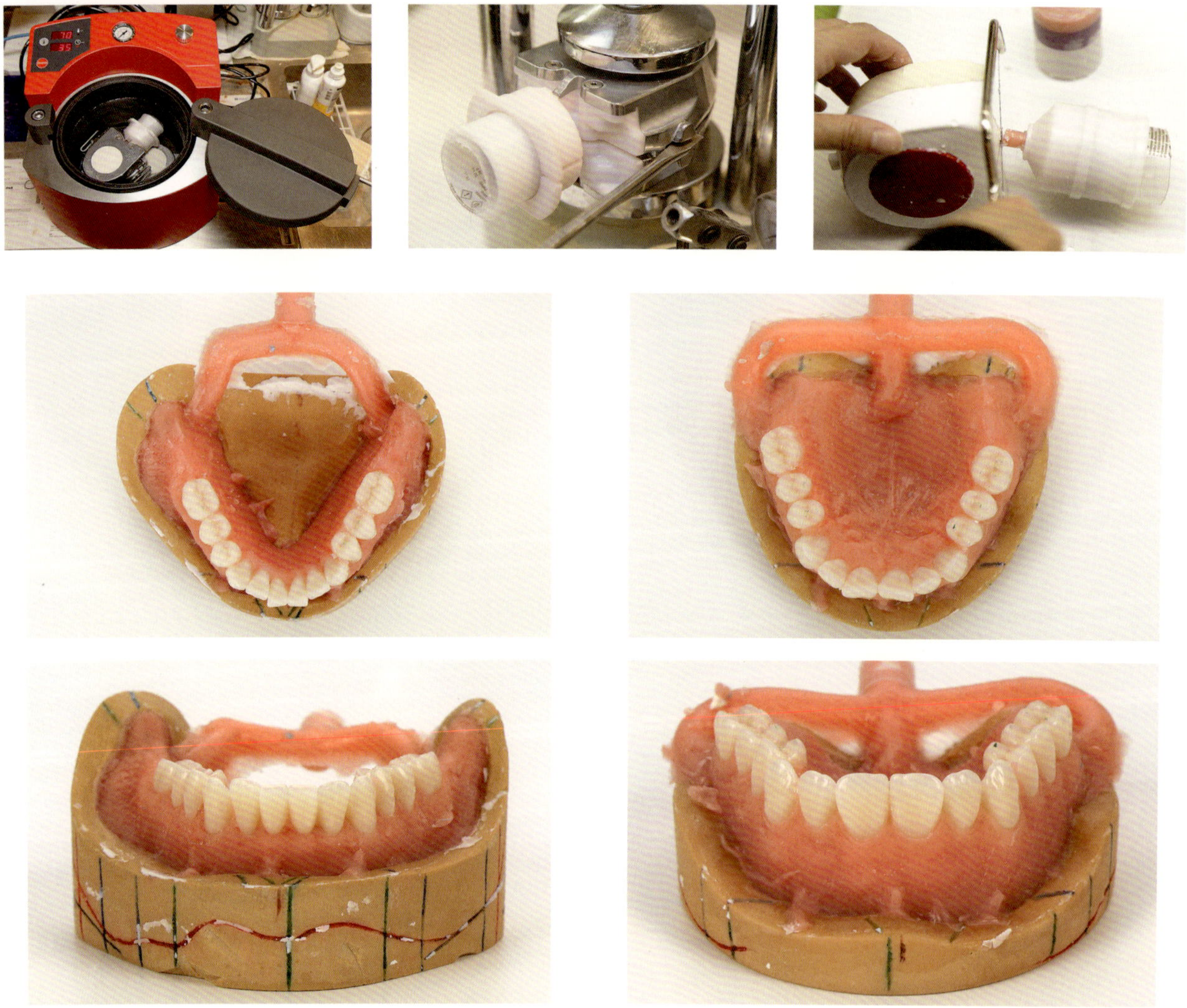

Fig75 Polemerization using the resin polymerizing apparatus IvoBase injector. IvoBase Hybrid Pink is used for the denture base resin at the author's (Iwaki) dental laboratory. This product is found to be superior in fit when it is compared to IvoBase High Impact, which has impact resistance, or Pink V-Implant, which is hybrid material. Additives in Pink V-Implant to cut off the base color are considered to be affecting the fit. The sprue for the maxilla should be placed outside as shown in the photo for better fit instead of being placed on the alveolar ridge crest or inside.

Occlusal adjustment after remount

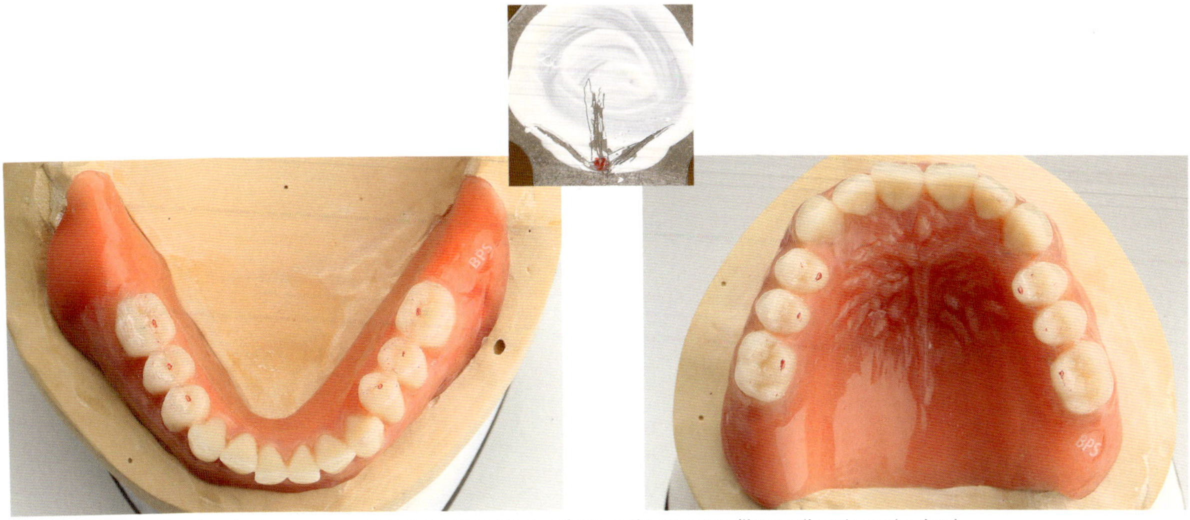

Step1 : Contacts in maximum intercuspation after adjustment (lingualized occlusion)

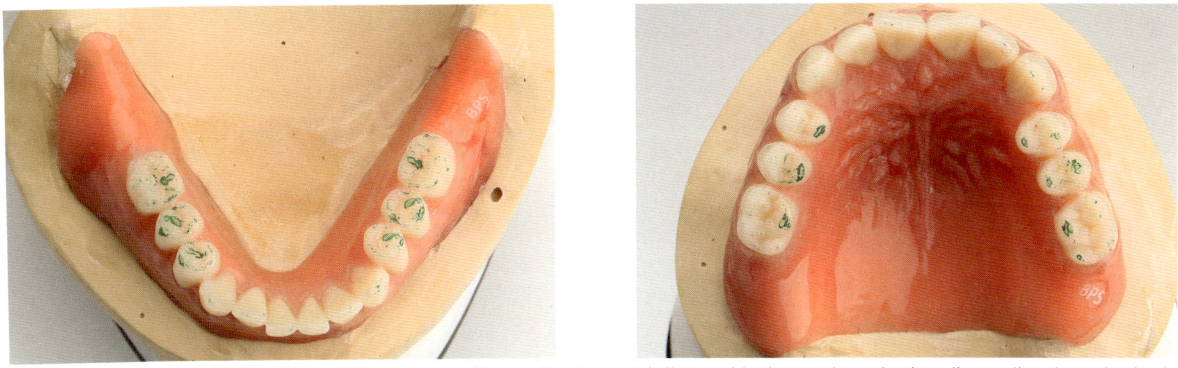

Step2 : Contacts during lateral excursion after adjustment (bilateral balanced occlusion, lingualized occlusion)

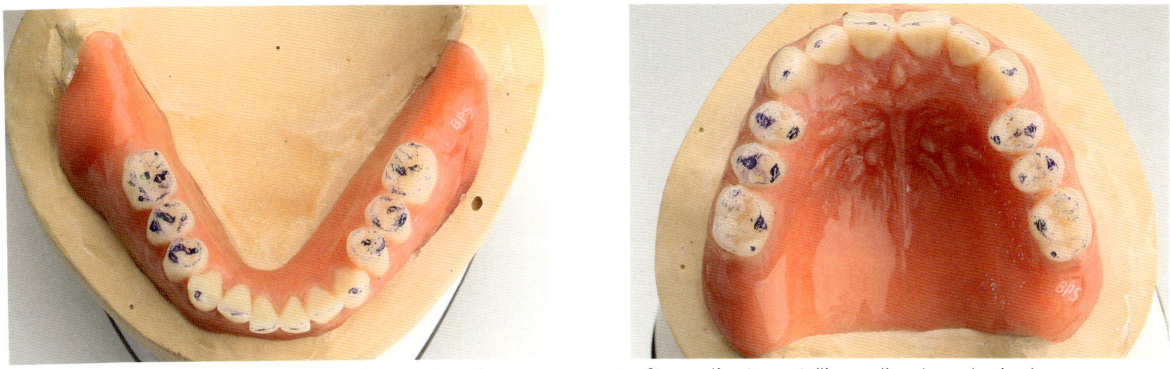

Step3 : Contacts during protrusive movement after adjustment (lingualized occlusion)

Fig76 Occlusion is adjusted at 1. maximum intercuspation, 2. lateral excursion (bilateral balanced occlusion), 3. protrusive movement, since there is no problem with temporomandibular joint function when the Gothic arch is drawn clearly as shown above.

20 Denture coloring (SR Nexco)

Denture coloring (Fig 77) is different between the female Difficult-to-Treat case and the male simple case (Part 4) especially in maxillary denture. There is not much difference in mandibular denture.

2 tones of base color are used (intensive gingiva3) to establish natural look since the distance between the cervical area to the denture border is rather long in maxillary anterior flabby ridge case.

Following is the specific coloring method for a female and a male patient by the dental technician.

(1) Female

- Stain red is applied on whole surface to express soft female characteristics and create three dimensionality.
- Liner2 was built up in root prominence area to increase value including denture border area and frenums as well.
- Gingiva2 was slightly applied to create femininity.
- Gingiva1 was slightly applied on the are of free gingiva for the same purpose as above.

(2) Male

- Larger amount of Gingiva2 and Gingiva34 were applied on denture border area irregularly to create masculinity.
- Gingiva1 was applied on attached and free gingiva.
- Larger amount of Liner2 was applied to emphasize the root eminence.
- Attached gingiva was emphasized by applying larger amount of Gingiva1 to the area of free gingiva and attached gingiva. As a result, orangish hue was created.
- Gingiva34 is the most suitable color to create the frenum and palatal rugae.
- Gingiva34 was aded on Liner2, which emphasized soot eminence, to make root surface look slightly orange for male simple case.

Coloring with consideration in gender

Class I for male (Part 4), Class II for female

Female

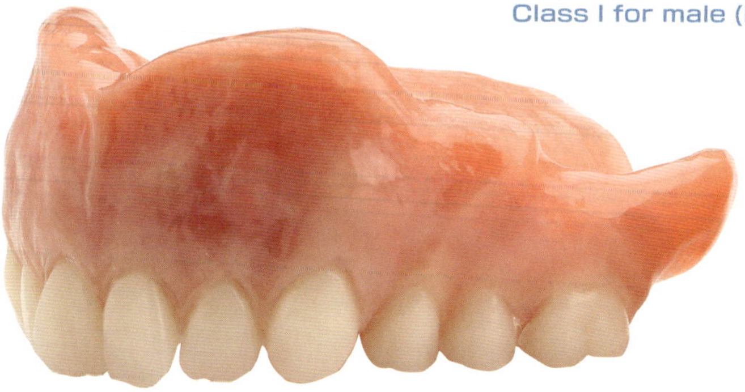

Male

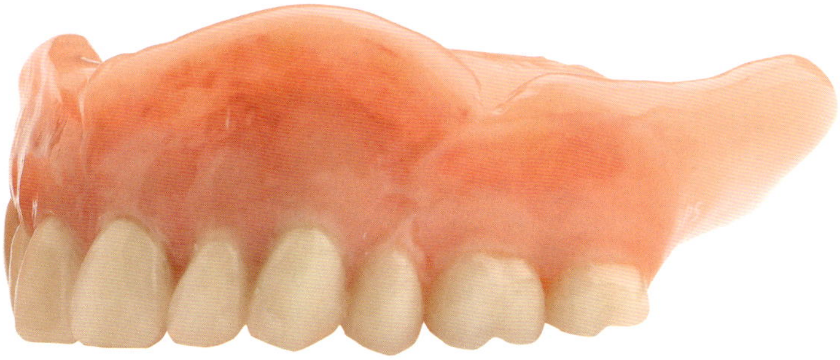

Male

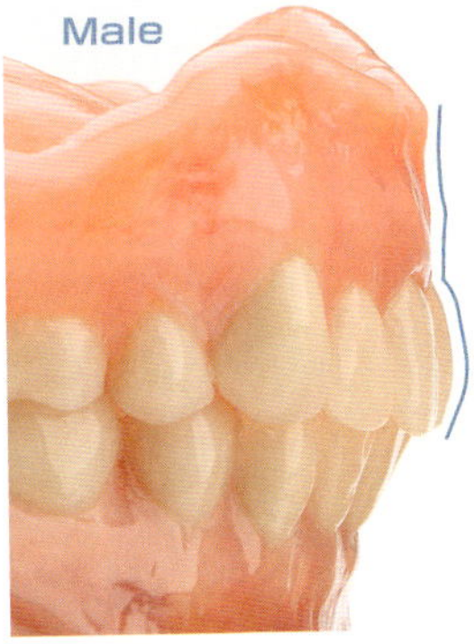

The denture tooth to gingival contour is not straight with rather prominent root contour for male

Female

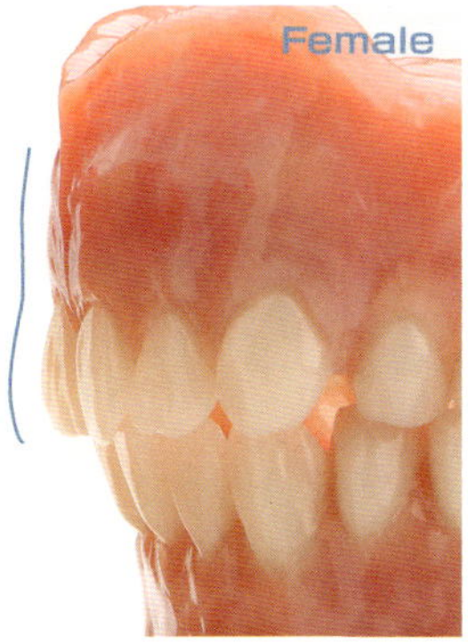

The denture tooth to gingival contour is formed rather straight for female

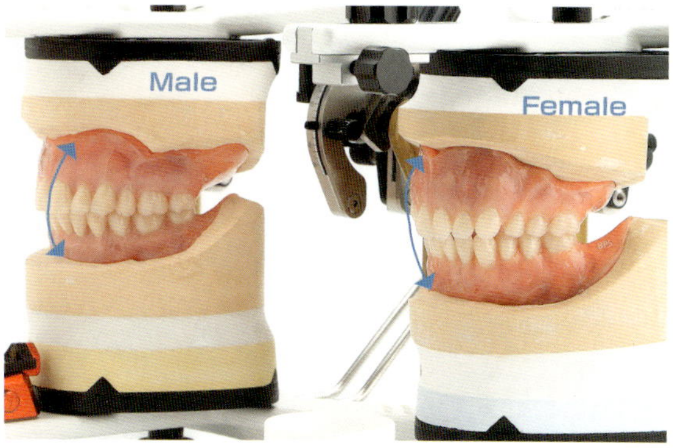

Male

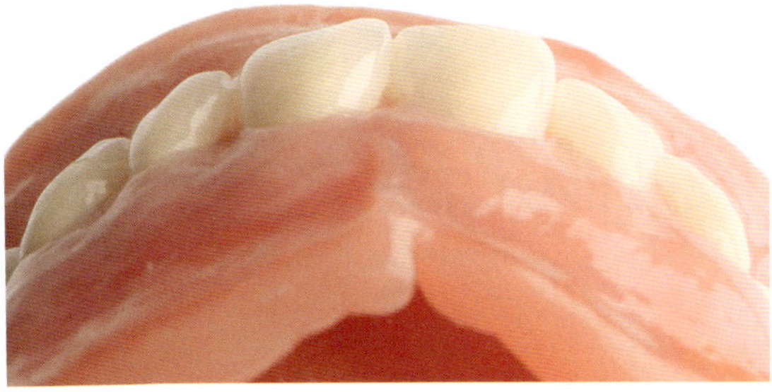

Female

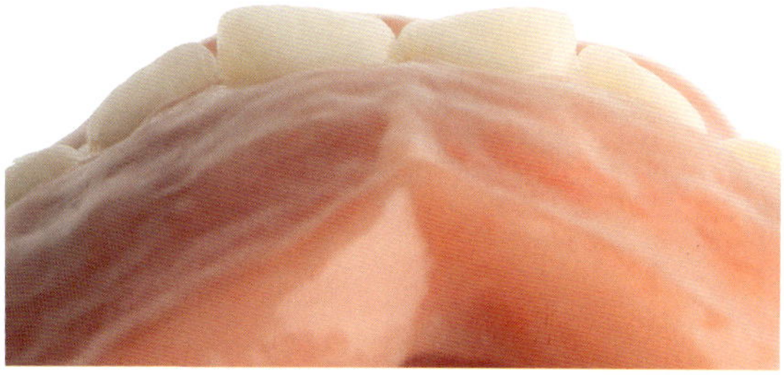

Fig78 The female case shown above is the case shown in this section and the male case shown above is the case for the simple case in Part 4. Denture coloring is thinly applied considering vessels running in alveolar mucosa area and from interdental papilla toward alveolar mucosa area.

Completed complete dentures

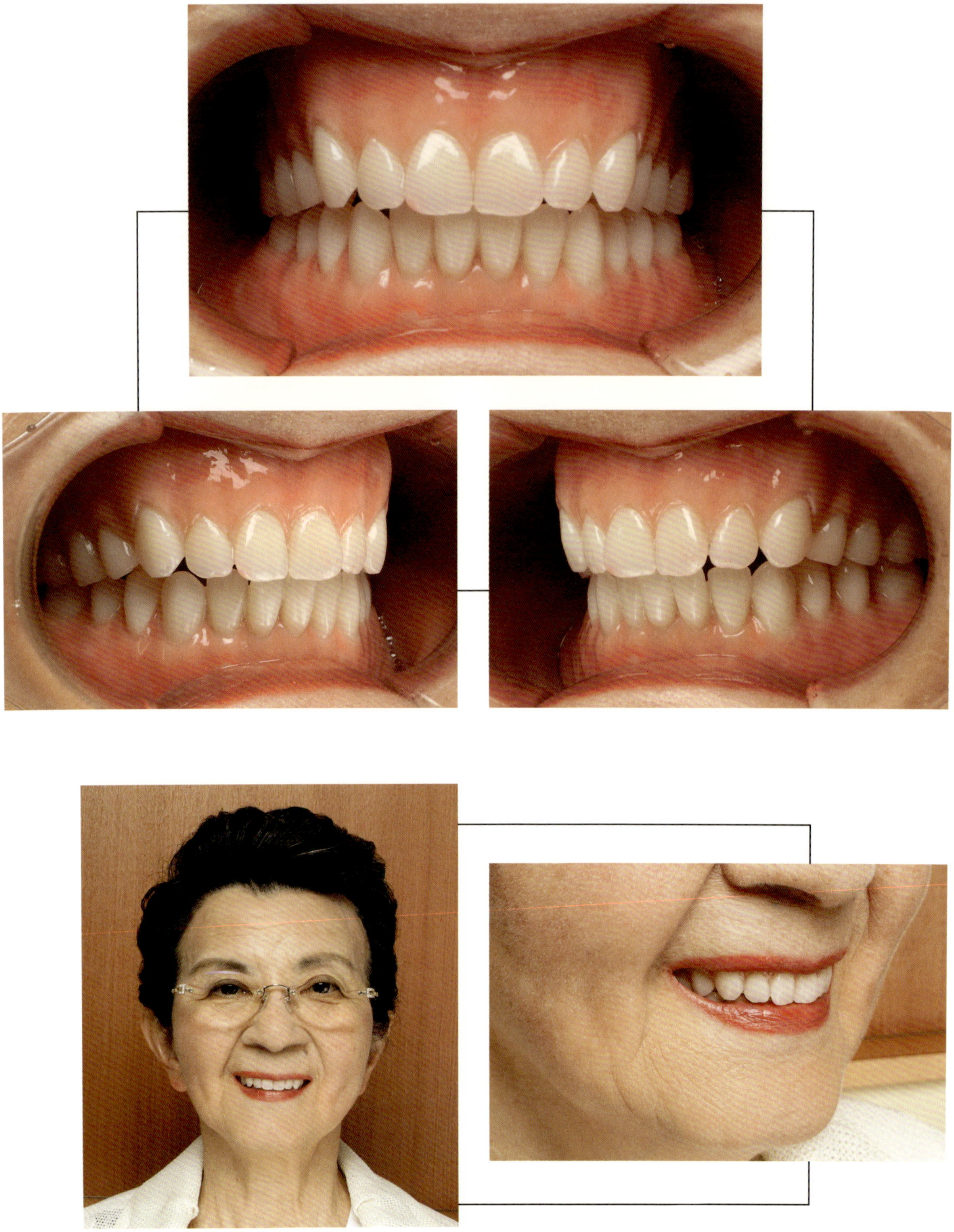

Fig79a Completed dentures inserted in the mouth.

Completed dentures to be expressed femininity

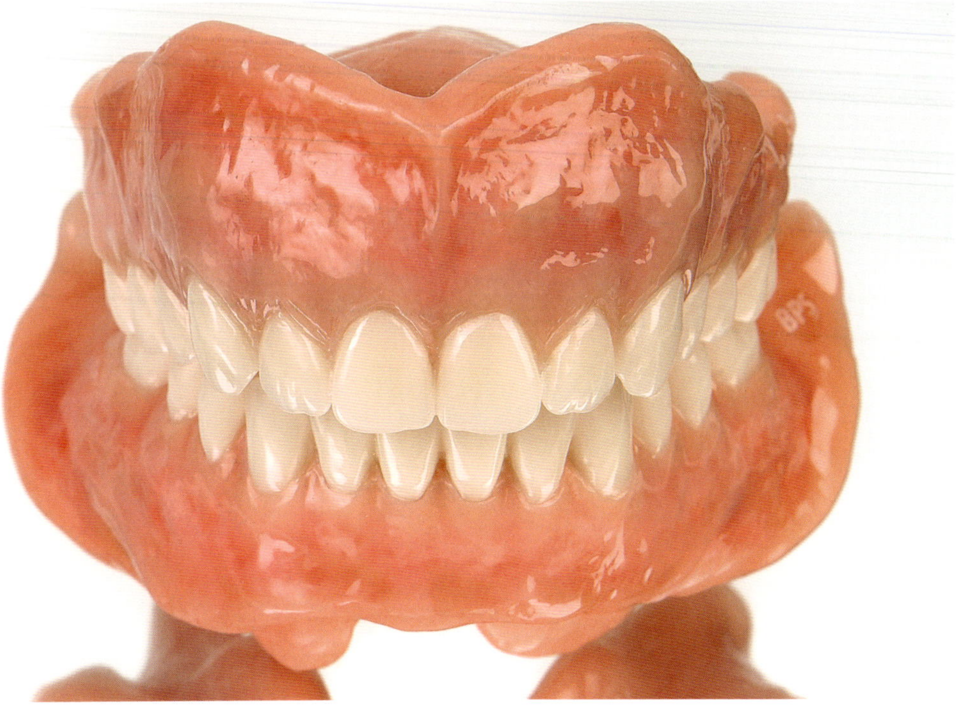

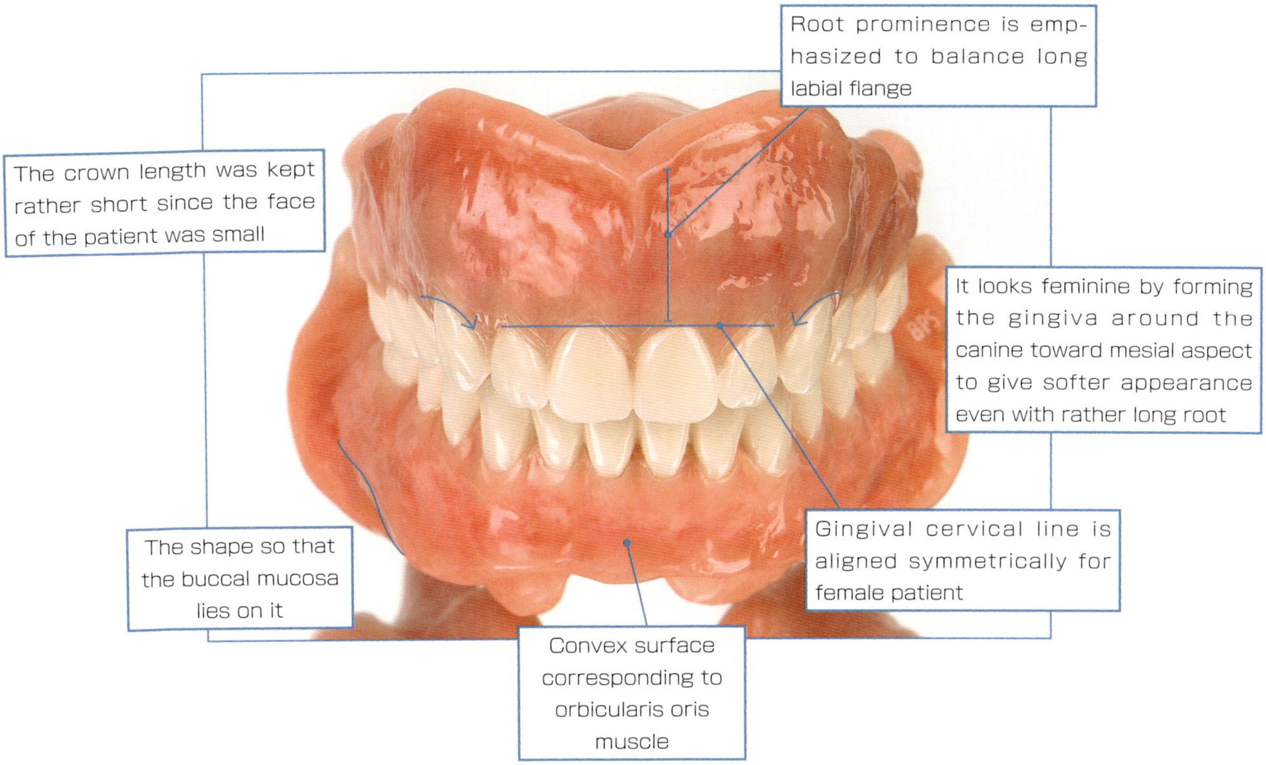

Completed complete dentures

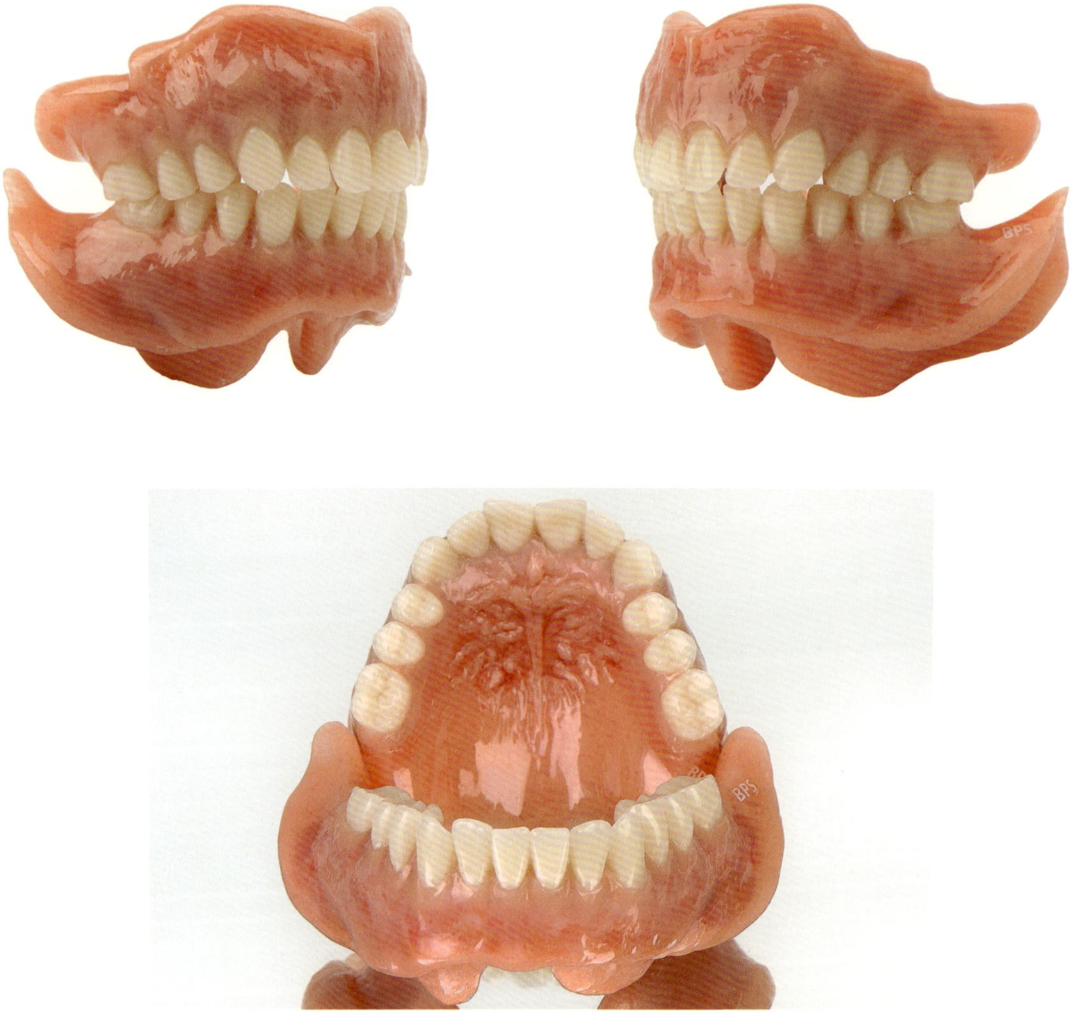

Fig79b Completed dentures in occlusion.

21 Summary

Completed maxillary and mandibular dentures are shown in Fig79. Various techniques are used in the dentures of Class 2-II Difficult-to-Treat case. This is a step up from the basic denture fabrication skills shown in Class 1. Close work relationship between the dentist and the technician is essential to achieve suction-effect, functional and esthetic satisfaction of the patient of this kind of Difficult-to-Treat case.

Part 6

Fabrication steps of the denture for Class II - division 1 case

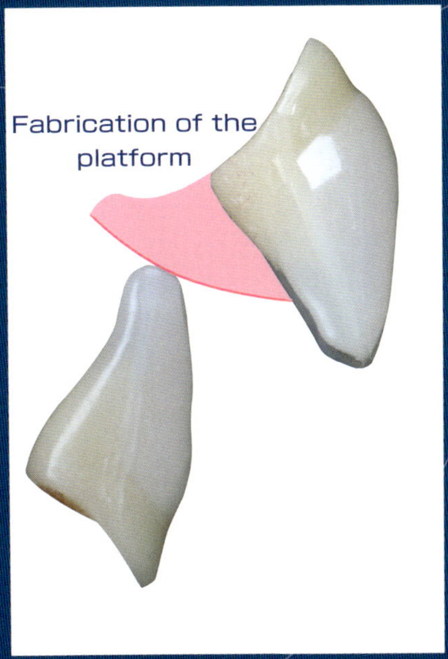

Dental Technician:
Kyoko Kokubo

1 Class II - division 1: maxillary prognathism case

Intra-oral photographs are shown in Fig 1 and the result of the examination for mandibular suction-effect complete denture is shown in Fig 2.

This case presents with severe ridge resorption, unfavorable retromolar pads and unstable mandibular position as well. Basic preliminary impression technique and simple bite registration technique using Centric Tray were carried out. Final impression using the custom tray was taken following the technique described in the treatment of Class I case in Part 4, since tongue retraction at opened mouth position was not so severe. The fabrication process of the conventional complete denture was followed for maxilla expecting loss of canines in near future even though enough retention was obtained from the O-ring attachments on canines.

The patient often suffers from persistent pain on mandibular alveolar mucosa from the denture with excessive over-bite with poor conditions for suction-effect. The cause of the problems is clarified and the solution is presented in this section.

2 Factors to lead to success with Class II - 1 case

Alignment of denture teeth provided with large over-bite and over-jet, which is

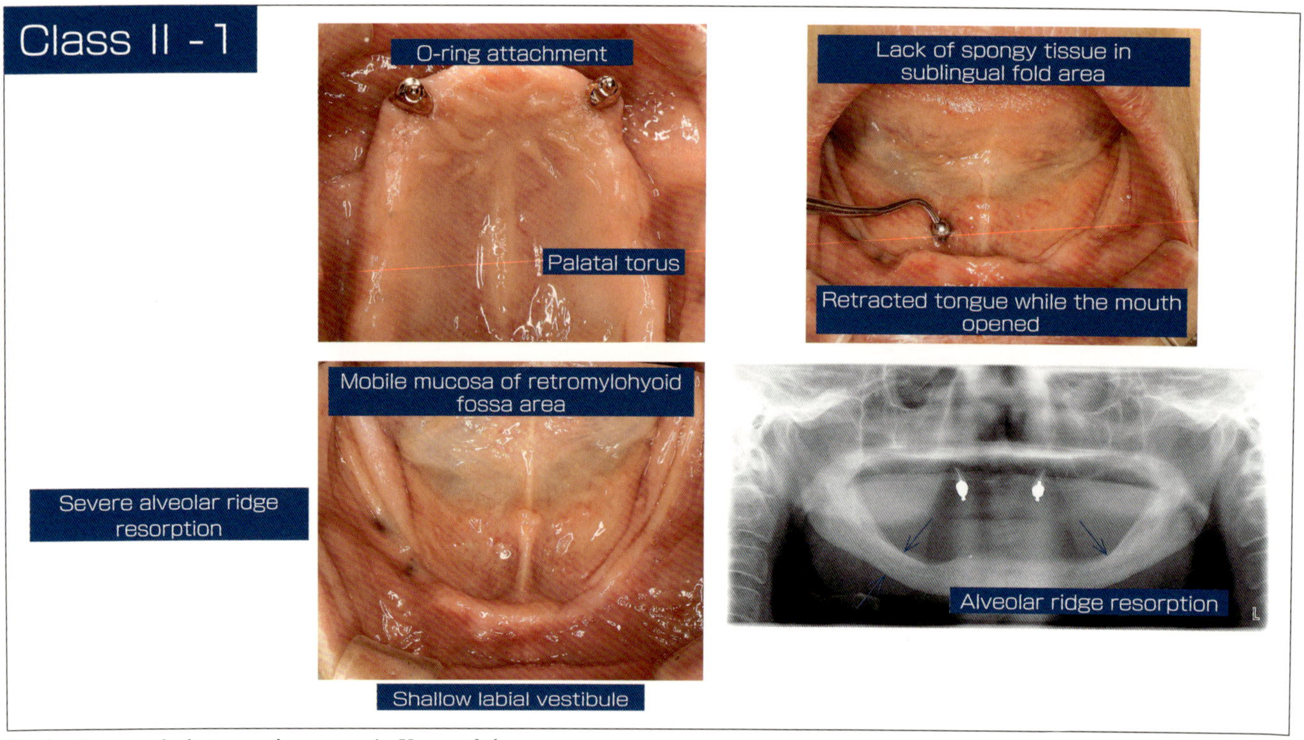

Fig 1 Intra oral photos and panoramic X-ray of the case.

Examination items for mandibular complete denture

Suction inhibiting factor	Right Good	Right Fair	Right Poor	Left Good	Left Fair	Left Poor
1. Ridge form			☑			☑
2. Spongy tissue in sublingual fold region		☑			☑	
3. Space for denture extension in retromylohyoid fossa region		☑			☑	
4. Pear-like shaped retromolar pad			☑			☑

Retromolar pad (one risk is ☑ as Fair, ☑ as Poor, if more than two risks are marked)

	Right	Left
1. The presence of firm fibrous tissue in anterior half	(Yes slightly No)	(Yes slightly No)
2. Size	(Large Moderate Small)	(Large Moderate Small)
3. Tilt angle	(Shallow Moderate Steep)	(Shallow Moderate Steep)
4. Change during open and close movement	(Small Moderate Large)	(Small Moderate Large)

5. Tongue retraction upon opening mouth	☐ Normal (less than 2cm)	☑ Further retraction (2~4cm)	☐ Even further retraction (more than 4cm)
6. Jaw relationship	☐ Class I	☑ Class II II -1	☐ Class III
7. Mandibular jaw position	☐ Guided position and habitual occlusal position coincide or within 2mm of discrepancy	☑ More than 2mm of discrepancy	☐ More than mm of discrepancy and unstable tapping point
8. Temporomandibular joint function	☑ Normal	☐ Disfunction	☐ Severe disfunction with pain

Special Note :
Wearing time of the denture, (Maxillary) Flabby tissue, Tori (Mandibular) Flabby tissue, Genial tubercle shallow labial vestibule in mandibular anterior region, etc

→ Shallow labial vestibule, abundant flabby tissue at retromylohyoid fossa area

Fig 2 The result of the intra-oral examination.

typical in Class II, is the factor to make mandibular denture unstable in Class II - division 1 (Class II - 1) case.

Maxillary premolars are aligned rather outside of the alveolar ridge crest with denture teeth setup according to general rule because maxillary anterior arch is pointy in many of class II - 1 cases. As a result, lateral force to sway the maxillary denture is generated upon chewing on premolars and the maxillary denture dislodges easily. Mandibular denture will also becomes unstable under function along with the maxillary denture.

The denture of Class II case tends to move and suction-effect tends to be broken easily since stability solely depends on mandibular molars without any contact on anterior teeth during function due to large over-jet. Solutions for these two problems are presented in this section.

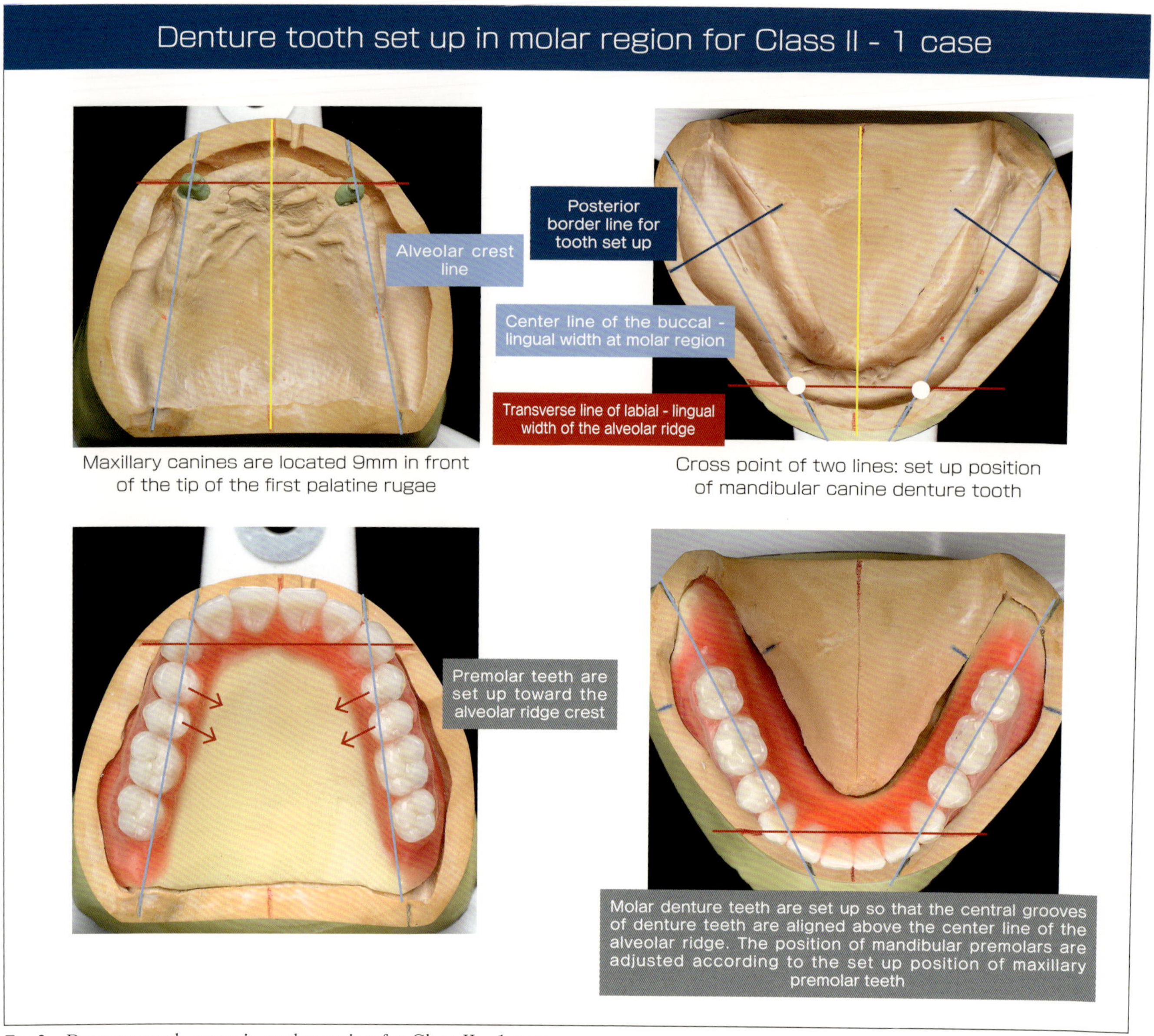

Fig 3 Denture tooth setup in molar region for Class II - 1 case.

(1)Denture tooth setup to prevent dislodgment of Class II - 1 maxillary complete denture

General rules for denture tooth set up for Class II - 1 was followed in this case according to the position of existing maxillary canines and patient's past photograph. Setting maxillary premolars towards alveolar ridge crest as much as possible without compromising esthetics is most important (Fig 3). Dislodgment of maxillary denture is prevented by minimizing the lateral vector of side-shifting. Esthetics is compensated by using larger size of the denture teeth or attaching the shell as shown in Fig 4 if it is compromised by setting maxillary first and second premolars too far inside.

Esthetics recovery in the case with large discrepancy between maxillary and mandibular arches

Esthetics is recovered by attaching the shell, shaved denture teeth, on top of first premolar teeth

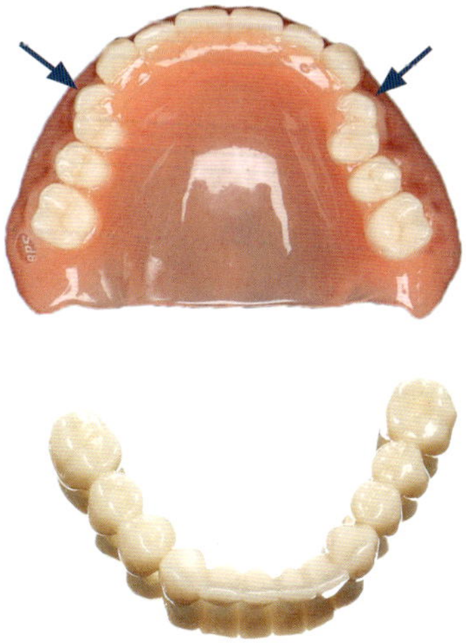

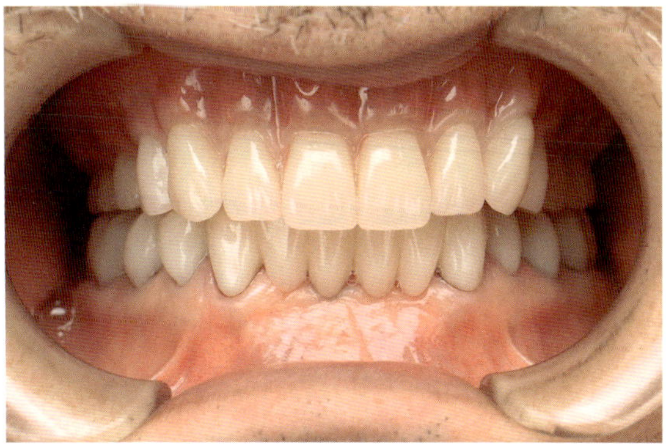

Fig 4 Compromised esthetics due to the first and second premolars positioned far inside is recovered by using larger denture teeth or attaching the shell as shown above.

Compensating curve provided in Class II - 1 case

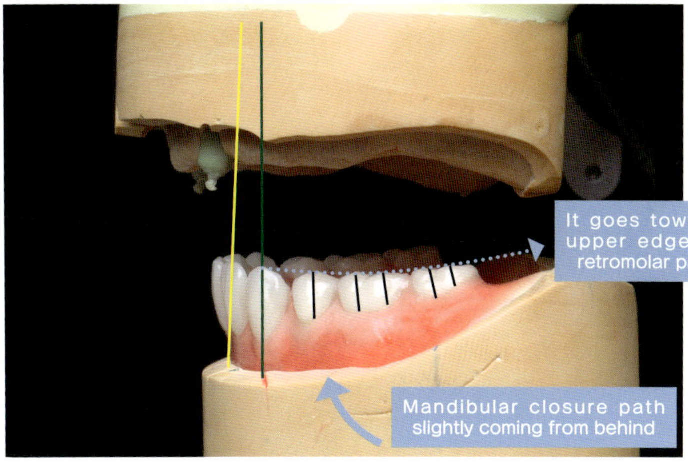

- Strong compensating curve is provided
- The occlusal plane goes up toward posterior (it goes up toward upper edge of retromolar pad from canine)

Fig 5 The mandibular closure path of Class II case starts from slightly behind to upward-forward direction compared to Class I case. Rather strong compensating curve is provided to avoid cusp interference according to the mandibular closure path.

(2) Denture tooth setup according to mandibular closure path in Class II - 1 case

Rather strong compensating curve is provided according to mandibular closure path in Class II - 1 case (Fig 5, 6). T - Type denture tooth (Ivoclar Vivadent) of Orthosit Orthotyp PE is designed larger than Normal type for Class I to establish occlusal relationship between buccal cusps with sharp angled buccal cusp incline

Providing Anterior clearance in Class II - 1 case

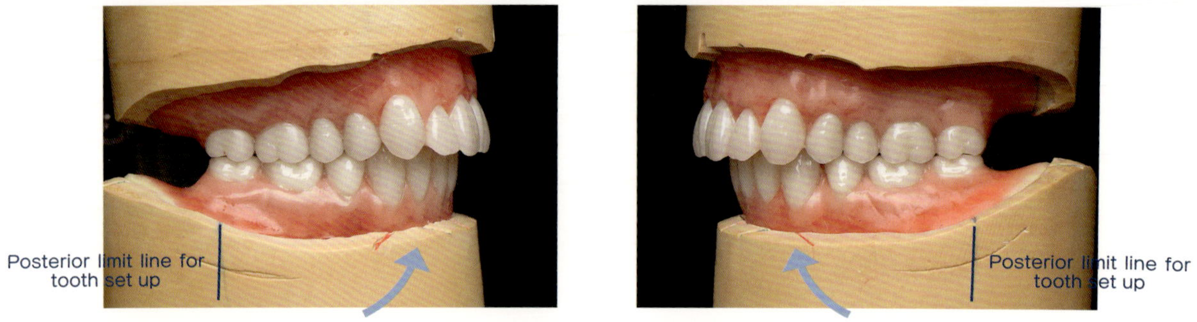

- Deep Over-bite is provided from maxillary first premolar to first molar
- Second molars are set up rather shallow to avoid cuspal interference during lateral and protrusive excursive movement due to strong compensating curve
- Mandibular first molars are omitted considering function and esthetics in this case. Canine relationship looks like Class I case

Fig 6 Denture tooth set up in Class II - 1 case.

Occlusal adjustment in Class II - 1 case

Cusps of maxillary first premolars are ground down accordingly so that they do not interfere during function

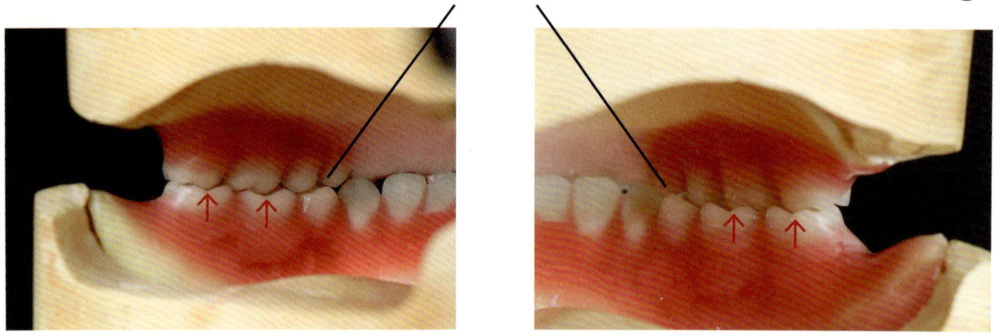

- Shallow occlusion of maxillary molar lingual cusps

Fig 7 Occlusal adjustment in Class II - 1 case.

in accordance with mandibular closure path, which comes in from the rear (Fig 7).

Mandibular molar buccal cusps are occluded tighter, since maxillary molar lingual cusps are occluded shallower (in order to avoid interference during function).

Fig 8 Large space between maxillary and mandibular anterior teeth in Class II - 1.

Large space between maxillary and mandibular anterior teeth in Class II - 1

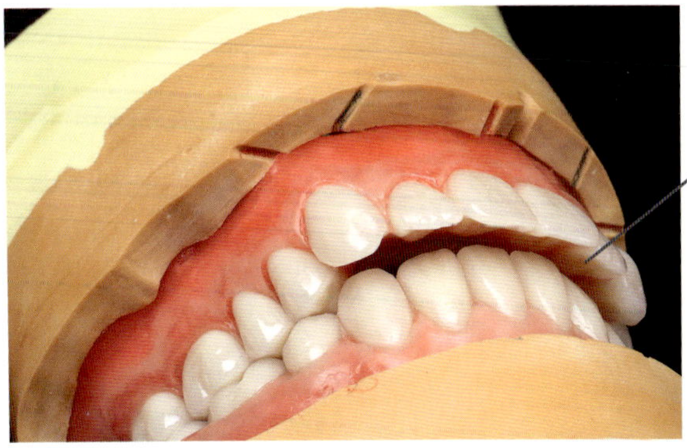

Large anterior clearance is generated

Fig 9 Tripod Contacts during chewing in class I.

The denture moves to function during chewing (Tripod Contacts during chewing)

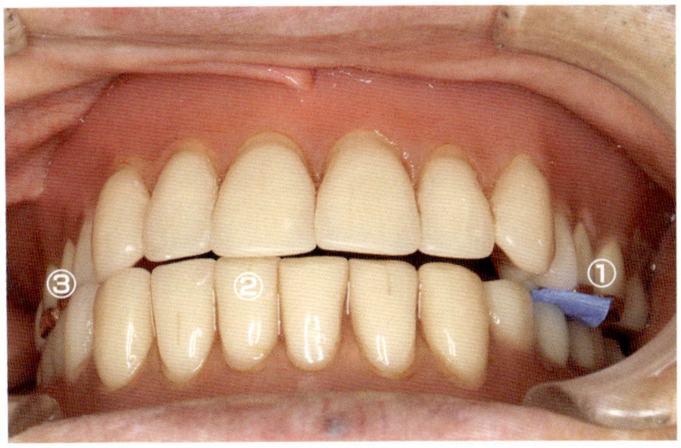

- Movement of the denture during chewing is decreased by establishing tripod contacts of ①piece of food, ②anterior teeth contact and ③balancing contact on the other side in class I
- Balance of the dentures during chewing is compromised due to 2-point contact in such class, which is the result of losing anterior teeth contact because of large space between maxillary and mandibular anterior teeth[83]

(3) The space between maxillary and mandibular anterior teeth in Class II - 1 case

Mandibular anterior tooth setup follows BPS guide line regardless of the position of maxillary anterior teeth. It results in large space between maxillary and mandibular anterior teeth (anterior clearance) since the base of mandibular teeth are aligned on the alveolar ridge (Fig 8).

Maxillary and mandibular space is just 0.1~0.2mm in natural teeth of healthy dentate people. Mandibular jaw movement is rather straight by keeping this space small. The movement of the denture is decreased by establishing Tripod Contacts of right and left molars (one side is with the piece of food inbetween) and somewhere in anterior region with the edentulous person in Class I relationship (Fig 9). Anteroposterior width of chewing rotation is larger in Class II - 1 patient due to large space between maxillary and mandibular anterior teeth. Lack of

Fabrication of the platform at the maxillary anterior palate area for the mandibular anterior teeth to contact

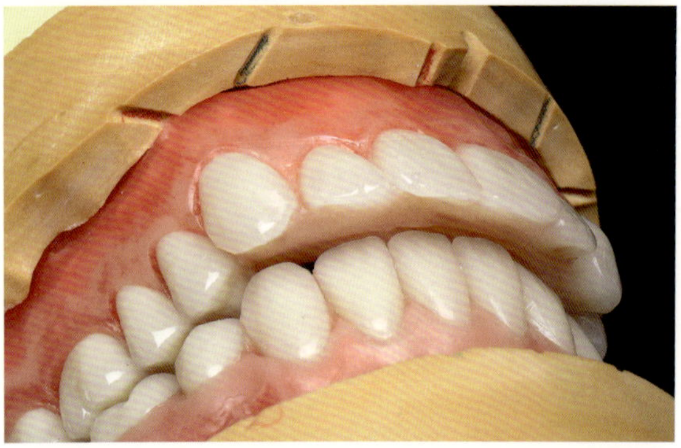

The platform is built up with wax for the mandibular anterior teeth to contact

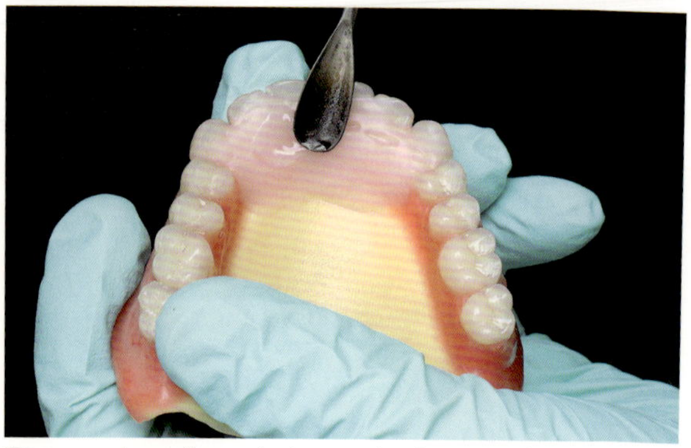

The wax is softened at wax denture try-in session and inserted in the mouth

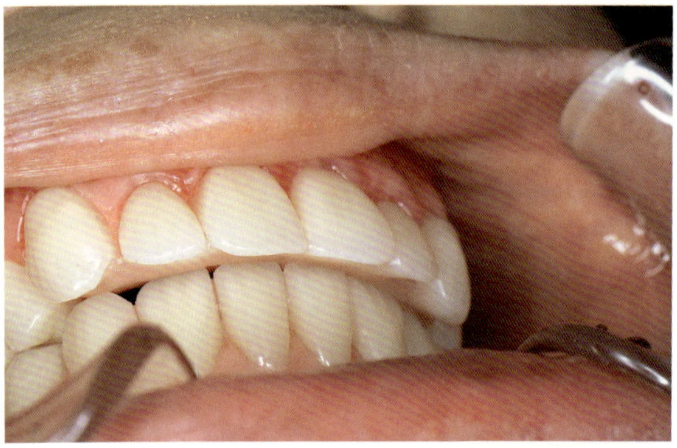

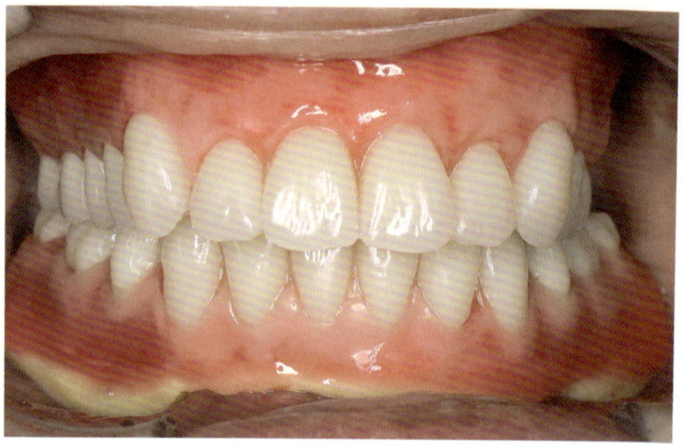

The patient is asked to do protrusive and lateral excursive movement

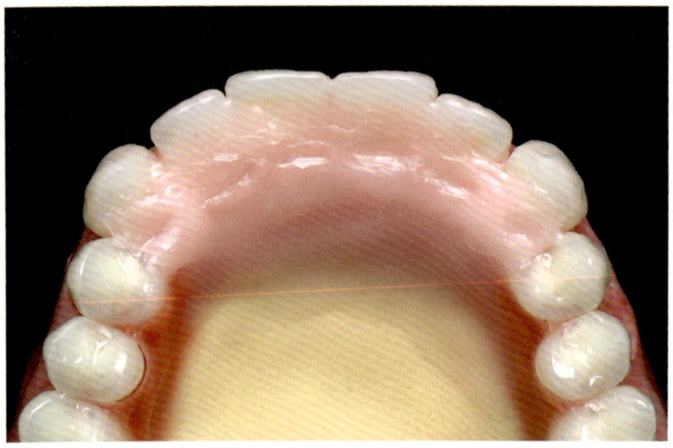

The wax is curved according to the movement shown above and the functional path is recorded on the platform. The bumpy wax is adjusted according to the shape of palatal torus and then replaced by resin

Fig 10 Fabrication of the platform at the maxillary anterior palate area for the mandibular anterior teeth to contact.

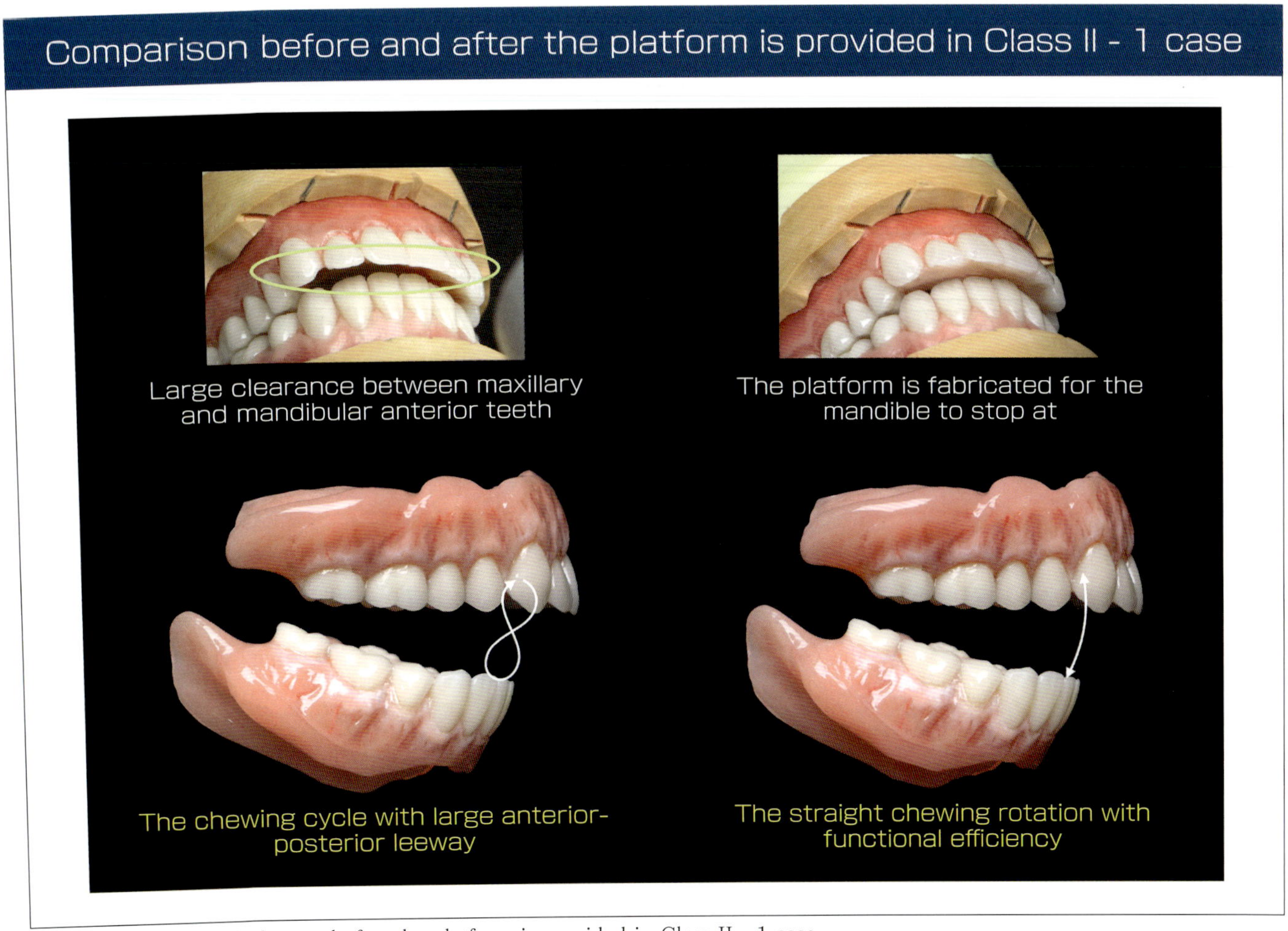

Fig 11 Comparison before and after the platform is provided in Class II - 1 case.

contact between maxillary and mandibular anterior teeth during occlusal function results in two points contact only in molars swaying the denture back and forth. Increased movement of the denture on the alveolar ridge causes denture stomatitis.

The platform, which creates contact to mandibular anterior teeth, is fabricated at maxillary anterior palatal region in order to solve this problem (Fig 10, 11). Mandibular jaw movement can be adjusted rather straight in Class II - 1 as it is in healthy dentate person by establishing the terminal point of the mandibular jaw movement (Anterior stop). Despite of the possibility of articulation disorder, the most important goal of denture fabrication is being able to eat normal. Restoring chewing ability should be the first priority of the treatment. It is conceivable that the influence of the platform on articulation disorder is different among languages. No influence of the platform on developing articulation disorder has been reported among Japanese patients in my clinical experience. Completed denture is shown in Fig 12.

Completed denture according to Class II - 1 relationship

Long buccal surface and short lingual cusp height is the characteristic of maxillary denture for Class II case

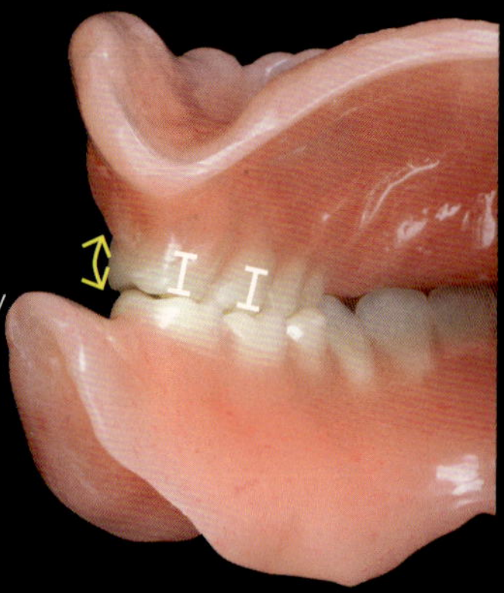

The denture tooth chosen (SR Orthosit PE T-Type, Ivoclar Vivadent)

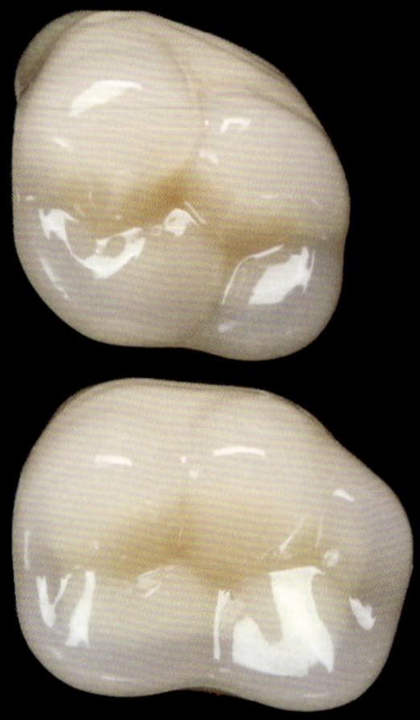

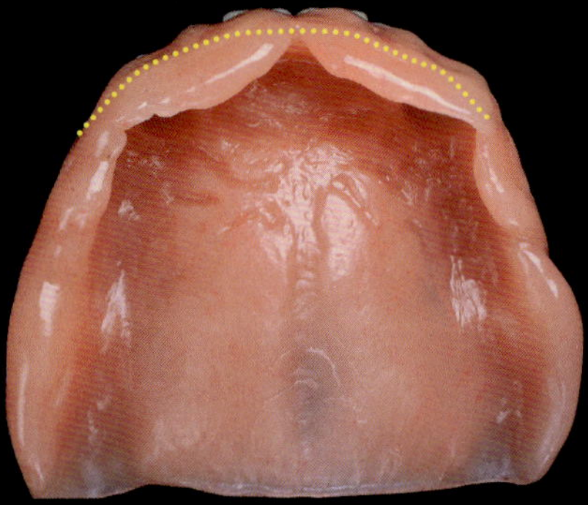

The ridge of maxillary anterior region observed on the model is square shape. It was diagnosed as Class II - 1 according to the patient's previous photos and position of remaining canines, even though pointy shaped ridge is typical for Class II - 1 case. Denture tooth setup was carried out as Class II - 1 case

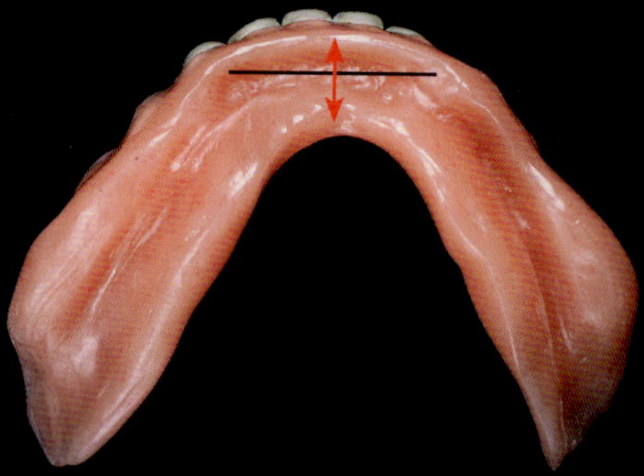

The base of mandibular denture teeth are aligned on the center of the alveolar ridge width according to the suction-effective denture concept

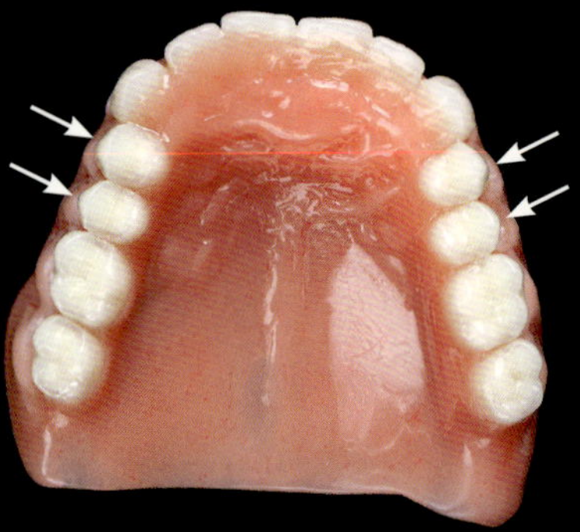

The first and second premolar teeth are set up closer to the alveolar ridge crest to prevent dislodgment of the denture

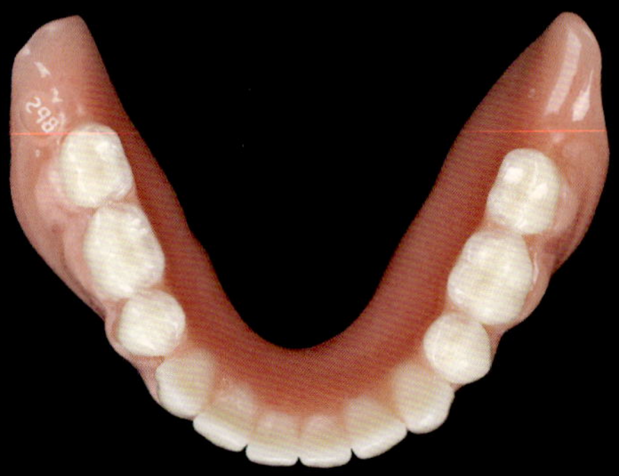

The area of outer slope of mandibular buccal cusp in Class II is wide with steep angle. The area of inner slope of lingual cusp is narrow with gentle angle

Fig 12 Completed denture according to Class II - 1 relationship and its characteristics.

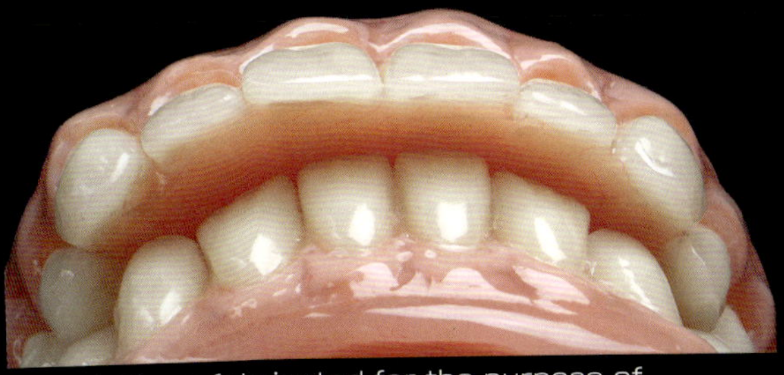

The platform fabricated for the purpose of establishing the anterior stop

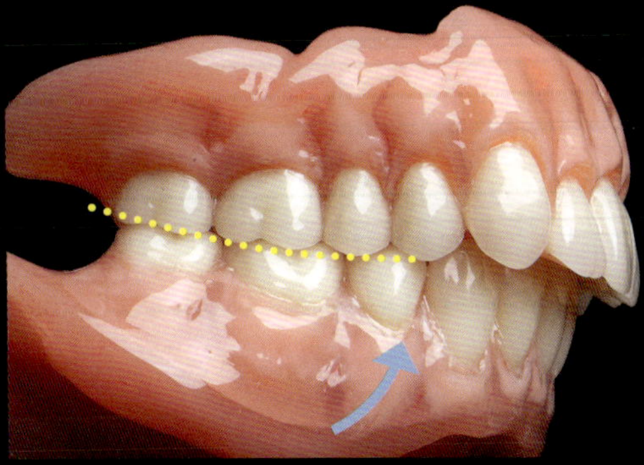

Strong compensating curve compared to Class I is provided according to the closure path, which is in posterior to up-forward direction. Occlusal relationship of maxillary molar buccal cusp against mandibular molar buccal cusp becomes shallower as it goes from anterior to the molar region

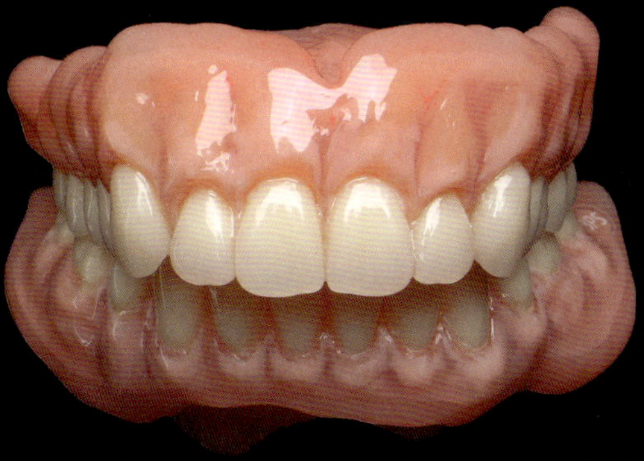

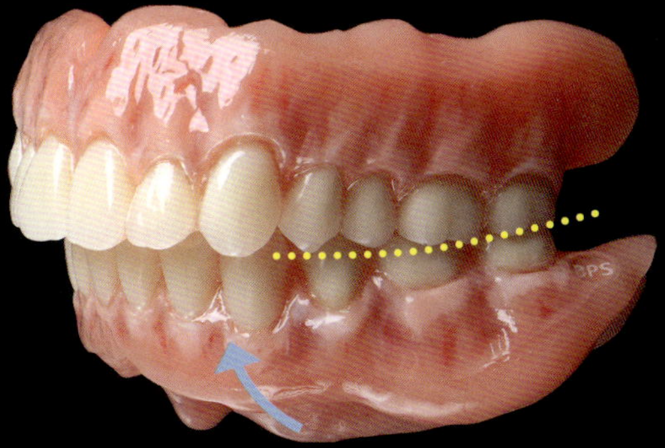

Large over-jet and over-bite in Class II - 1 case

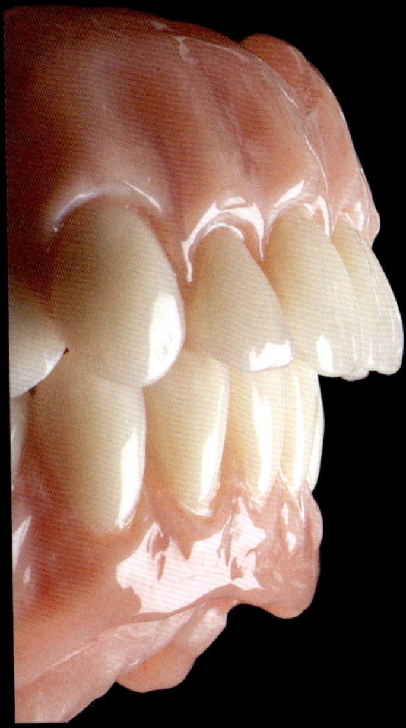

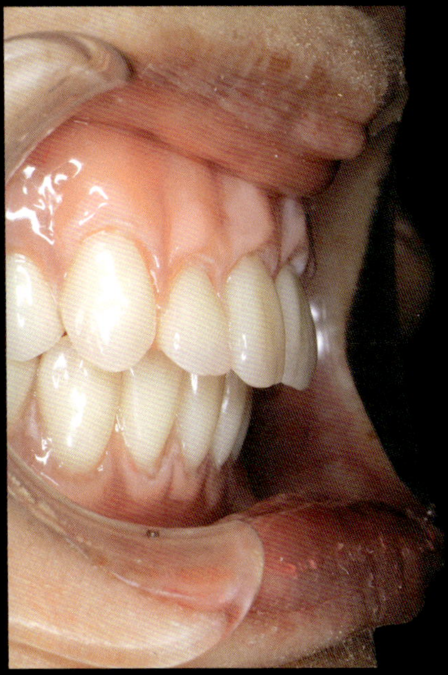

Completed denture for Class II -1 with esthetic consideration

3 Summary

The problem, we encounter while setting up denture teeth for Class II - 1 deep over-bite case, is that the mandibular jaw movement or mandibular denture becomes unstable due to large anterior clearance between maxillary and mandibular anterior teeth. The platform, fabricated on the palate of maxillary anterior region to overcome this problem, makes the mandibular movement straighter to provide reasonable chewing ability with minimum mandibular denture movement. Dislodgment of maxillary denture caused by large size discrepancy between maxillary and mandibular ridge form is prevented by setting maxillary first and second premolar teeth closer to the alveolar ridge crest. Thus, maxillary denture is stabilized and suction-effect of the mandibular denture is maintained.

Part

7

Denture fabrication method of Class III patient with TMD

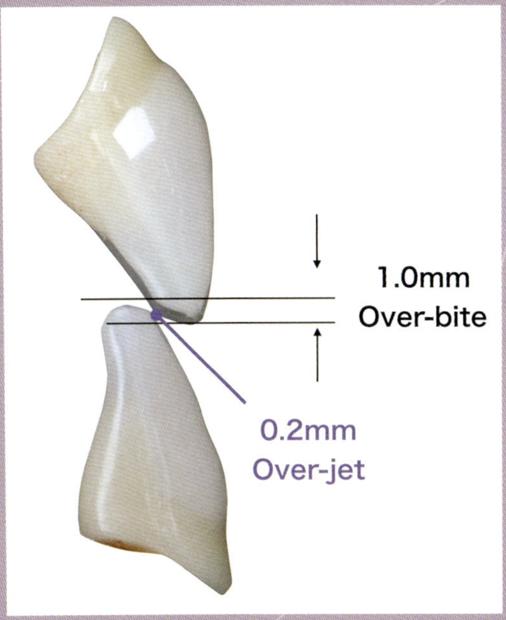

Dental Technician:
Tetsuya Sudo

1 Difficult Class III case

As intra-oral photographs are shown in Fig 1,2, this class III patient has problems with TMD, both of maxillary and mandibular denture dislodgment caused by maxillary flabby tissue, mandibular ridge resorption and the excessive mentalis contraction which lifts the mandibular denture up when the mouth opens.

Especially, TMD with unstable mandibular jaw position including clicking sound and uneven condylar movements is the worst inhibiting factor to generate the mandibular denture lifting since the denture easily shifts away in odd direction in the opened mouth.

The solution of these problems is presented through this section. In general, most of the Class III patients want to have a facial appearance of Class I individual. Due to this reason, maxillary anterior teeth are set up more anteriorly on top of the maxillary alveolar ridge position ; therefore, it is difficult to acquire the denture stability. The clinician faces a challenge to fabricate stable dentures in this situation since it is difficult to have great stability on both arches together.

VDO has been raised 8mm in this case during the fabrication in order to find the comfortable mandibular jaw position for the patient, as a result, the mandibular jaw position was changed due to the new elevated VDO and the improvement of the holizontal mandibular jaw position even after new dentures were issued. The method of remounting and occlusal adjustment method are also explained in this chapter as well.

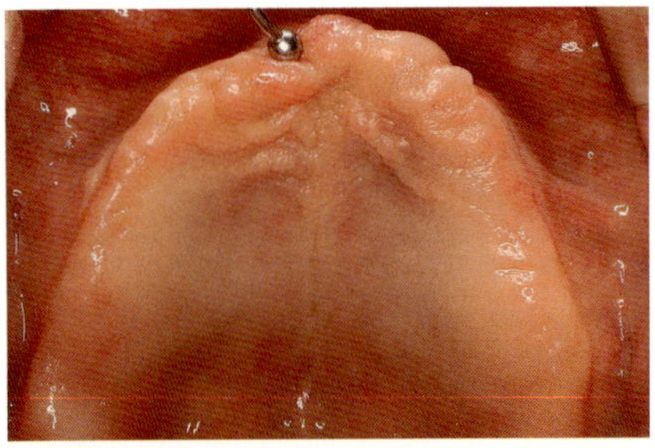

Maxillary anterior mild flabby gum
(the ball instrument is pushing the flabby gum)

▶ ClassIII
▶ Maxillary Flabby Gum
▶ Mandibular alveolar ridge resorption

More Difficult Case

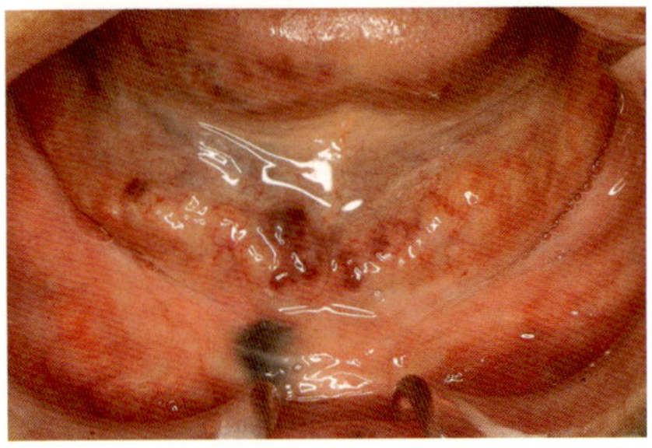

Severe molar area alveolar resorption anterior alveolar ridge is flat, there is almost no buccal and lingual flange

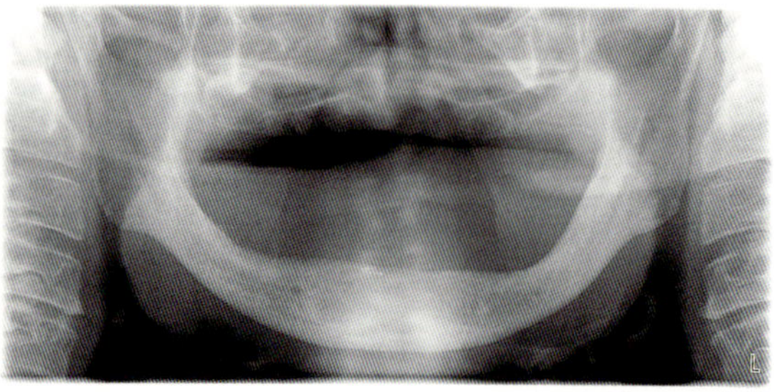

Even though panoramic X-ray shows enough alveolar ridge, the clinical view is completely different. This is the typical Class III case appearance

Fig 1 Clinical intra oral pictures and panoramic x-ray of the featured case.

Examination items for mandibular complete denture

Suction inhibiting factor	Right			Left		
	Good	Fair	Poor	Good	Fair	Poor
1. Ridge form		☑				☑
2. Spongy tissue in sublingual fold region			☑			☑
3. Space for denture extension in retromylohyoid fossa region		☑			☑	
4. Pear-like shaped retromolar pad		☑				☑

Retromolar pad (one risk is ☑ as Fair, ☑ as Poor, if more than two risks are marked)

	Right	Left
1. Is there firm fibrous tissue in anterior half	(Yes slightly No)	(Yes slightly No)
2. Size	(Large Moderate Small)	(Large Moderate Small)
3. Tilt angle	(Shallow Moderate Steep)	(Shallow Moderate Steep)
4. Change during open and close movement	(Small Moderate Large)	(Small Moderate Large)

5. Tongue retraction upon opening mouth	☐ Normal (less than 2cm)	☑ Further retraction (2〜4cm)	☐ Even further retraction (more than 4cm)
6. Jaw relationship	☐ Class I	☐ Class II	☑ Class III
7. Mandibular jaw position	☐ Guided position and habitual occlusal position coincide or within 2mm of discrepancy	☑ More than 2mm of discrepancy	☐ More than mm of discrepancy and unstable tapping point
8. Temporomandibular joint function	☐ Normal	☐ Disfunction	☑ Severe disfunction with pain

Special Note :
Wearing time of the denture, (Maxillary) Flabby tissue, Tori (Mandibular) Flabby tissue, Genial tubercle shallow labial vestibule in mandibular anterior region, etc

→ Anterior flabby gum, Shallow labial and lingual vestibule spaces. Left TMJ has clicking sound during opening and closing mouth movement.

Fig 2 Examination result with examination table of the treating case.

2 Manipulation of centric tray can become challenging (Fig 3)

Single step of double arch bite registration technique using the centric tray for the simple case was explained previously. However in this Class III case, first of all silicone putty impression on the mandible was done and then the hard alginate impression on the maxillary flabby gum ridge was done (Refer : Part 5, page 90, Fig 14).

3 Class III case custom tray fabrication (Fig 4, 5)

One of the features of Class III patient is the mandibular closure path runs more anterior than that of the class I patient's. Therefore occlusal plane tends to be inclined posteriorly. Once the occlusal plane is created towards to

Initial bite registration with the centric tray (Twice method)

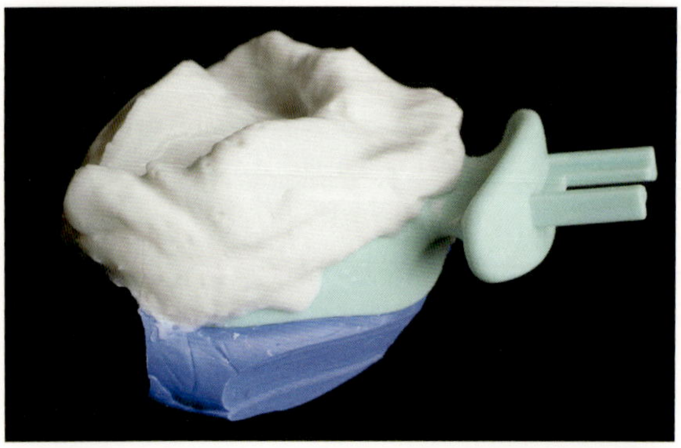

Combination initial bite registration method by using heavy body type alginate material on maxilla and silicone material on mandible. (Refer : Part 5 page 90, Fig 14)

Fig 3 Initial bite registration with the centric tray (Twice method).

Custom tray fabrication for Class III case

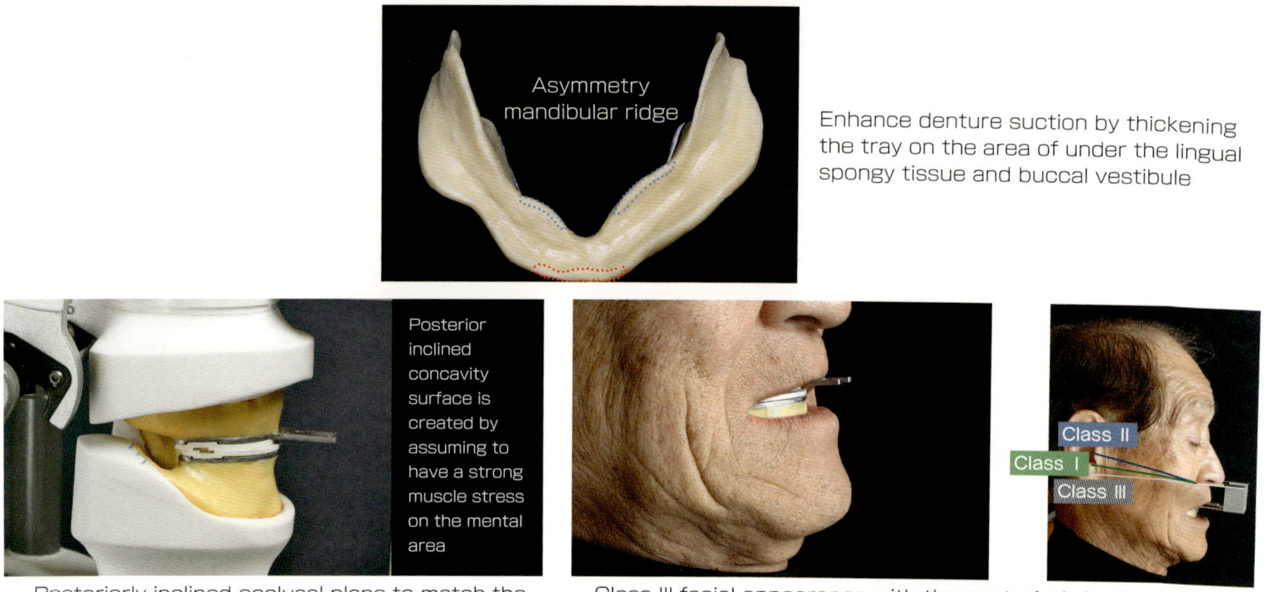

Posteriorly inclined occlusal plane to match the opening and closing path of Class III case

Class III facial appearance with the posteriorly inclined mentalis muscle attachments area

Fig 4 Custom tray fabrication for Class III case.

anterior 1/3~1/2 of the retromolar pad, both arch's cusps can occlude into maximum intercuspation without interferences. Class III patient tends to have strong muscle contraction around the mentalis area during mouth opening. Therefore, the denture labial polished area should be inclined posteriorly to prevent denture dislodgment from the lip contraction force. Since the mandibular alveolar ridge locates anterior to the maxillary alveolar ridge, the mandibular bite rim mount (white mounting plate) is positioned slightly anterior to the maxilla.

Class III tray try in and adjustment

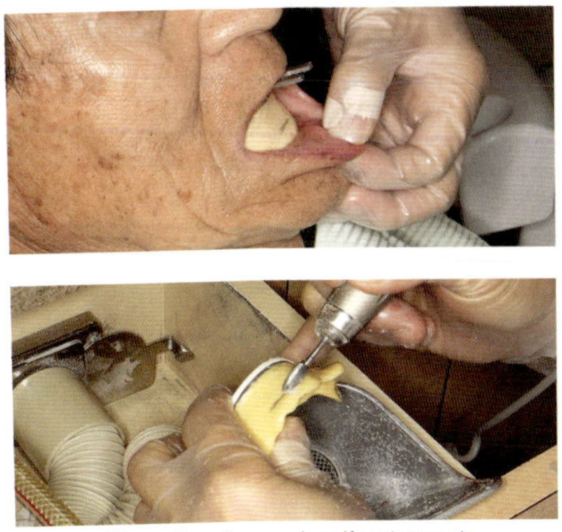

Tray try in and adjustment
Mark the strong touching area with lower lip intra-orally, then make concavity surface until the tray wouldn' t come out by the lower lip pressure while opening the mouth.

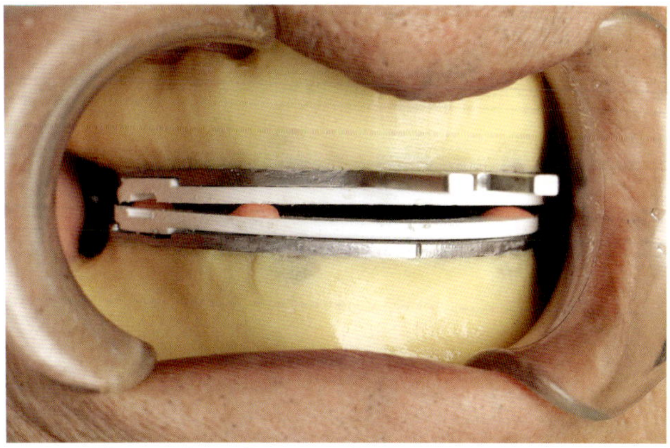

Bite registration error is checked with wax
There was an uneven space between maxillary and mandibular plates, so the final impression was carried out by leaving wax as it is. This wax allows the custom tray to be pressed evenly.

Fig 5 Class III tray try in and adjustment.

Final impression and Gothic arch tracing for Class III case

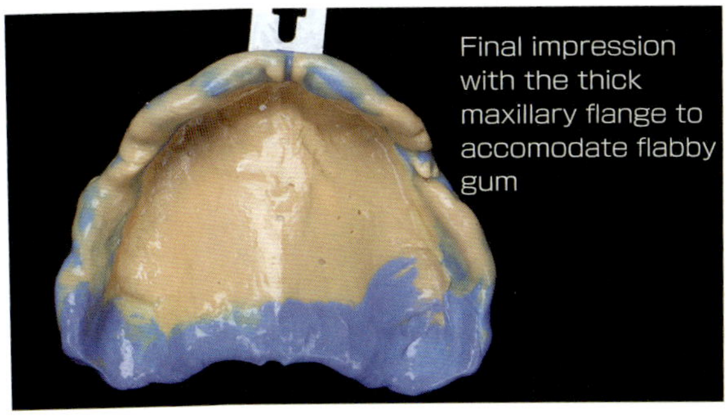

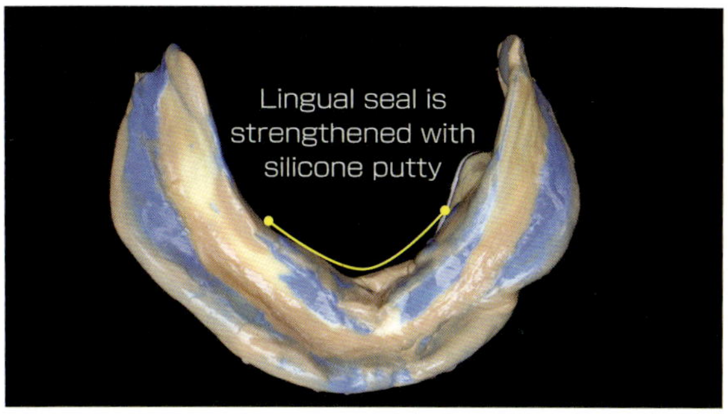

Since this case has a mild flabby gum,the optional impression technique with putty that was introduced with Class II-2 case wasn't used. The border molding was done with heavy body impression material and the final impression was taken with the light body material. After the completion of maxillary and mandible final impressions, the posterior palatal seal was well sealed with the functional postdam technique (virtual monophase)

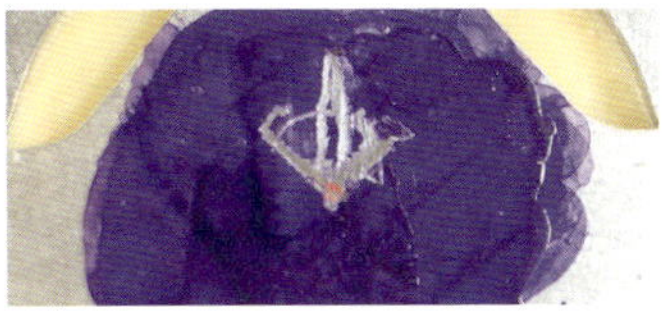

The small gothic arch appearance that implies the functional disorder. The mandibular position deviation can be suspected after the final denture insertion

After lingual seal is strengthened with the silicone putty, the border molding is carried out with the heavy body material.
The final impression was done with the light body material. There is a narrow space on the labial vestibule. However, adding the thickness to the tray would cause more dislodging effect by the lower lip that is the typical feature of the Class III case, so the tray periphery thickness has been altered without adding putty material (Refer: Part 5,Page112~114)

Fig 6 Final impression and Gothic arch tracing for Class III case.

4 Maxillary final impression (Fig 6)

The impression method of flabby gum ridge using silicone putty that is introduced with Class II Div 2 case wasn't carried out to this case, since flabby gum condition wasn't too severe.

Denture teeth set up with Class III case : At the time of mounting on the articulator

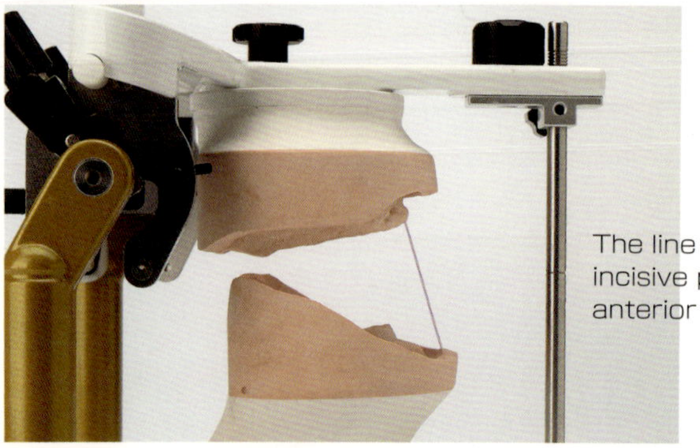

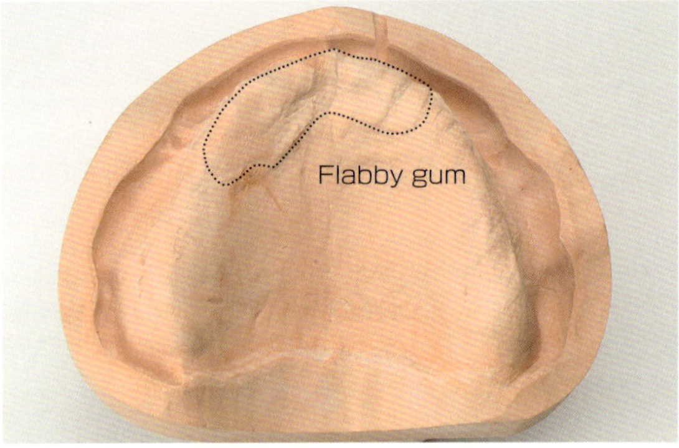

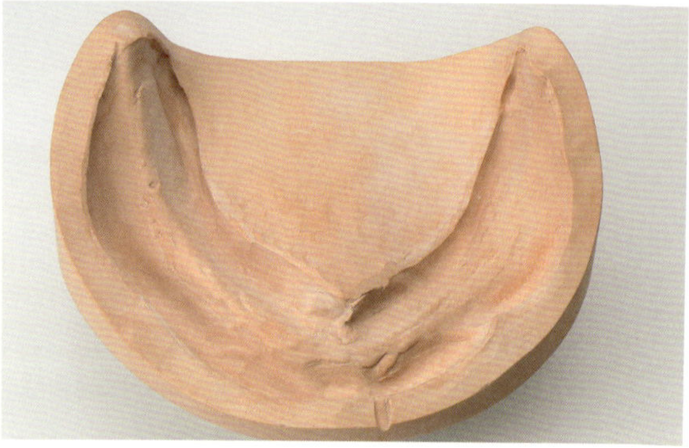

Extensive mandibular alveolar ridge resorption

Fig 7 The master casts of Class III case.

Good clinical judgement and decision making skill are well required to handle the difficult cases.

5 Mandibular final impression (Fig 6)

If the shallow labial vestibule space was observed, lip support should be enhanced with the putty material. However in this particular case, since the lower lip force for the denture dislodgment can be increased for the Class III patient, the tray border was simply thickened in stead of applying putty on the tray.

6 Gothic arch (Fig 6)

Even though apex and tapping points are matching together, the range of the mandibular functional movement is extremely small and the clicking sound of left temporomandibular joint during opening and closing movement has a big influence to the entire jaw functional movement. Therefore, detailed occlusal adjustment on the new dentures are going to be required due to the slight jaw relationship changes or functional movement after the insertion.

Class III denture teeth set up : marking the design lines

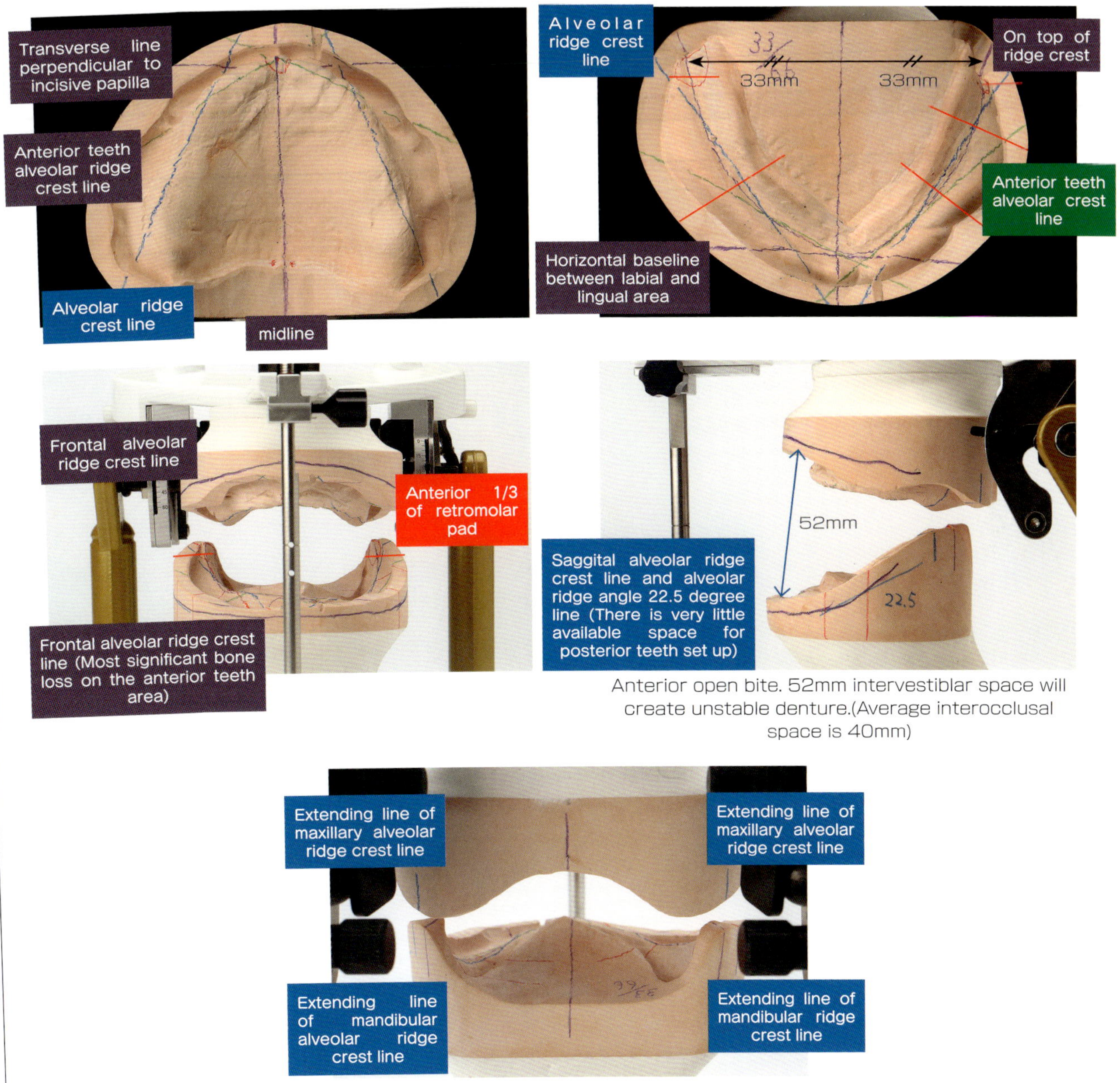

Fig 8 Marking the design lines.

7 Class III denture tooth setup

Class III has a feature that usually the mandible is larger than the maxilla; therefore, the teeth setting becomes cross bite[84] (Refer Part 4 for the model analysis, Fig 8).

Class III denture tooth set up : Maxillary anterior tooth set up

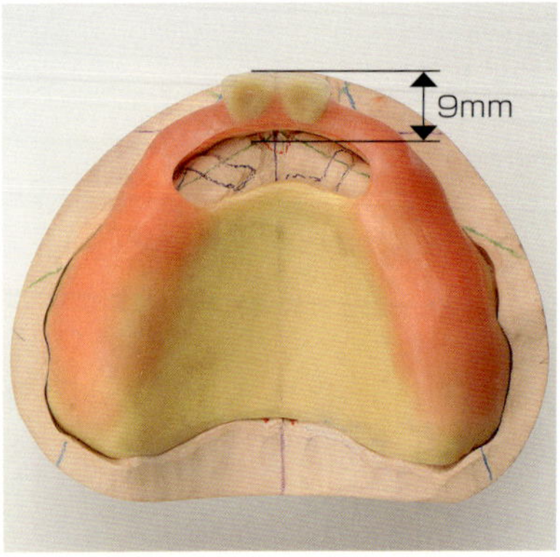

Maxillary incisors are set up by the reference of the incisive papilla location

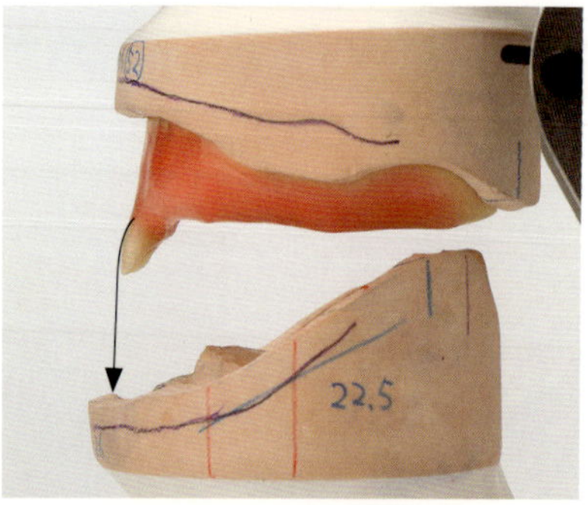

The suggital inclination of the maxillary central incisors is set so that the incisal edges are directed toward to the mandibular labial vestibule for the esthetic

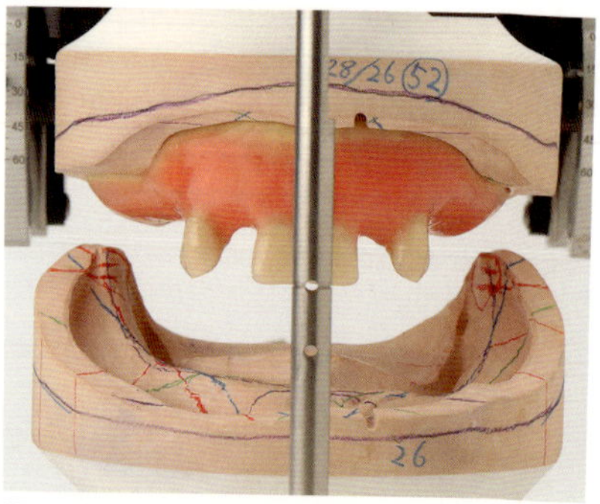

The canines are positioned in line with the first large pair of transverse palatine rugae. The intervestiblar distance is 52mm. The intervestiblar middle point is 26mm. (Maxillary incisors' incisal edge position should be 28mm from the mucogingival junction by adding 2mm overbite)

Fig 9 Maxillary anterior tooth set up.

Class III denture tooth set up : Mandibular canine set up

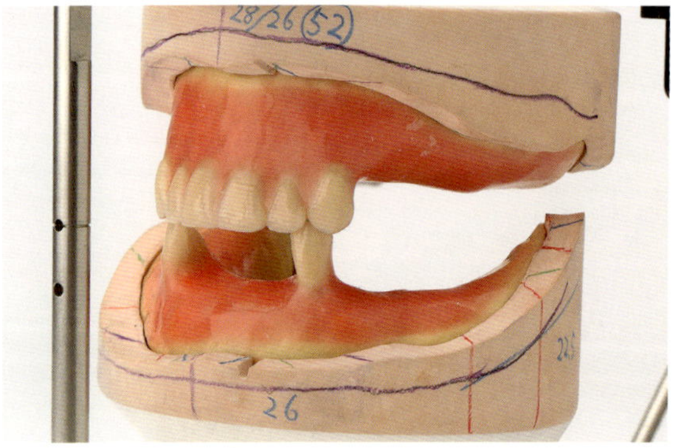

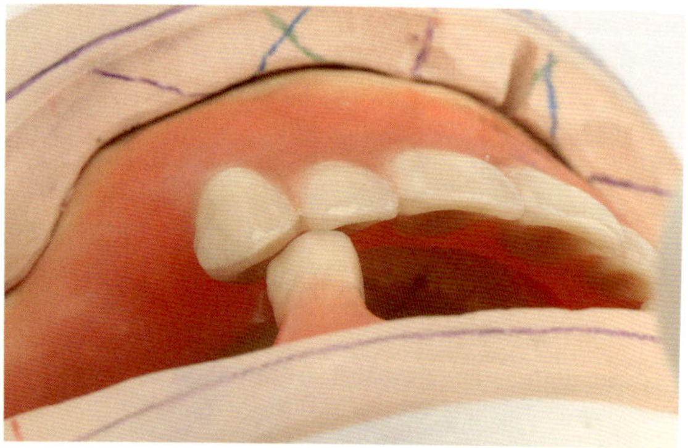

The cusp tip of the mandibular canine is positioned near the inter proximal contact between the maxillary canine and lateral incisor, slight over-jet is applied

Fig 10 Mandibular canine set up.

Class III's Sagittal condylar path angle is smaller than that of Class I in general. On the adjustable articulator, that should be set 15 degree angle and anteroposterior space between maxillary and mandibular anterior teeth should be 0~1mm (The smaller is the better). Over-bite should be arranged for 0.5~1mm edge to edge.

Usually tips of mandibular center incisal teeth should be located at half the intervestibler distance measured in the midline. Finally, in this case, mandibular anterior teeth contacted each other 2mm of overbite was applied. After adjusting protrusive and lateral functional movement on the articulator, 1mm over bite, 0.2mm anterior clearance were applied.

Class III denture tooth setup : Mandibular premolar and molar setup

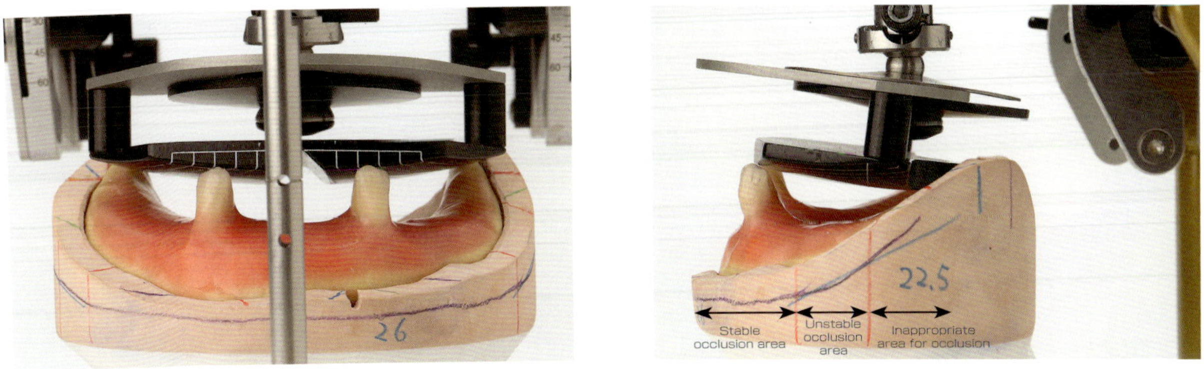

This case's occlusal plane posterior reference point should be 1/3 of the hight of the retromolar pad (Slightly posteriorly inclined)

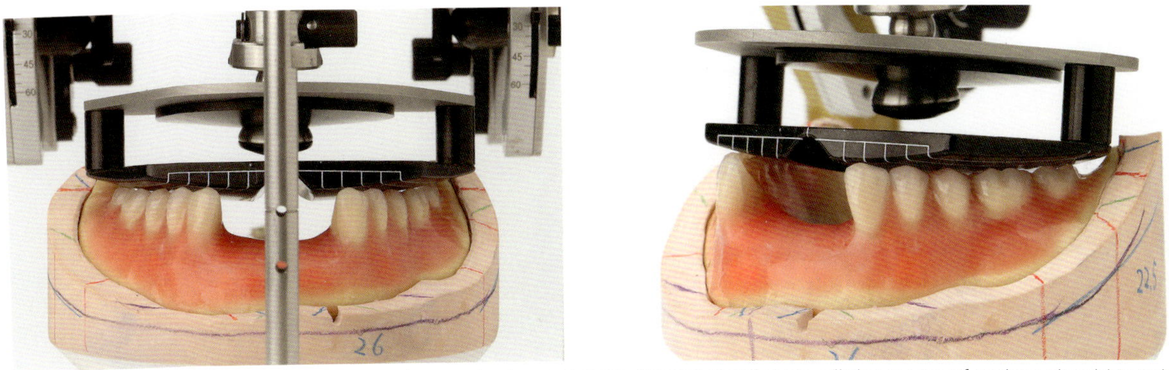

The first premolar buccal cusp, second premolar buccal cusp, lingual distal cusp, all the cusps of molars should touch to the 3D template

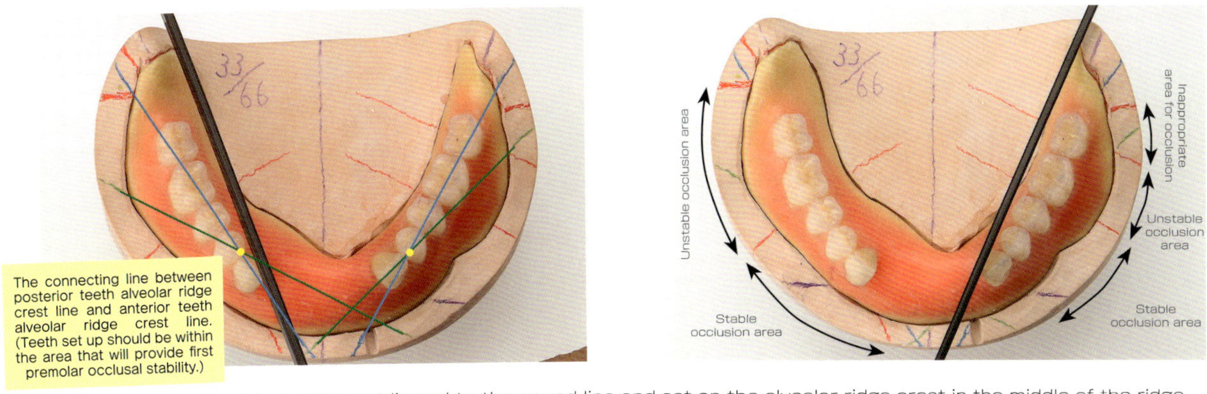

Denture teeth should never be set lingual to the pound line and set on the alveolar ridge crest in the middle of the ridge. Left last molar is set within the inapproproiate occlusion area, however, molars are very important to acquire the denture stability for Class III case. Therefore, the dentist should perform the dislodging test intra-orally

Fig 11 Mandibular premolar and molar setup.

In this case, Orthosit K type (Cross bite, Ivoclar Vivadent) are selected for the posterior set up. This is the only posterior denture teeth designed for Class III cross bite case on the market. SR Vivodent are selected for the anterior teeth set up.

Central incisors are positioned anteriorly at 9mm from the middle of incisive papilla and their contours are directed toward to the mandibular muco-gingival junction (Fig 9). Vivodent mandibular canine tooth position should be set on the

Class III denture tooth setup : Maxillary first molar setup

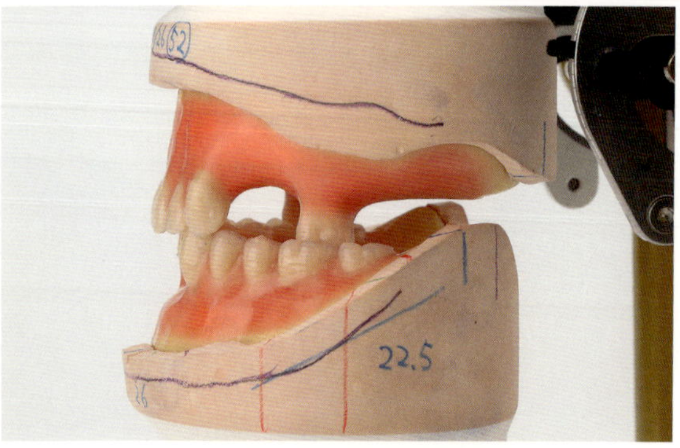

Maxillary first molar was set with cross-bite to prevent dislodgment since the maxillary arch is small. The difficult ridge case : The alveolar ridge incline is more than 22.5 degree

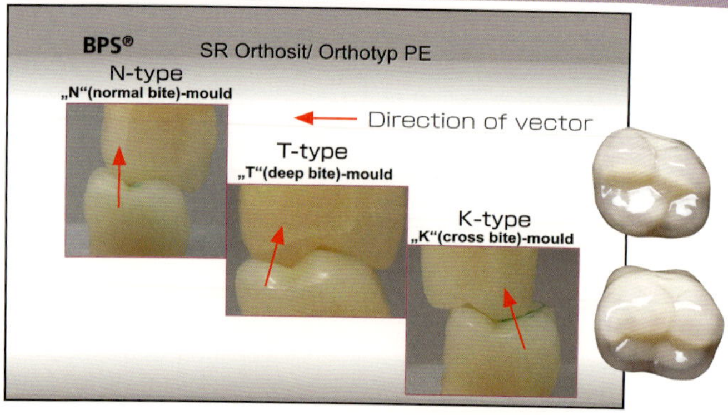

Orthosit PE cross bite K type is the particular denture teeth that the broad surface of mandibular molar' s buccal incline pushes maxillary buccal outer incline towards to palatal direction in order to stabilize maxillary denture

Fig 12 Maxillary first molar set up.

Class III denture tooth setup : Maxillary molars setup

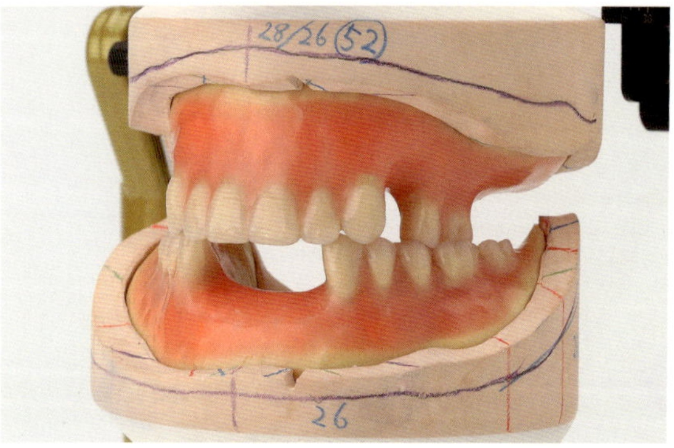

(Deflection point)Maxillary second premolar is set with edge to edge as a starting point of cross bite of premolars and molars

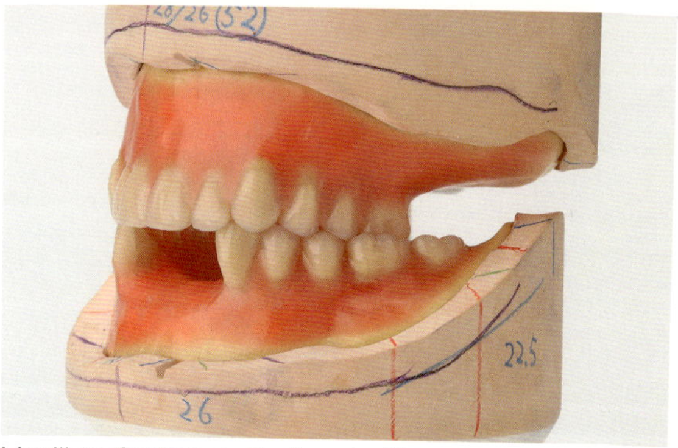

Maxillary first premolar is set with normal over jet and over bite by considering a nice esthetic transition from the canine

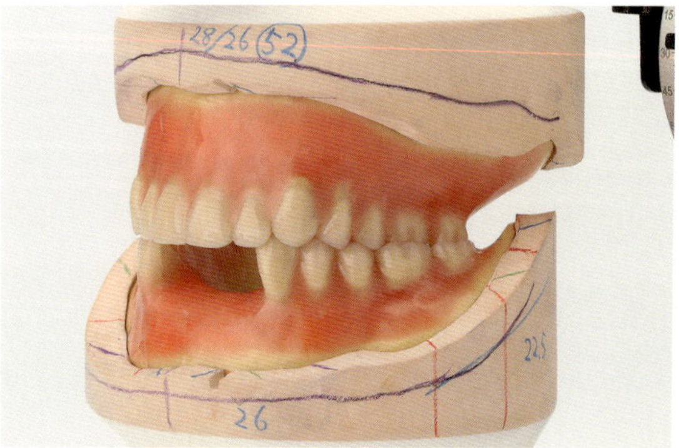

Maxillary second molar is set with cross bite. Orthosit teeth are designed to have plane contact and guiding plane for lateral and protrusive movements. Molars should be set appropriately in cross bite

Fig 13 Maxillary molars setup. If the sagittal alveolar ridge's teeth setting angle is more than 22.5°, the need for setting the second molar should be evaluated with the denture stability test performed by the dentist. 22.5° theory is just a concept so it's not mandatory to follow. If it is more than 22.5°, it can be adjusted by applying a compensating curve.

Class III denture tooth setup : Maxillary molars setup

Class III mandibular anterior tooth set up should be done with slight over jet and over bite even though anterior occlusion should be either cross bite or edge to edge relationship. Also, cervical area should be set with lingual inclination by considering the strong pressure from the orbicularis oris muscle as same as for the Class I, II

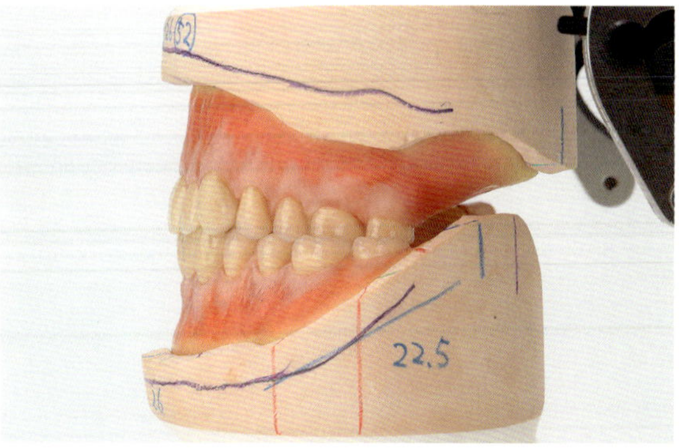

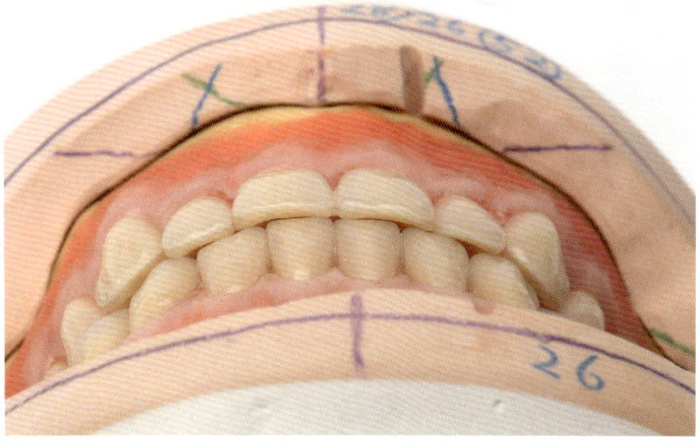

0mm clearance between maxillary and mandibular anterior teeth. After applying full balanced occlusion with posterior teeth on the articulator, anterior clearance 0.5mm and over-bite 0.5～1.0mm are created on the anteriors

Fig 14a Mandibular anterior teeth set up. Maxillary and mandibular anterior teeth are contacting prior to the occlusal adjustment. It can be appreciated that cervical part of the mandibular anterior teeth are slightly inclined lingually. During the Class III tooth set up and gingival wax up, It is important to take the strong orbicularis oris muscle pressure into consideration.

location of between maxillary lateral and canine mesial corner with minimum over jet since posterior teeth should be set as a cross bite with Class III case. (Fig 10)

For the Class III case, occlusal plane posterior reference point should be 1/3 of the height of the retromolar pad and slightly posteriorly inclined. Orthosit K type teeth's cusps should touch the template and teeth should be set perpendicular to the template curvature. Denture teeth should be set in the middle of the alveolar ridge width and outside of the Pound line (the line connected between inner line of retromolar pad and the corner of canine) with the good occlusal stability (Fig 11).

Maxillary first molars are set in cross bite with mandibular teeth. (Fig 12) Second premolar should be set in edge to edge as a starting point of cross bite of premolars and molars. First premolar should be set in a normal occlusion in consideration of the esthetic transition from canines. Maxillary second molars should be set in cross bite (Fig 13).

Mandibular anterior tooth set up follows, mandibular anterior teeth should be se-

Class III denture tooth setup technique

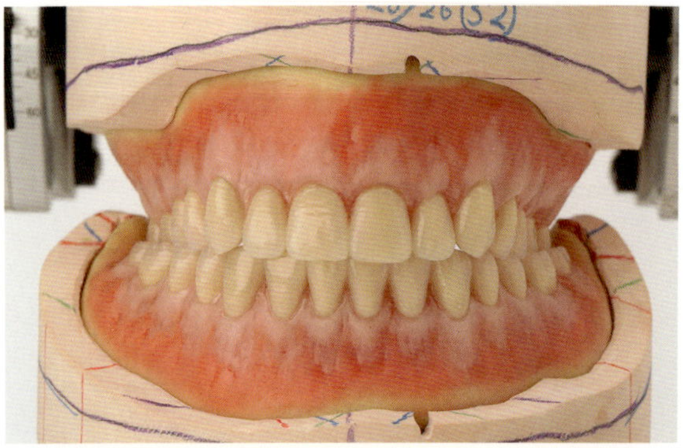

When dentures are inserted in the mouth, usually only premolars can be seen from the outside, therefore even though posterior teeth are set up with cross bite, there shouldn't be an esthetic concern

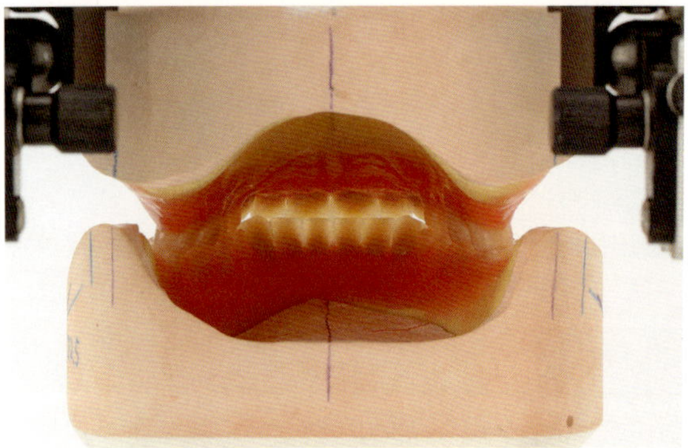

Lingual view. It is appreciated that maxillary arch is smaller than mandibular arch. Molars are set with cross bite and the denture stability is acquired by mandibular denture teeth pushing maxillary denture teeth palatally. Normal over jet and over bite are applied to the first premolar in order to keep the esthetic appearance and lateral movement guidance. But the second premolar should be set with edge to edge relationship to be the starting point of the posterior cross bite setting with the lateral movement guidance

Fig 14b Class III denture tooth set up technique.

lected according to the canine to canine distance (Fig 14). Fig 14b shows the technique of Class III denture teeth set up.

Maxillary and Mandibular anterior teeth should contact together at the time of the tooth setup. Side view of mandibular anterior teeth, teeth's cervical area is situated slightly inward. Class III tooth setup should be carried out with the consideration of dealing with the orbicularis oris muscle pressure as same as Class I, II setup.

8 Adjustment of Class III Denture tooth setup

First premolars should be set in normal occlusion. Second premolars should be set in edge to edge position in order to set molars in cross bite. Therefore, mandibular teeth appears to have a nice arch form but in the maxillary arch, there is a gap between second premolar and first molar. If the gap is large, this may cause negative

Maxillary second premolar is set with cross bite. But an appropriate over bite should be kept in order for the patient not to have tongue biting. The teeth setting with premolars normal set up and molars cross bite creates a large gap between premolars and molars. Orthosit K type denture teeth allow to create minimum gaps between premolars and molars by adjusting maxillary second molar to edge to edge setting

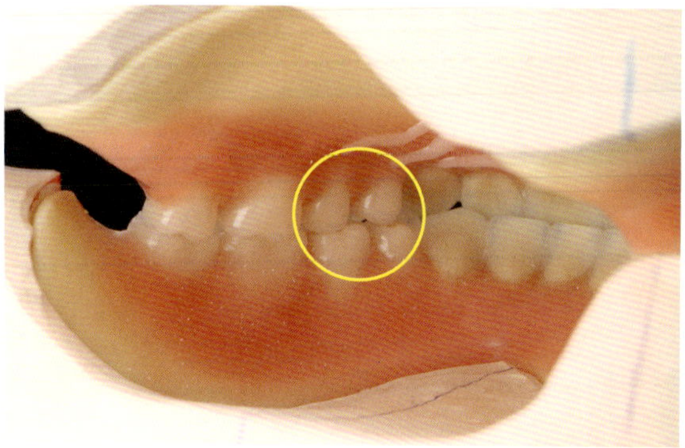

A gap appears around the first molar area since the cross bite setting starts from there. However less gap can be created by setting the distal area of second premolar slightly lingually and the mesial area of the first molar with the rotation in order not to create the tongue discomfort or food impaction

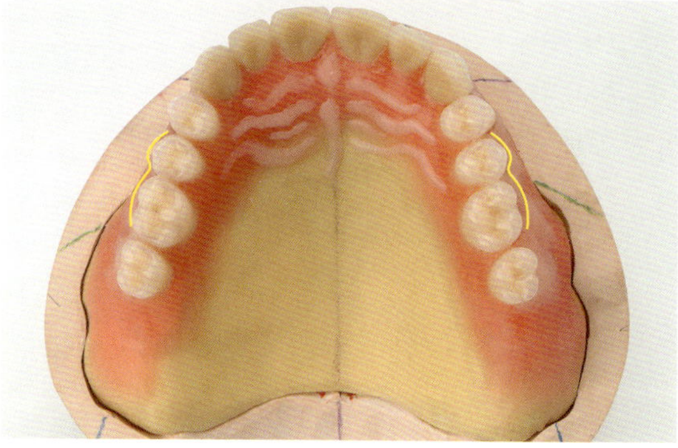

effect such as a food impaction. So the tooth setting adjustment is done in order not to have a large gap.

During working side in lateral movement, mandibular premolar distal incline glides against maxillary premolar mesial incline, and maxillary and mandibular molars disclude at the same time. At the non-working side, mandibular buccal inner incline glides against maxillary buccal outer incline. This is the semi-balanced occlusion (Fig 15).

During protrusive movement, maxillary first premolar distal incline glides against mandibular second premolar mesial incline. Maxillary second premolar distal incline glides against mandibular first molar mesial incline. Consequently, over-bite 1mm and antero posterior space 0.2mm on the anteriors are created.

9 Class III denture coloring (Candulor)

The Class III case usually has chopping type jaw movement that is different from

Class III denture tooth setup : Occlusal adjustment

Red : Post occlusal adjustment (Maximum intercuspation)

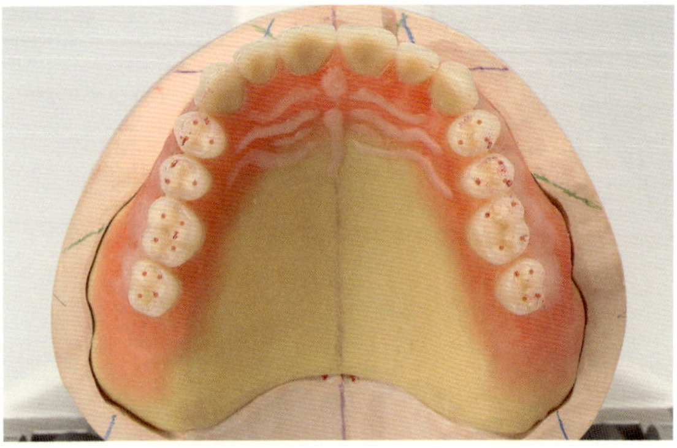

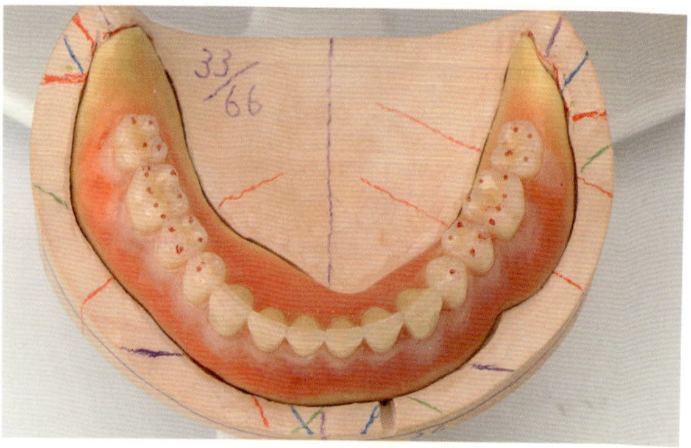

Orthosit is the denture teeth that is designed to have the guiding planes of lateral and protrusive movements. This planes slide during the functional movement and it is designed to have a point contact during the maximum intercuspation. If K type teeth are selected, since maxillary arch is smaller, maxillary premolar palatal cusp should be in contact. Molars are set in cross bite, buccal cusps should be in contact in order to direct mandibular molar's occlusal force towards to palatal direction effectively

Blue :Post occlusal adjustment (Semi-balanced occlusion)

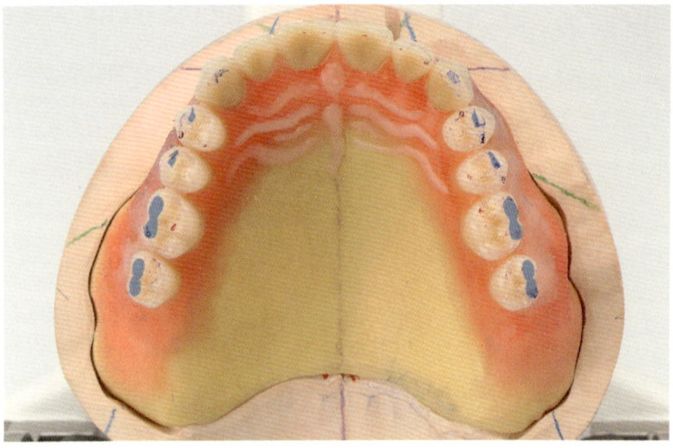

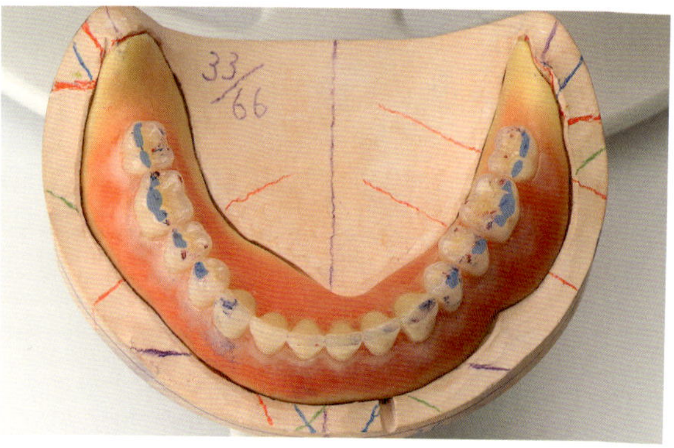

During the lateral movement, maxillary denture will become stable by sliding mandibular premolar distal incline and maxillary premolar mesial incline together. Canine should slide together with premolar during the lateral movement, however, if the denture becomes unstable, this sliding movement of canine should be eliminated. The non-working side movement should be that mandibular molar buccal inner incline and maxillary buccal outer incline slide together. This is different from full balanced occlusion. Less adjustment is required to this semi-balanced occlusion[7]

Green :Post occlusal adjustment (Protrusive movement)

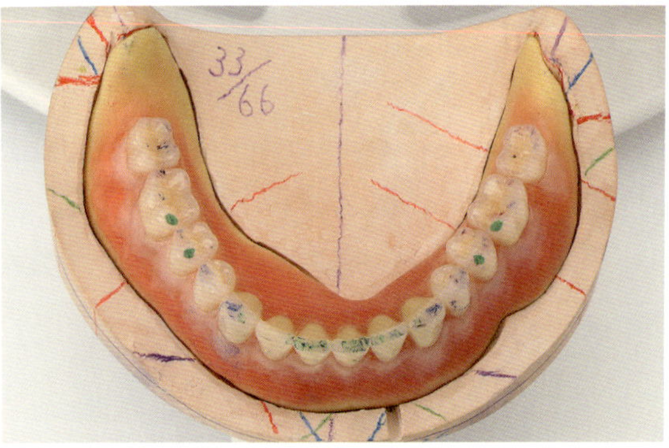

During the protrusive movement, maxillary first molar distal incline and mandibular second premolar distal incline, maxillary second premolar distal incline and mandibular first molar mesial incline should slide together and at the same time maxillary and mandibular anterior teeth should slide together. After the adjustment, over-bite 1mm and over-jet 0.2mm were observed

Fig 15 Occlusal adjustment.

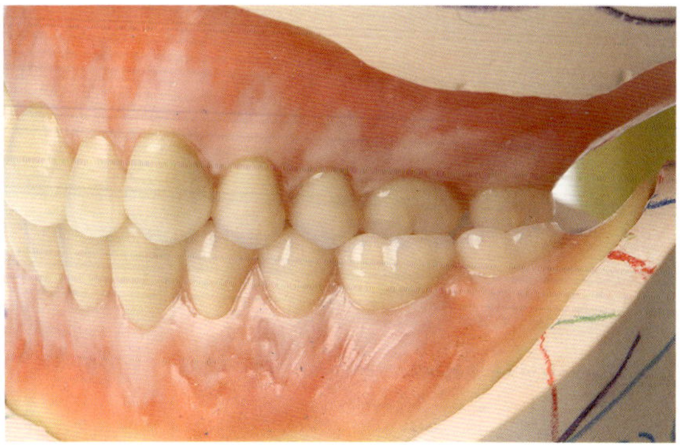

Class III is chopper type, therefore, even though Orthosit denture teeth that is designed to have plane type contacts, this wouldn' t give interference

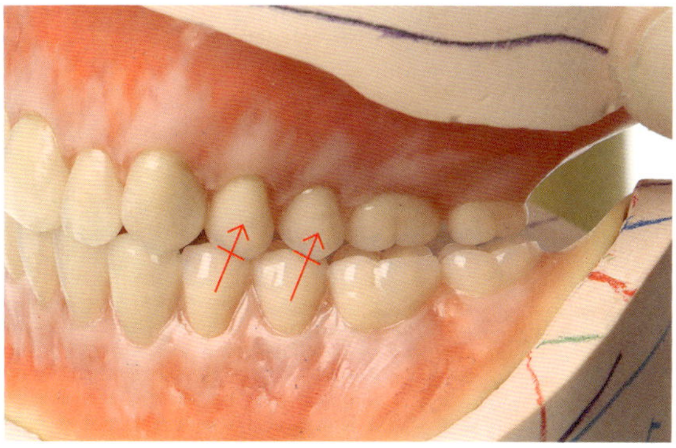

During the lateral movement, molars are discluded by guiding movement by the maxillary and mandibular premolars together. At the same time on the non-working side, premolars are discluded and molars are guiding

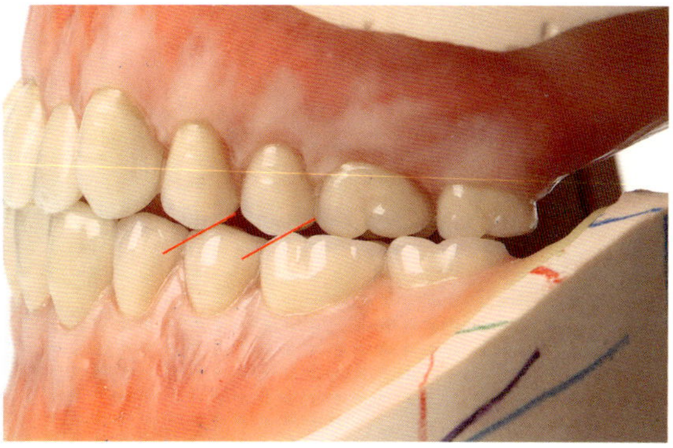

During the protrusive movement, anterior guidance should be applied according to the posterior guidance. For the Class III case, since the occlusal plane is posteriorly inclined, molars are not guiding but maxillary second premolar and mandibular first molar should be sliding together

Class III denture tooth setup : Confirmation of denture tooth position

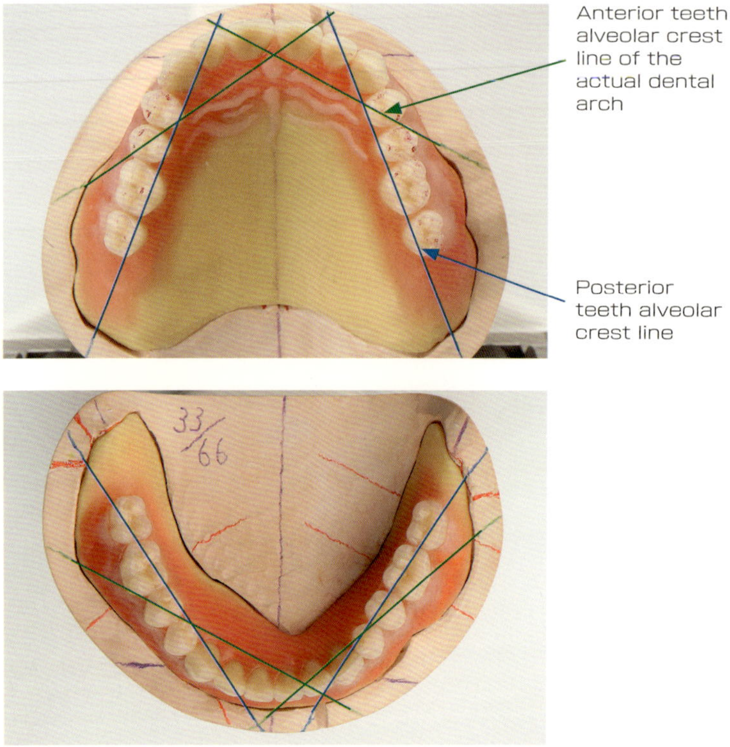

Fig 16 Regarding to the maxillary posterior teeth setting up, premolar's functional cusps should be positioned on the alveolar crest, but molar's buccal cusps (since cross bite is applied, maxillary molar's buccal cusps become functional cusps) should be positioned slightly buccally from the alveolar crest. The force vector from mandibular molars to maxillary molars directs towards to inner side of the alveolar crest due to the cross bite and compensating curve; therefore, the movement of the denture can be minimized. However since maxillary anterior tooth set up can occur too far labially, the first premolar set up can locate off from the alveolar crest ridge and then become unstable. The first premolar should be set up within the connecting lines between the line of anterior teeth crest ridge line and the line of posterior teeth ridge crest in order to keep the denture teeth stability.

Class III denture tooth set up completion

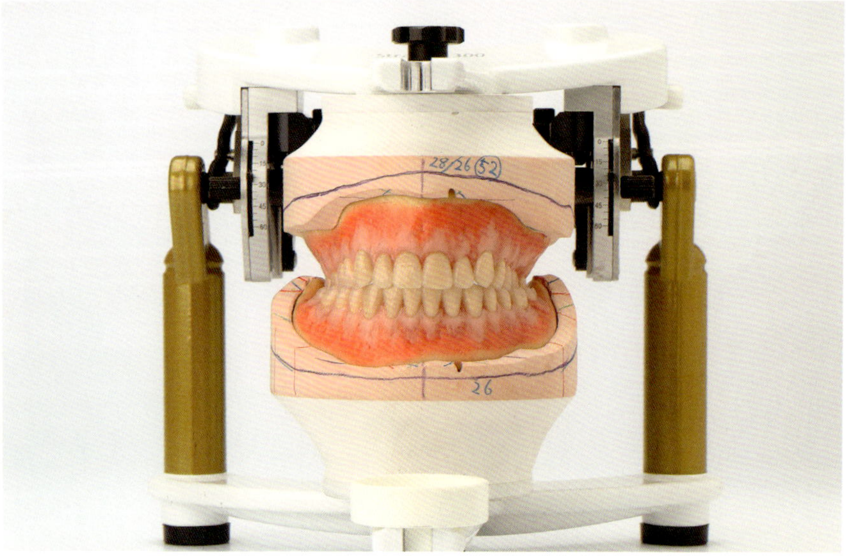

Fig 17 Class III denture tooth setup completion.

Denture coloring sequence ①

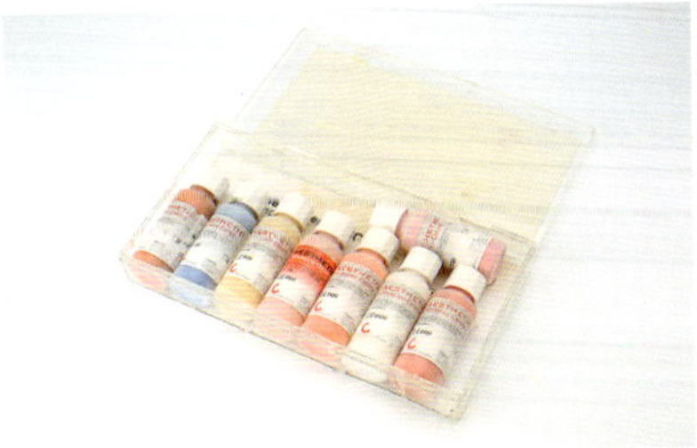

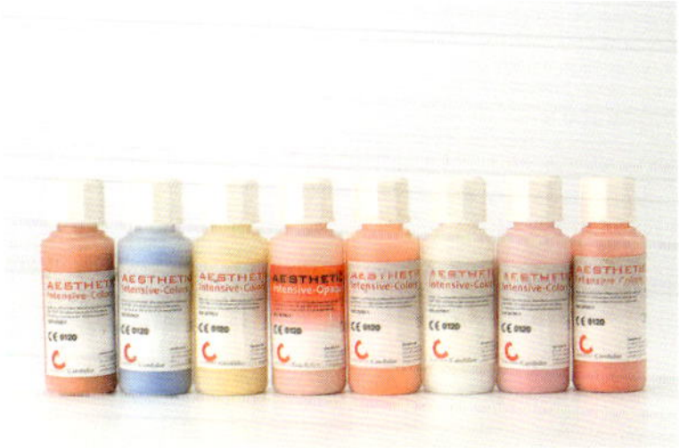

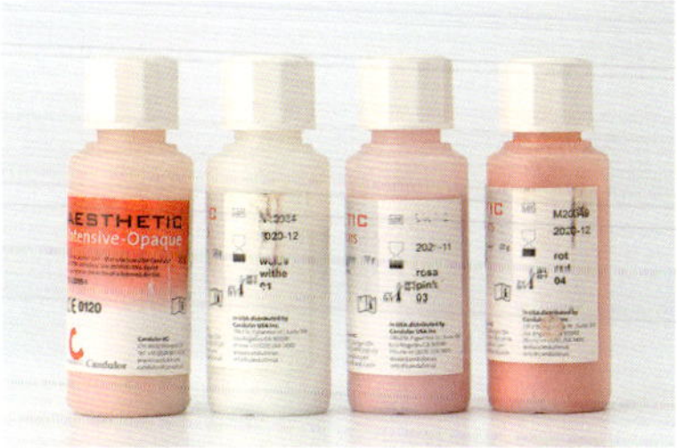

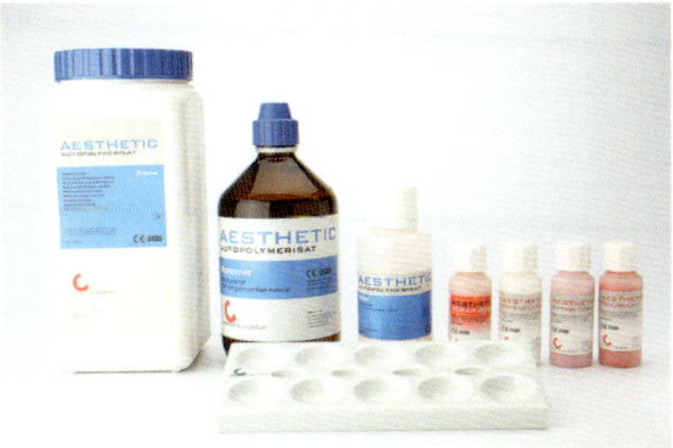

Step1 : For this case, esthetic resin polymer #34, esthetic resin monomer, esthetic resin polymer #53, esthetic intensive color set: intensive opaque, white, pink, red are used.(Candulor, Rinkai) Red fiber (Nisshin) are also used

Step2 : After flasking, dichloromethane is applied for the better adhesion of the denture teeth and coloring resin. Then the contact primer (Kulzer) is applied to enhance more adhesion

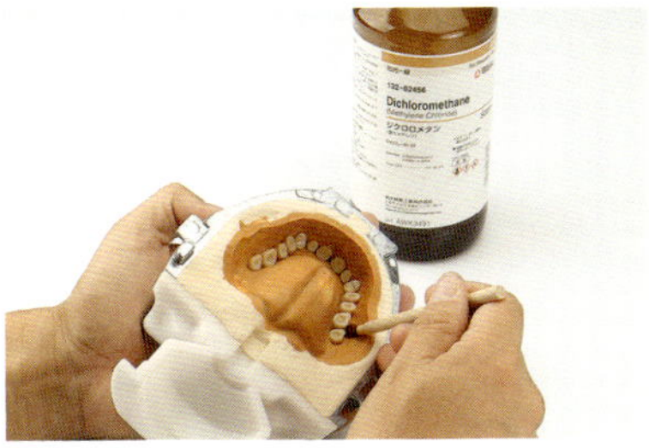

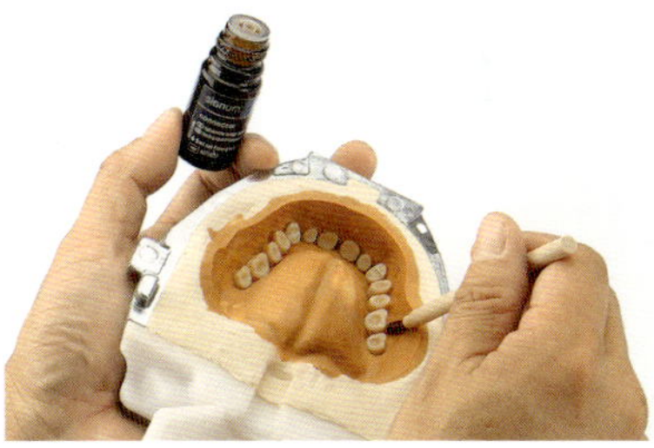

Step3 : In this case, gingival coloring was done with 4 kinds of colors. #53 and #34 are placed individually in 2 separate places on the palette. Opaque and white are mixed individually with #34 to create 2 different colors

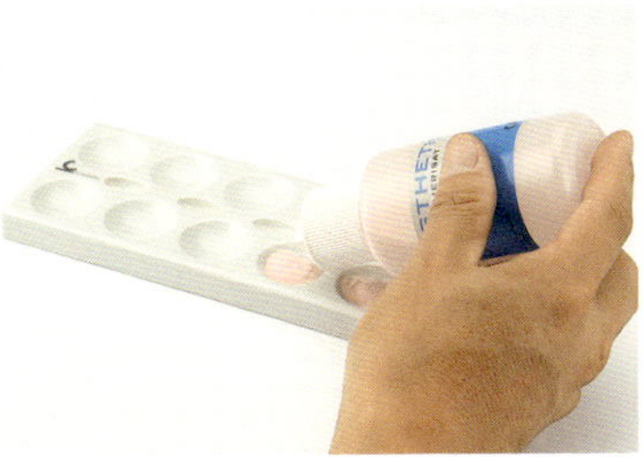

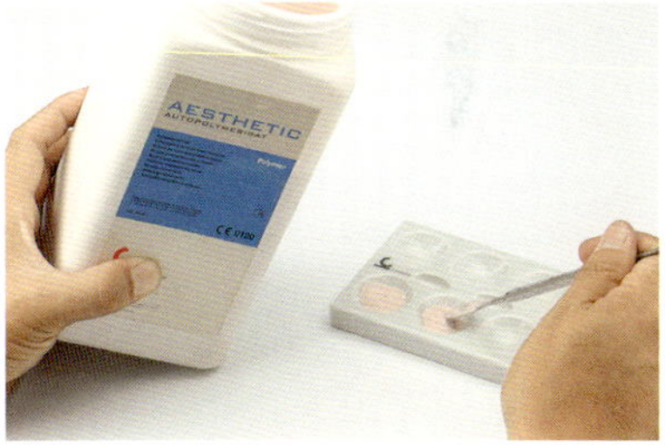

Fig 18a Denture coloring sequence①.

the Class I, Class II movement. Therefore, once the careful attention for the occlusal plane and tooth set up arrangement is paid, the stable occlusal force can be created by the dentures (Fig 16,17).

The sequence of Class III denture coloring technique are explained as follows (Fig 18).

Denture coloring sequence ②

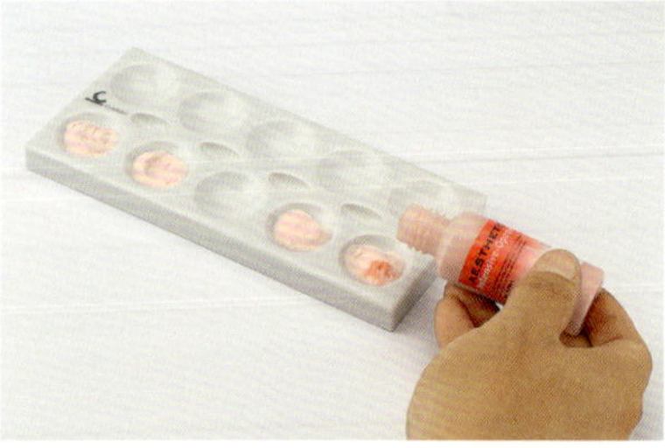

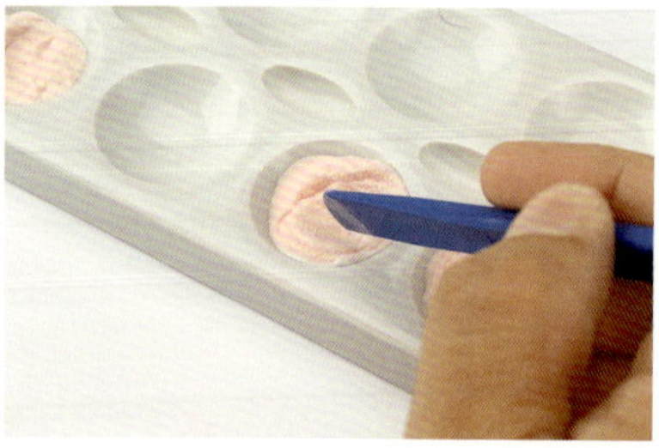

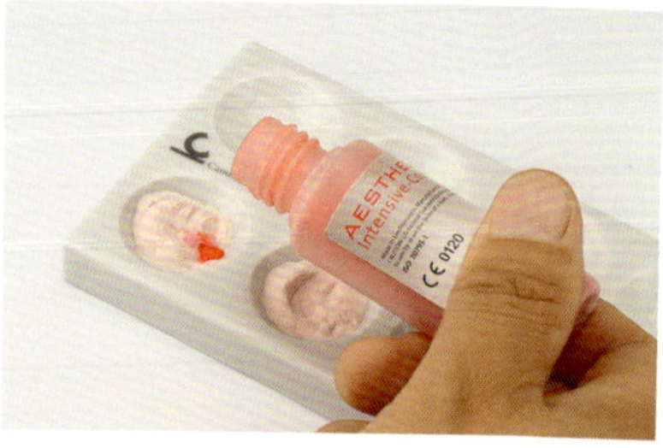

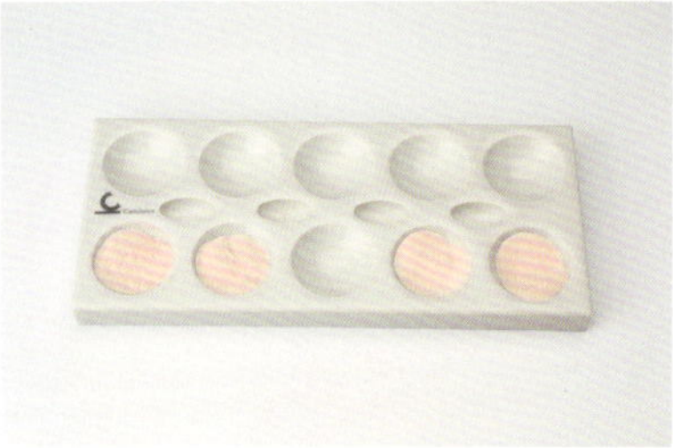

Step4 : One of #53 is used by itself and the other one of #53 is mixed with pink and red

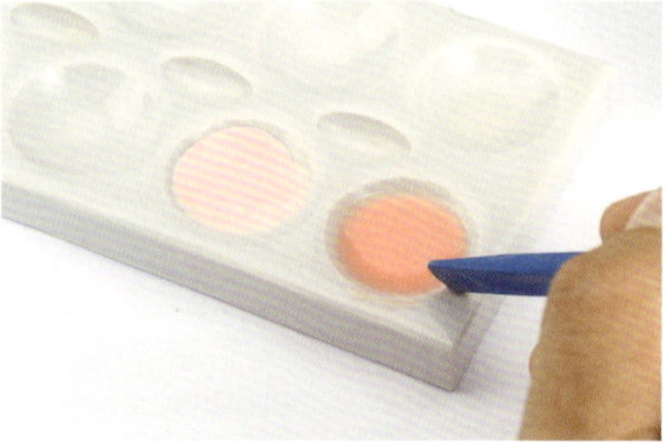

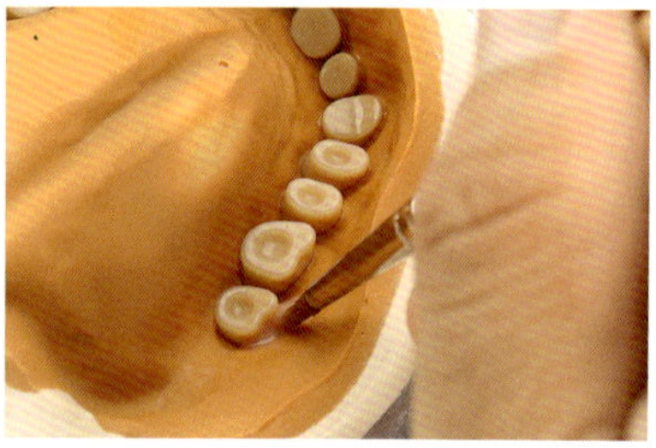

Step5 : Attached gingiva area : #34 and intensive opaque polymer are well mixed without bubble. This needs to be applied 2-3mm thickness layers on the denture teeth before contact primer is drying out. The resin layer should be thin around cervical area and papilla area in order to create a nice gradation to the next resin layer

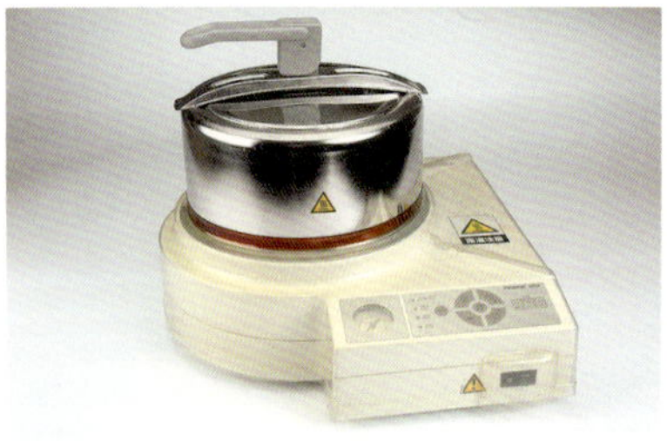

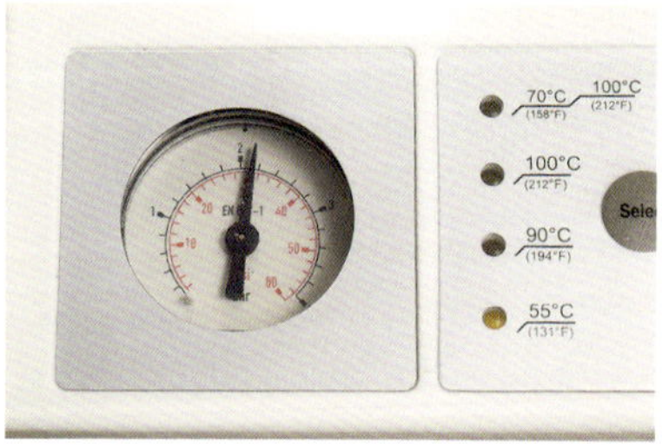

Step6 : Palamat elite (Kulzer), compressive air polymerizing unit is used for resin polymerization under 2 atm 55℃ to avoid porosity

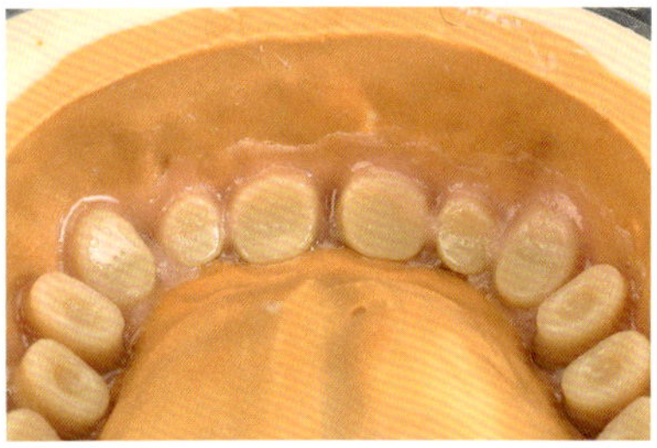

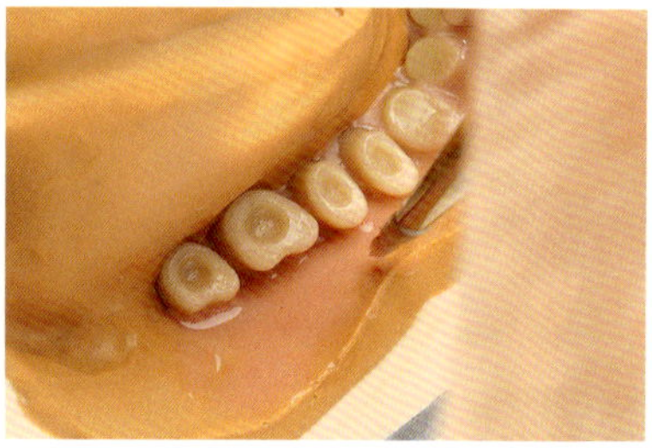

Step7 : After polymerization, contact primer is applied again for the next resin layer, then #53 is applied with thin coat

Fig 18b Denture coloring sequence ②.

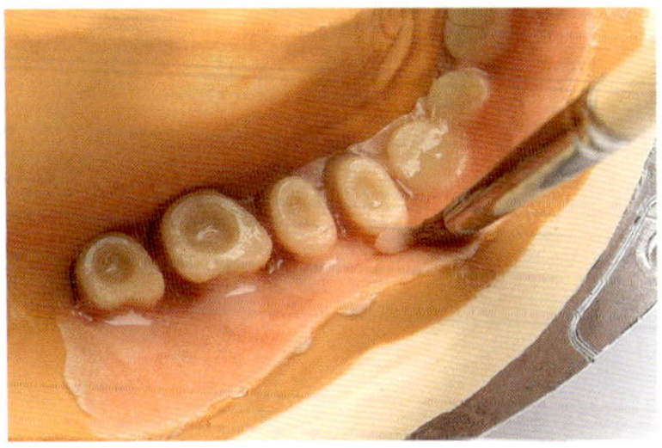

Step8 : #53 application on the surface allows to cover the coloring resin during the polishing and have a great effect to enhance the coloring resin gradation

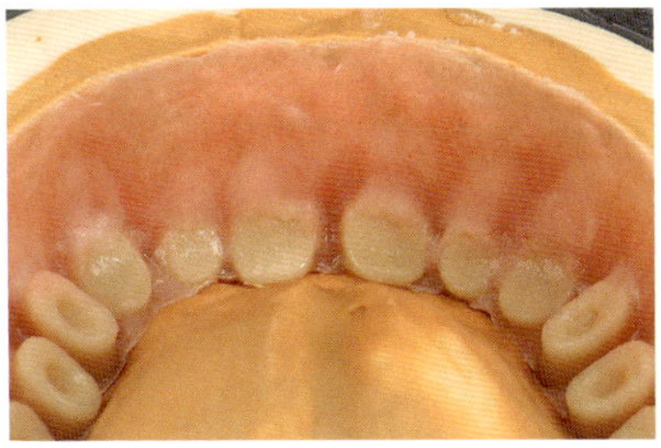

Step9 : #34 and white mix is applied on the root surface and is creating a gradation effect

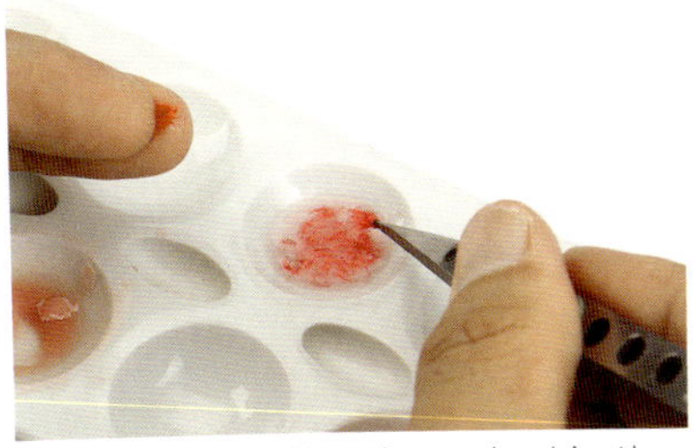

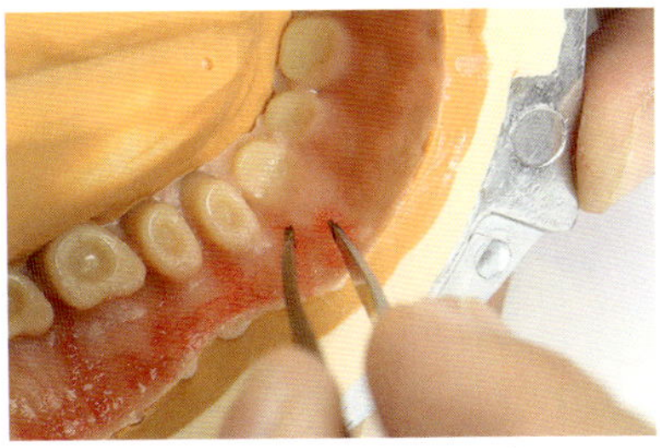

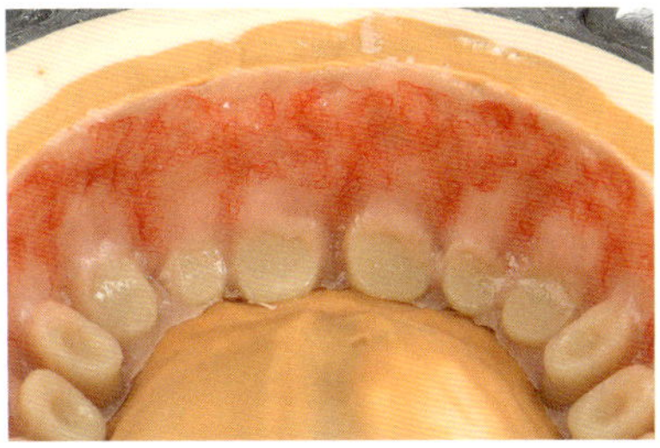

Step10 : Red fiber is soaked in the resin primer and is applied on the mucogingival area by the tweezers after the contact primer application

Step11 : #53 and pink and red mix is applied thinly on the entire surface, then polymerized under 2 atm 55℃ . It is important to polymerize resin every step by step with the compressive air polymerizing unit in order to eliminate any air bubbles and achieve complete polymerization. Otherwise, the unwanted staining may occur and plaque accumulation on the rough surfaces may occur, eventually this can be one of the origins for the aspiration pneumonia

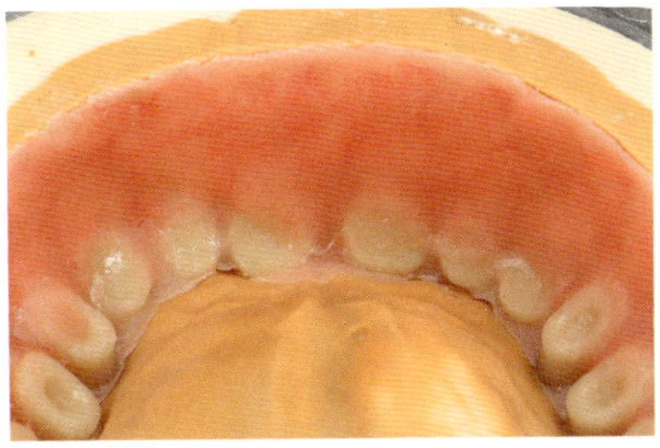

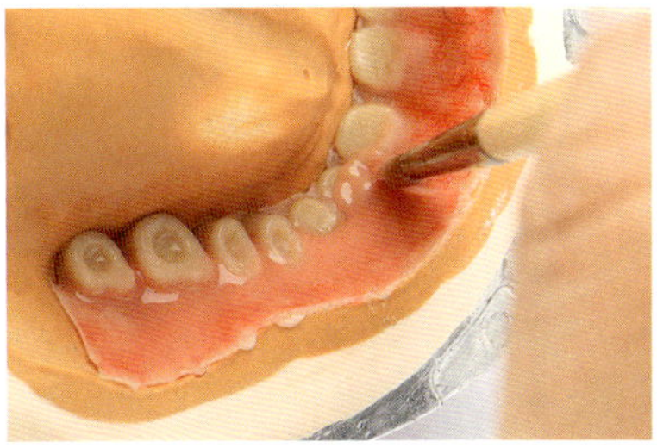

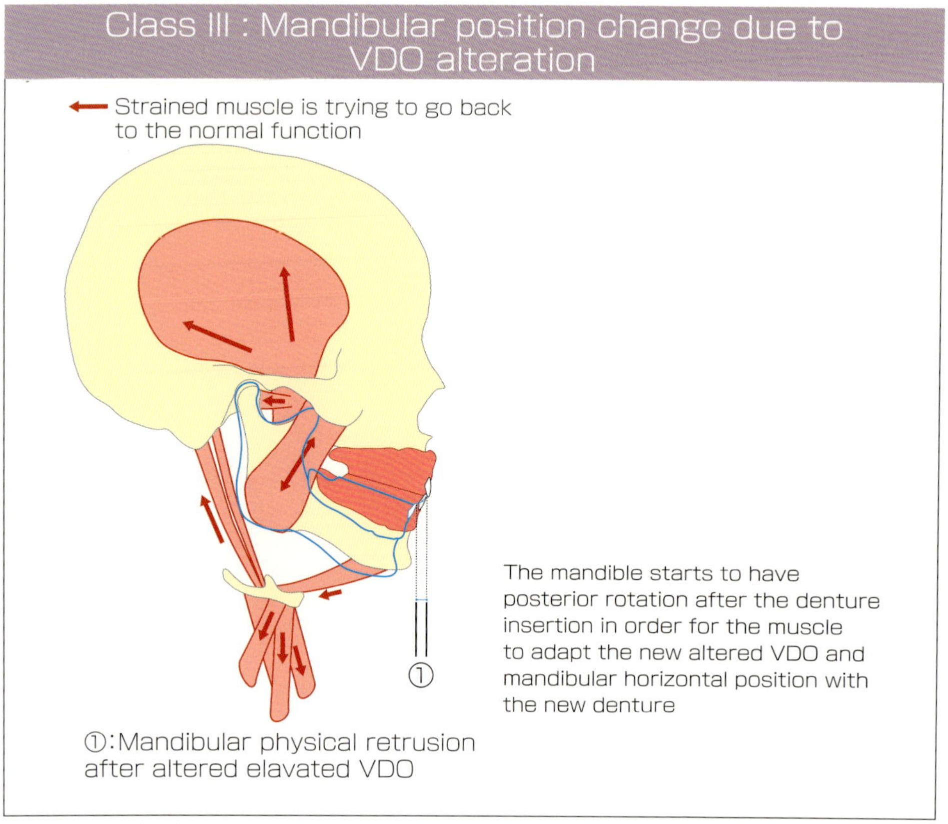

Fig 19 Mandibular position change due to VDO alteration.

10 Adjustment after the remount (Muscle rehabilitation after the denture insertion)

Even though the mandibular denture suction was acquired successfully at the time of the denture insertion, there is a case that the patient comes back with pain and denture dropping and lifting caused by mandibular jaw position change, especially when the patient has the mandibular functional movement disorder.

This phenomenon may happen by the joint in a clockwise rotation of the mandible after the denture insertion since unused muscle is activated by the elevated new VDO and improved horizontal jaw position with the new denture (Fig 19). It is obvious to lose the denture suction by having the denture instability that is caused by the premature contacts during the functional movement since the mandibular position has been completely changed even after the new dentures insertion.

However It is very difficult to find the small premature contacts with the articulating paper during the functional movement since there is no denture stability during the adjustment. Therefore, the remounting procedure on the articulator will allow for the clinician to perform the more accurate occlusal adjustment (Fig 20,21). The remount will allow for the clinician to achieve occlusal

Class III : Predicted post operative mandibular position change

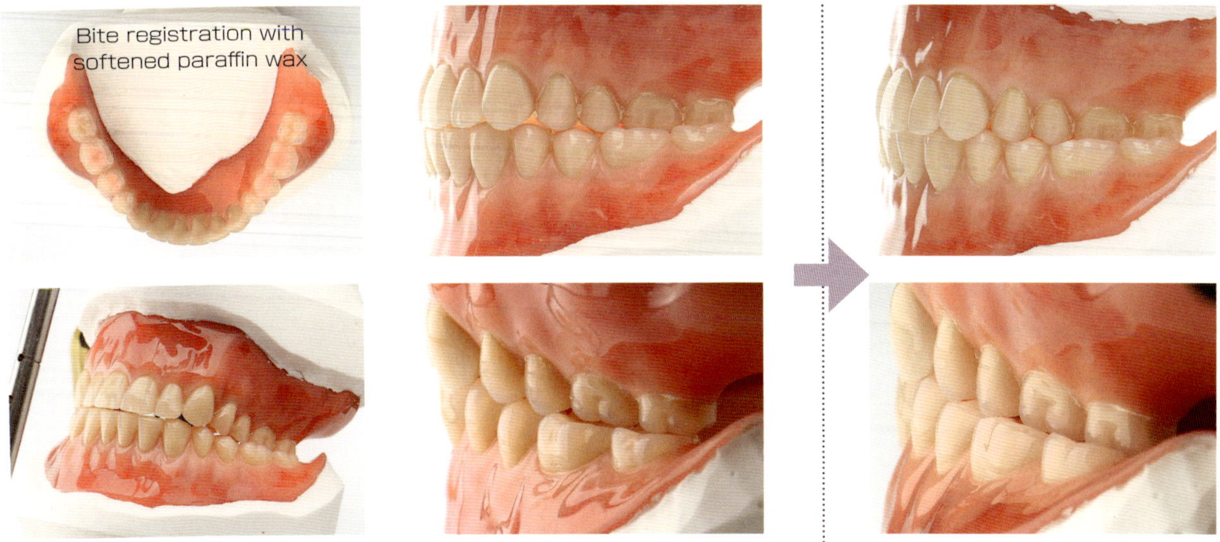

After the denture insertion, premature contacts were detected. Remount was done by acquiring a new bite registration with softened paraffin wax on the molars. This can be explained that after the new denture insertion, the mandibular position has been altered with posterior rotation

Prior to the adjustment
There is no even contacts on the molars and maxillary and mandibular teeth are not in good contacts

Post adjustment
There is even occlusal contacts on all the denture teeth

Fig 20 Post operative mandibular position change.

Adjustment after remounting

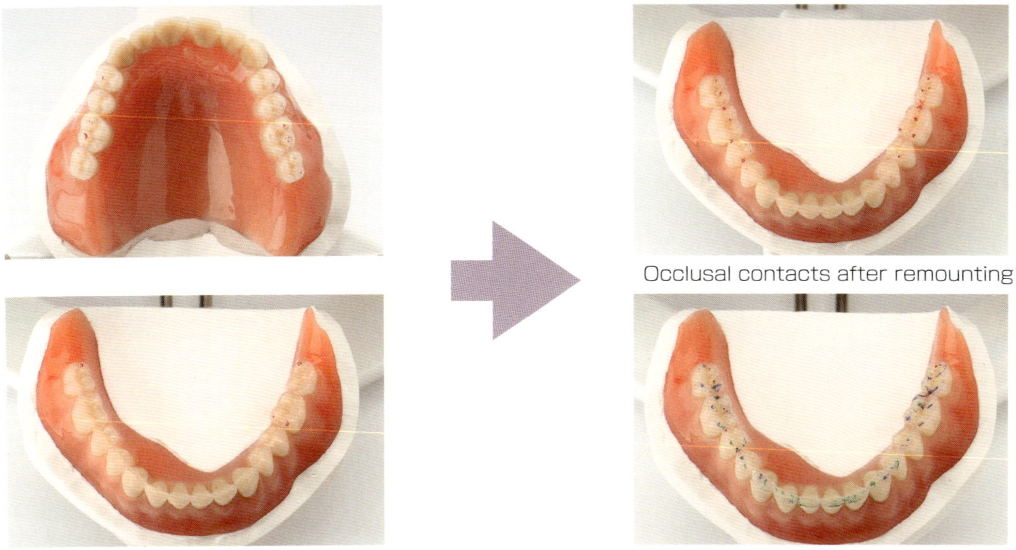

Occlusal contacts right after remounting

Occlusal adjustment with protrusive and lateral movements (full balanced occlusion)

Fig 21 Adjustment after remounting.

adjustments in the maximum intercuspal position, full balanced occlusion in function during lateral and protrusive movements on anterior and posterior teeth in the laboratory.

Complete the denture fabrication

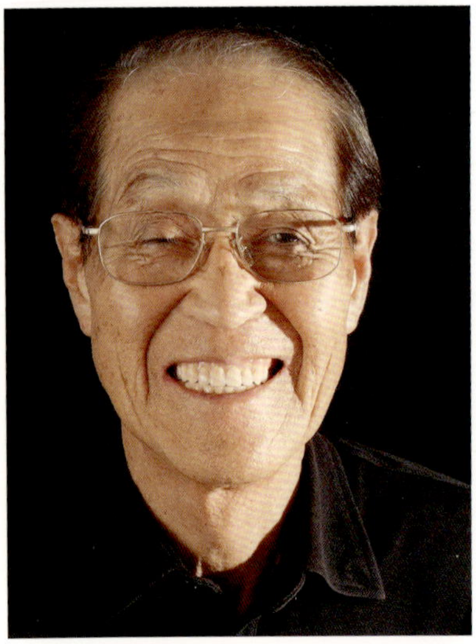

Denture coloring was done in flask

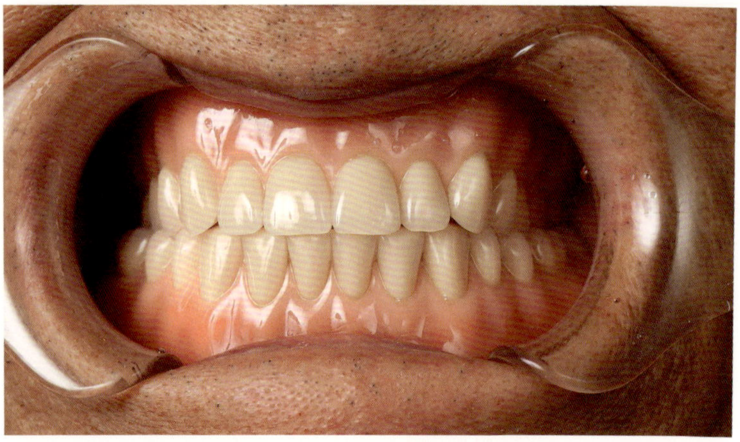

Anterior tooth interference during functional movement can be avoided by reducing overjet. Also overbite was given slightly so maxillary and mandibular anterior teeth are allowed to have contacts. This has a purpose to prevent the post insertion mandibular position change

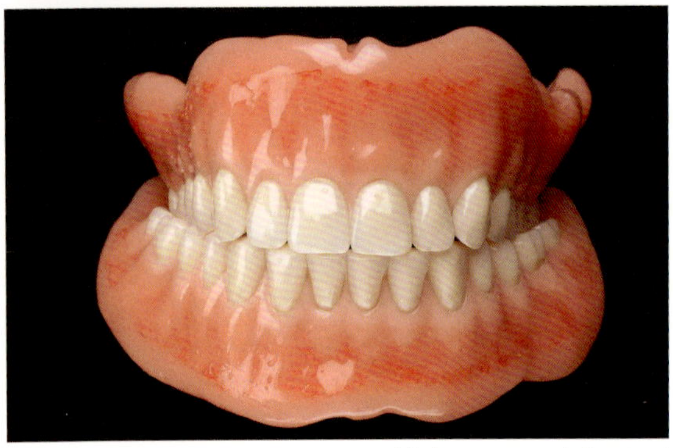

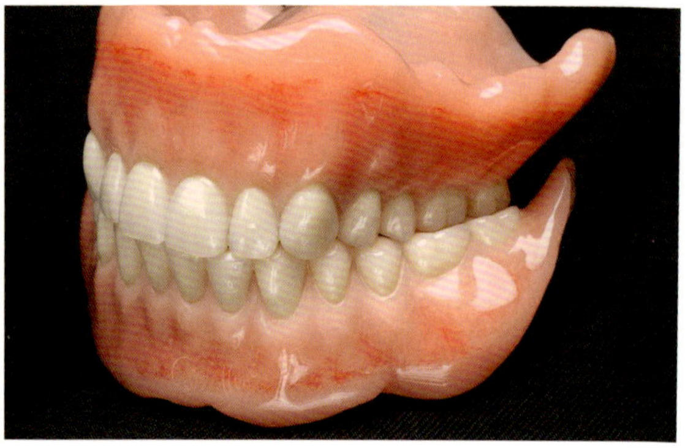

Molars cross bite and polished surface morphology

Fig 24 Complete the denture fabrication.

11 Summary

Class III case's features and denture fabrication method were discussed in this chapter (Fig 22). The extremely high level of the clinician's diagnostic skill, technical skills and patient's management skill is required to treat those extremely difficult maxillary and mandibular denture case. As explained in this chapter the required skill levels satisfying this class III patient with our dentures are quite different from the Class I, Class II div 2 and Class II div 2 cases that have been already explained. Also the phenomenon of mandibular position change after the new dentures insertion happens often to the cases that required to change an large VDO and a horizontal mandibular position[85]. The difference between the easy case and the difficult case is that for the difficult case, there may be a patient's big disappointment coming from the pain after new dentures insertion with the denture movement. The more difficult and challenging the case is, the more important for the clinician to have the strong patient's management and communication skill[86,87].

At the conclusion

CAD/CAM denture fabrication sequence

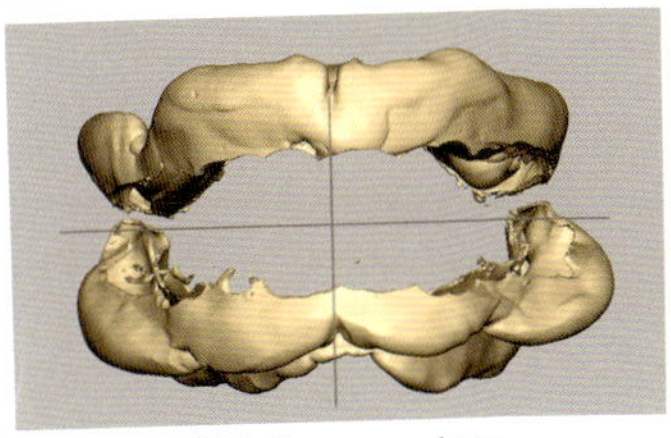

①Full scanning

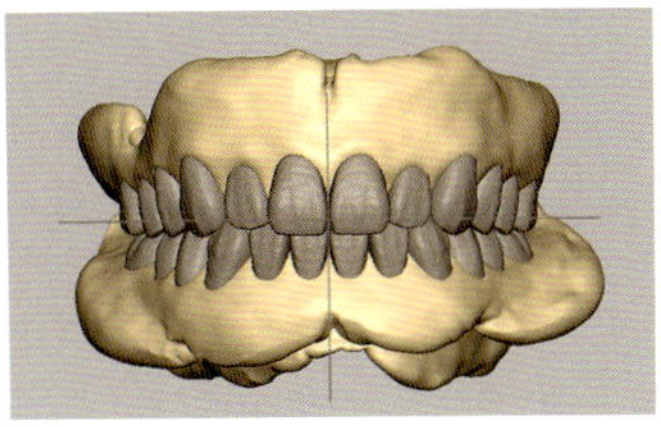

②Teeth set up on the computer

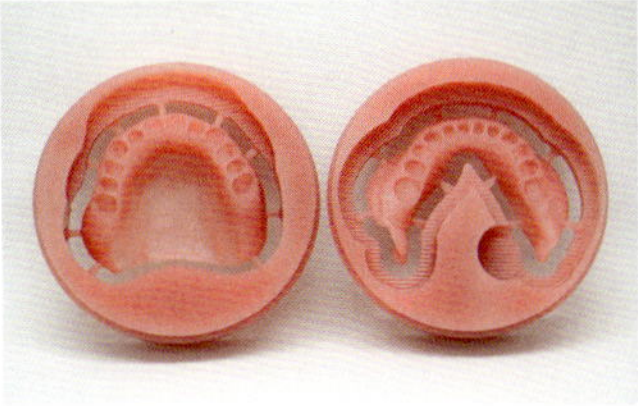

③Devesting from the resin disks

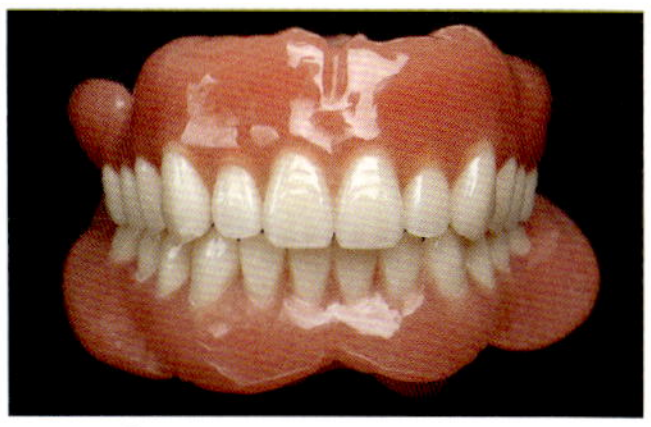

④CAD/CAM denture fabrication completion

For the longest time, the denture fabrication process hasn't had a big changes until now. But recently, the new invention of the denture fabrication method with CAD/CAM has been developed efficiently and rapidly. Globally, a lot of the dental vendors started to develop and introduced the CAD/CAM fabricated denture method and it is becoming quite popular internationally.

The biggest advantage of the digital denture fabrication is that the laboratory fabrication material error such as the model distortion induced by the stone expansion, the mounting error induced by the expansion of the mounting stone, the denture base resin curing shrinkage and thermal distortion of the master cast can be avoided or improved[88]. Denture teeth set up and denture polished surface modification can be accomplished on the computer within 30-45min. Once the starting button is pushed, resin will be milled automatically. Therefore, the entire denture fabrication process time will be dramatically cut short and it is extremely efficient.

However, even though the laboratory process will be changed by the digital fabrication, the clinical process such as impression or bite registration processes wouldn't changed. Inappropriately acquired final impression or interocclusal record will create ill fitting and unfunctional denture. Therefore, unless the clinician has a high level of clinical skill, this digital technique wouldn't be utilized as effective as it should be[89]. No matter where the clinician practices dentistry, the highest goal of the clinician should be "Fabricating the best denture ". Once the concept of the suction effective dentures, systematic BPS system are incorporated into the digital dentistry, the more accurate and well designed CAD/CAM denture should be fabricated in the future.

To achieve this outcome in the future, it is very important to have skilled and experienced educators and well trained CAD/CAM dental technicians.

We surely need to make more effort to make our patients happy.

Jiro Abe 2017 Fall

Part 1

1. Abe J, Kokubo K, Sato K. 4 Steps from Start to Finish Mandibular Suction-Effective Denture and BPS: A Complete Guide(English Ed.). Tokyo: Quintessence Publishing, 2012.
2. Yuda A. My clinical experience: [Staring - Game functional impression] for denture fabrication at home - visit dental treatment - what I have learned through 135 cases of complete denture cases-(in Japanese). The Nippon Dental Review 2012; 72(11) : 125-133.
3. Yuda A, Kobayashi S. Risk control of the denture at home- visit dental treatment: In order to use the denture safely under high risk environment (in Japanese). The Nippon Dental Review 2013 : 73(11) : 105-112.
4. Endo Y. New approach to OSAHS. Application of the intra oral device for the obstructive sleep apnea-hypopnea syndrome patient with missing teeth (in Japanese). the Quintessence 2012; 31(12): 96-109.
5. Endo Y. Paradigm shift of mandibular complete denture impression (first part) (in Japanese). QDT 2016; 41(6); 16-38.
6. Endo Y. Paradigm shift of mandibular complete denture impression (second part) (in Japanese). QDT 2016; 41(7): 14-31.
7. Schaffner T. Hand book of complete denture prosthetics. Liechtenstein; Ivoclar Vivadent, 1994.
8. Fiedler K. BPS-Totalprothetik mit System zum Ziel. München: Neuer Merkur, 2003.
9. Frick H, Abe J. BPS Complete denture fabrication system, which is recognized world wide - Recognize the difference from clinical complete denture in Japan-(in Japanese). Dental Outlook 2006; 108(6): 1101-1128.
10. Abe J, Sato K, Kokubo K. Achieving suction effect of the mandibular complete denture (in Japanese). QDT 2008; 33(1-8): 13-42, 48-57, 56-63, 44-55, 52-61, 36-46, 48-59, 50-62.
11. Boucher C, Hickey JC, Zarb GA. Prosthodontics treatment for edentulous patients. St Louis: CV Mosby, 1970.
12. Matsuda K, Maeda Y. Bibliography of clinical complete denture The 4th Final impression (General discussion) (in Japanese). The international journal of dental technology 2015; 43(4): 458-465.
13. Matsuda K, Yoshinobu Maeda. Bibliography of clinical complete denture The 5th Final impression (Detailed discussion) (in Japanese). The international journal of dental technology 2015; 43(5): 570–579.
14. Abe J, Nukazawa S. Difference between the conventional mandibular preliminary impression technique and the preliminary impression technique for the purpose of achieving suction-effect of mandibular complete denture (in Japanese). Practice in Prosthodontics 2010; 43(5): 510-524.
15. Sato K. What is Suction Denture? (in Japanese). Tokyo: Dental Diamond, 2014.
16. Abe J. Suction-effect of mandibular complete denture for everybody (in Japanese). Tokyo; Hyoron Publishers, 2004.
17. Abe J. Monthly Publication Jiro Abe ~ Mandibular complete denture•the road to suction-effect~ (in Japanese). Tokyo: Dental Diamond, 2007.

Part 2

18. Abe J. Agreed, once we know!! Tricks and crucial points for complete denture treatment 1. Diagnosis for suction-effect of mandibular complete denture (in Japanese). Dental Diamond 2016; 41(7): 102-107.
19. Abe J. What is most important in complete denture treatment? Summary (in Japanese). The Nippon Dental Review 2016; 75(12): 66-69.
20. Ii H. Retrospective study about inhibitory factors for suction-effect of mandibular complete denture(in Japanese). The journal of the Academy of Clinical Dentistry 2016; 36(3): 184-191.
21. Ii H, Abe J. What is suction-effect of mandibular complete denture affected by? - The investigation in regards to inhibitory factors for suction-effect -(in Japanese). The Nippon Dental Review 2017; 77(5): 91-99.
22. Honda T. Agreed, once we know!! Crucial points for complete denture treatment. Seal at sublingual fold area(in Japanese). Dental Diamond 2016; 41(12): 88-93.
23. Sato K. Feature. What is most important in complete denture treatment? [Position of the tongue] is most important!(in Japanese). The Nippon Dental Review 2015; 75(12): 55-60.
24. Wright CR, Swartz WH, Godwin WC. Mandibular denture stability. Ann Arbor: Overbeck, 1961.
25. Wright CR et al. A study of the tongue and its relation to denture stability. J Am Dent Assoc 1949; 39(3): 269-275.
26. Kamijo Y. Oral anatomy Vol. 5 Splanchnology (Clinical ed.) (the fifth edition) (in Japanese). Tokyo: Anatome Co., 1969:1491-1492.
27. Ichikawa M. The report regarding the design of outline of mandibular complete denture base based on the result of measurement experiment of denture base withdrawal traction force. The first report: study of retentive force according to the different amount of coverage of retromolar pad by the denture base(in Japanese). The journal of the Academy of Clinical Dentistry 2012; 32 (1, 2 merger issue): 57-64.
28. Ichikawa M. The design of denture base border around retromolar pad considering suction-effect of the mandibular complete denture(in Japanese). Practice in Prosthodontics 2012; 45(5): 550-559.
29. Ichikawa M. Special article What is most important in complete denture treatment? [Retromolar pad] is most important!(in Japanese). The Nippon Dental Review 2015; 75(12): 29-35.
30. Ichikawa M. Agreed, once we know!! Tricks and crucial points for complete denture treatment Denture base border shape of suction-effective mandibular complete denture Retromolar pad (in Japanese). Dental Diamond 2016; 41(9):86-93.
31. Abe J. Treatment of edentulous patient Difference in mechanism of correcting mandibular position between anatomical denture teeth and flat table denture teeth(in Japanese). The journal of the Academy of Clinical Dentistry 1999; 20(1): 62-70.
32. Abe J. Mandibular position in the treatment of edentulous patient III•complete Clinical use of the treatment denture(in Japanese). The Nippon Dental Review 2001; 61(5): 109-116.

Part 3

33. Fenlon MR, Sherriff M. An investigation of factors influencing patients' satisfaction with new complete dentures using structural equation modeling. J Dent 2008; 36(6): 427-434.
34. Alfadda SA. The relationship between various parameters of complete denture quality and patints' satisfaction. J Am Dent Assoc 2014; 145(9): 941-948.
35. Matsumaru Y. Why dentures fabricated by different approaches are still accepted by a single patient? - A study of the clinical research-(in Japanese). (In.) Abe J (Chief author). QDT Art & Practice Special edition Dr. Abe J and 5 dental technicians present equally valid and effective different approaches to fabricate dentures for the same case. Tokyo: Quintessence Publishing Japan, 2013: 112-123.
36. Saito Y. Special article What is most important in complete denture treatment? [Occlusion] is most important!(in Japanese). The Nippon Dental Review 2015; 75(12):36-41.
37. Matsumaru Y. Special article What is most important in complete denture treatment? A study of "Acceptable complete denture by the patient" through literatures(in Japanese). The Nippon Dental Review 2015; 75(12):61-65.
38. Matsuda K, Kurushima Y, Maeda Y, Enoki K, Mihara Y, Ikebe K. Crossover trap for comparing the bifunctional prosthetic system with conventional procedures. Eur J Prosthodont 2015; 3(3):64-70.
39. Matsumaru Y. Knowledge and clinical key points to improve complete denture impression technique. Clinical Key points for closed-mouth impression technique(in Japanese). Dental Outlook 2016; 128(6): 1137-1143.
40. Abe J, Kyoko Kokubo. Relationship between the amount of anterior clearance and movement of complete dentures after insertion(in Japanese). Practice in Prosthodontics 2009; 42(5): 552-563.
41. Yoshitomi N. Influence of anterior occlusal contacts of complete dentures upon chewing on mandibular movement(in Japanese). J stomata Soc Jpn 1997; 64(3): 436-453.

Part 4

42. Abe J. How to use the new snap impression tray [Frame Cut Back tray] - The first step to achieve suction-effect of mandibular complete denture-(in Japanese). Dental Magazine 2010; 133: 38-41.
43. Abe J. Clinical biomaterial seminar Mandibular edentulous impression tray -frame Cut Back tray-(in Japanese). The Nippon Dental Review 2010; 133: 38-41.
44. Abe J. Difference between the conventional mandibular preliminary impression technique and the preliminary impression technique for the purpose of achieving suction-effect of mandibular complete denture Introduction to the Frame Cut Back tray impression system(in Japanese). Practice in Prosthodontics 2010; 43(5): 510-524.
45. Aizawa M. Bite registration for suction-effect of mandibular complete denture. Simplified bite registration technique using Centric Tray(in Japanese). Dental Diamond 2016; 41(15): 108-115.
46. Omori A, Kamijo Y, Wakatsuki E et al. A study of chewing cycle using X-ray television movie(in Japanese). Shikwa gakuho. journal of the Tokyo Dental College Society 1975; 75: 87.
47. Takano K. Change in buccal mucosa during chewing using X-ray television movie(in Japanese). Shikwa gakuho. journal of the Tokyo Dental College Society 1979; 79: 1361-1453.
48. Omori A. Change in movement of buccal mucosa using X-ray television movie(in Japanese). Shikwa gakuho. journal of the Tokyo Dental College Society 1979; 79: 1757-1813.
49. Abe J. Clinical steps of denture fabrication to achieve suction-effect of mandibular complete denture -improvement of posterior border seal around retromolar pad-(in Japanese). J Jpn Prosthod Soc 2011; 3(3): 220-230.
50. Yamazaki F. A survey on the outline of denture base of bilateral extension mandibular removable partial denture(in Japanese). The journal of the Academy of Clinical Dentistry 2013; 33(3): 195-201.
51. Nozawa K. A survey among dental technicians on complete denture fabrication steps and anatomical land mark(in Japanese). The journal of the Academy of Clinical Dentistry 2013; 33(1-2): 23-30.
52. Someya S. A report of "sinew" found at distal to mandibular second molar and the area of anterior border of retromolar pad(in Japanese). The journal of the Academy of Clinical Dentistry 2018; 28(1-2): 14-20.

53. Miyake H. Agreed, once we know!! Tricks and crucial points for complete denture treatment Denture base border of suction-effective mandibular complete denture (3) "Someya's sinew" and "Retromylohyoide fossa"(in Japanese). Dental Diamond 2016; 41(11): 90-96.

54. Abe J, Saito Y, Ono T, Kokubo K. The record base to minimize operator's mistakes & custom impression tray with suction-effect(in Japanese). Tokyo: GC, 2007.

55. Iwaki K. Reconsideration of complete denture fabrication steps by BPS (1~4) (in Japanese). ZERO 2015, 2016; 14(2,3,4), 15(1): 32-43, 24-32, 48-58, 58-71.

56. Aizawa M, Iwaki K. Clinical steps to facilitate suction-effect of mandibular complete denture -the system to achieve ideal shape of complete denture in harmony with biology(in Japanese). Practice in Prosthodontics 2015; 48(6): 626-638.

57. Sudo T. Laboratory steps by 4 dental technicians who are JDA instructors to achieve suction effective functional complete denture -basic knowledge and technique to satisfy the patient 1. Fabrication of a custom tray to lead to successful suction-effect(in Japanese). the international journal of dental technology 2016; 44(9): 1083-1094.

58. Abe J. How should the edentulous area be treated I. Adaptation of oral mucosa in neglected edentulous area(in Japanese). The Nippon Dental Review 2002; 62 (8): 129-142.

59. Nukazawa S. My clinical experience, change from conventional impression technique to suction-effective impression technique for mandibular complete denture(in Japanese). Practice in Prosthodontics 2010; 43(5): 525-535.

60. Watt DM. MacGregor AR. Designing Complete Dentures. Philadelphia; WB Saunders, 1976.

61. Pound E. Conditioning of denture patients. J Am Dent Assoc 1962; 64: 461-468.

62. Sudo T. Precise and effective denture teeth set up according to the clear guide line -development of [Laser marker stand] and its various use. 7. Fabrication of a complete denture with consideration of future implant overdenture(in Japanese). The international journal of dental technology 2015; 43(4): 474-485.

63. Morinaga J. Laboratory steps by 4 dental technicians who are JDA instructors to achieve suction effective functional complete denture -basic knowledge and technique to satisfy the patient 5. Polished surface shape to support suction-effect(in Japanese). The international journal of dental technology 2017; 45(2): 255-265.

64. Abe J, Kokubo K. Denture a la carte(in Japanese). Tokyo: GC, 2008.

Part 5

65. Someya S, Sato K. Clinical discussion/ management of maxillary flabby ridge(in Japanese). (In.) Murakami H, Watanabe N, Enomoto K (Eds.). How to climb up to the summit called 'complete denture' Seeking the best clinical rout. Tokyo: Ishiyaku Publishers Inc, 2009: 179-195.

66. Abe J. Jiro Abe's Difficult-to-Treat complete denture case Clinical reality, which everybody wants to know(in Japanese). Tokyo: Ishiyaku Publishers, 2013.

67. Kelly E. Changes caused by a mandibular removable partial denture opposing a maxillary complete denture. J Prosthed Dent 1972; 27(2): 140-150.

68. Nozawa K. A survey among dental technicians on complete denture fabrication steps and anatomical land mark(in Japanese). The journal of the Academy of Clinical Dentistry 2013; 33(1-2): 23-30.

69. Iwaki K. Laboratory steps by 4 dental technicians who are JDA instructors to achieve suction effective functional complete denture -basic knowledge and technique to satisfy the patient 6 (Last part) Occlusal adjustment to minimize denture adjustment and improve suction-effect(in Japanese). The international journal of dental technology 2017; 45(3): 392-398.

70. Sudo T. Laboratory steps by 4 dental technicians who are JDA instructors to achieve suction effective functional complete denture -basic knowledge and technique to satisfy the patient 2. Closed-position functional impression and registration of mandibular position to achieve suction-effect -the custom tray with wax rim and BPS Gnathometer(in Japanese). The international journal of dental technology 2016; 44 (10): 1236-1245.

71. Saito Y. Analysis of Gothic arch and tapping point recording as part of bite registration for complete denture - relationship between quantitative assessment of the tracing and morphological evaluation of Gothic arch score-(in Japanese). The journal of the academy of Clinical Dentistry 2009; 29(4): 252-265.

72. Saito Y. Bite registration for suction-effect of mandibular complete denture 2 Gothic arch (GoA)(in Japanese). Dental Diamond 2016; 41(16): 98-105.

73. Yaegashi H, Endo Y, Kodama K, Mushimoto E, Tanaka H. The effect of perception of periodontal ligament on deprogramming of masticatory muscle(in Japanese). Summary of Japanese society of stomatognathic function 8th meeting, 1995, 14-15.

74. Wise MD. Occlusion and restorative dentistry for the general practitioner(in Japanese). Part 2 - Examination of the occlusion and fabrication of study casts. Br Dent J 1982; 152(5): 160-165.

75. Downs DH. An investigation into condylar position with gauge and bimanual manipulation. J Gnathology 1988; 7(1): 75-81.

76. Mizokami T, Sakurai K. Utilization of Tapping•Point for bite registration(in Japanese). The Dental; 1(3): 243-250.

77. Mizokami T, Nanami T, Sakurai K, Omatsu M. Bite registration with Gothic arch tracing method utilizing Tapping•Point(in Japanese). Dental Outlook 1988; 71: 826.

78. Sakurai T, Fukamizu K, Tsutsumi K, Nakao K. Learn about "Painless denture" by Sakurai method(in Japanese). Practice in Prosthodontics 1990; 23(6): 593-628.

79. Ono J, Kato T, Tsutsumi T (eds.). the international journal of dental technology Supplement Atlas Complete denture Learn from the model(in Japanese). Tokyo: Ishiyaku Publishers Inc., 1994: 88-101.

80. Endo Y. A study of recording method of horizontal mandibular position for complete denture patient(in Japanese). Comparison and Active method and Passive method. The Journal of the Japan Prosthodontic Society 1996; 40•95th special edition: 184.

81. Baba E. A clinical trial research of Gothic arch apex and terminal hinge position(in Japanese). Odontology 1973; 61(2): 434-447.

82. Matsumaru Y. Influence of mandibular residual ridge resorption on objective masticatory measures of lingualized and fully bilateral balanced denture articulation. J Prosthodont Res 2010; 54(3): 112-118.

Part 6

83. Saito Y. A complete denture moves while in function -Fabrication of a complete denture to minimize the movement-(in Japanese). the Quintessence 2010; 29(6): 141-148.

Part 7

84. Odagaki T. Laboratory steps by 4 dental technicians who are JDA instructors to achieve suction effective functional complete denture -basic knowledge and technique to satisfy the patient 4. Difference in denture teeth set up among Angle Class I and II and III(in Japanese). the international journal of dental technology 2017; 45(1): 116-129.

85. Abe J. Chair side adjustment of a complete denture at insertion appointment(in Japanese). (In.) Hideaki Muraoka (edit). Dental Diamond Special issue. Treatment of edentulous patient -learn from others- table clinic in the journal. Tokyo: Dental Diamond, 1998: 115-126.

86. Palla S. Occlusal considerations in complete dentures. (In.) McNeill C (Ed.). Science and practice of occlusion. Chicago: Quintessence Publishing 1997, 457-467.

87. Carlsson GE, Omar R. The future of complete dentures in oral rehabilitation. A critical review. J Oral Rehabil 2010; 37(2): 143-156.

88. Orii Y, Abe J, Sasaki K. CAD/CAM Complete denture fabrication with human sensibility in search for the better fit (in Japanese). The Nippon Dental Review 2015; 75(3): 91-98.

89. Abe J. What will change or remain after introduction of CAD/CAM denture? -digital denture and current edentulous denture treatment (in Japanese)- (In.) Abe J, Amakawa Y, Amano A, Ishikawa T, Ishitani N, Ito A, Ushikubo T, Urano S, Oka K, Obama T, Kihara T, Kubota T, Komiyama Y, Sugiyama S, Tanaka M, Tsuchiya K, Nikaido M, Hayashi M, Hidaka T, Hosomi H, Horiuchi K, Mizukami T, Mitsuhashi A, Miyazaki M, Waki M, Watanabe H. Anticipation in 31 topics. The compass of clinical dentistry 2017. Tokyo: INTERACTION, 2017: 128-133.

List of materials used

			(Page)
Part 1			
Mandibular preliminary impression tray	Frame Cut Back Tray	YDM, Morita	11
Part 4			
Alginate impression material & tray	AccuDent XD Alginate Impression system	Ivoclar Vivadent	34
Mandibular preliminary impression tray	Frame Cut Back Tray	YDM, Morita	35
Simplified bite registration tray	Centric Tray	Ivoclar Vivadent	36
Semiadjustable articulator	Stratos 200	Ivoclar Vivadent	38
Model transfer jig	Horizontal guide	Ivoclar Vivadent	38
Gothic arch tracing kit	Gnathometer M	Ivoclar Vivadent	42
Alveolar ridge shape imprint device	Profile Compass	Candulor, Rinkai	53
Denture tooth setup template	2D Template	Ivoclar Vivadent	56
Denture tooth setup template	3D Template	Ivoclar Vivadent	56
Face bow	UTS3D Universal Transfer Bow	Ivoclar Vivadent	56
Denture teeth	SR-Phonares	Ivoclar Vivadent	62
Hard resin	SR Nexco	Ivoclar Vivadent	62
Carbide burr	#8	Emesco	62
Carbide burr	HP699	Emesco	62, 67
Carbide burr	Shofu FissureCarbaHP	Shofu	63
Primer	Contact Primer	Kulzer, Kulzer Japan	63
Primer	Signum Connector	Kulzer, Kulzer Japan	63
Curing light	Evolution Max	Dreve, Rinkai	63
Sponge for removal of inhibited layer	Disposable sponge	Ivoclar Vivadent	65
Vacuum curing light	Visio Beta Vario	3M Japan	67
Carbide burr	HM77MF 023HP	Meisinger, GC	67
Part 5			
Mandibular preliminary impression tray	Frame Cut Back Tray	YDM, Morita	80, 81, 82
Alginate impression material	Accudent Tray Gel	Ivoclar Vivadent	86
Model transfer jig	Horizontal guide	Ivoclar Vivadent	91
Gothic arch tracing kit	Gnathometer M	Ivoclar Vivadent	124, 125
Occlusal plane plate	Y.N. occlusal plane plate	Senjo, Morita	102
Fit checker	GC Fit checker	GC	105
Face bow	UTS3D Universal Transfer Bow	Ivoclar Vivadent	128
Semiadjustable articulator	Stratos 200	Ivoclar Vivadent	128
Denture tooth setup template	3D Template	Ivoclar Vivadent	128, 135
Upper lip length ruler	Papilla meter	Candulor, Rinkai	131
Resin polymerization system	IvoBase system	Ivoclar Vivadent	140
Pressure polymerization unit with high temperature and high pressure	Polymax 5	Dreve, Rinkai	72
Part 6			
Denture teeth	SR Orthosit PE	Ivoclar Vivadent	153, 158
Part 7			
Simplified bite registration tray	Centric Tray	Ivoclar Vivadent	162, 164
Denture teeth	SR Orthosit PE K-type	Ivoclar Vivadent	169, 170
Denture coloring material	Esthetic resin	Candulor, Rinkai	177
Denture coloring material	Red fiber	Nissin	177
Organic solvent	Dichloromethane	Wako Pure Chemical Industries	177
Primer	Contact Primer	Kulzer, Kulzer Japan	177
Fixed temperature pressure polymerization unit	Palamat Elite	Kulzer, Kulzer Japan	178

*Virtual (Ivoclar Vivadent) was choice of material for silicone putty and impression material unless specified.
*Laser Marker Stand (Pages : 51, 53, 59) is not on the market for sale. Please refer to Takashi Tsusumi. Serial publication precise and effective denture teeth set up according to the clear criteria - Development and its various use of [Laser Marker Stand]. 1. General remarks: History of development of Laser Marker Stand. the international journal of dental technology 2014; 42(10): 1116-1131.(in Japanese) for the history of the product.

Quintessence Publishing Co., Ltd.
3-2-6, Hongoh, Bunkyo-ku, Tokyo 113-0033, JAPAN
Tel: +81-3-5842-2270
Fax: +81-3-5800-7597
URL: www.quint-j.co.jp
Printing and Binding: Sun Art Printing Co., Ltd. Osaka
Printed in Japan
ISBN 978-4-7812-0676-9 C3047